Advances in Cancer Stem Cell Biology

Roberto Scatena • Alvaro Mordente
Bruno Giardina

Editors

Advances in Cancer Stem Cell Biology

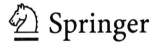

Editors
Roberto Scatena
Department of Laboratory Medicine
Catholic University
00168 Rome, Italy
r.scatena@rm.unicatt.it

Bruno Giardina
Department of Laboratory Medicine
Catholic University
00168 Rome, Italy
bgiardina@rm.unicatt.it

Alvaro Mordente
Institute of Biochemistry
and Clinical Biochemistry
Catholic University
School of Medicine
00168 Rome, Italy
alvaro.mordente@rm.unicatt.it

ISBN 978-1-4614-0808-6   e-ISBN 978-1-4614-0809-3
DOI 10.1007/978-1-4614-0809-3
Springer New York Dordrecht Heidelberg London

Library of Congress Control Number: 2011935366

© Springer Science+Business Media, LLC 2012
All rights reserved. This work may not be translated or copied in whole or in part without the written permission of the publisher (Springer Science+Business Media, LLC, 233 Spring Street, New York, NY 10013, USA), except for brief excerpts in connection with reviews or scholarly analysis. Use in connection with any form of information storage and retrieval, electronic adaptation, computer software, or by similar or dissimilar methodology now known or hereafter developed is forbidden.
The use in this publication of trade names, trademarks, service marks, and similar terms, even if they are not identified as such, is not to be taken as an expression of opinion as to whether or not they are subject to proprietary rights.

Printed on acid-free paper

Springer is part of Springer Science+Business Media (www.springer.com)

Preface

The classic hallmarks of cancer are a poorly differentiated phenotype, and a cellular and genetic heterogeneity. In the past, the cellular diversity of cancer has mostly been attributed to the genetic instability of its cells. As the tumor cell population expands, individual cells pick up random mutations, and their molecular identity starts to diverge. By the time the cancer is detected, the millions of cells that make up the tumor have become as different from each other.

Cancer stem cells (CSCs) or, as defined by other authors, tumor-maintaining cells or cancer stem-like cells are a subpopulation of cancer cells that acquired some of the characteristics of stem cells to survive and adapt to ever-changing environments. These include the ability to self-renew and the capacity to produce progenitors that differentiate into other cell types.

It has been originally hypothesized that CSCs could potentially arise from normal stem or early progenitors. Now, the longstanding notion that fully committed and specialized cells might de-differentiate over the course of tumor initiation and progression to originate CSCs has been reevaluated. At present, data emerge to indicate that cancer cells that resemble stem cells need not be part of the original tumor but rather may emerge during later stages of tumor development. The observed tumor heterogeneity is probably a combination of growing genomic instability and epigenetic instability associated with the acquisition of a stem cell-like phenotype. These instability promote a new a fundamental peculiarity of CSCs, i.e., genetic plasticity.

CSCs represent the ideal justification for a lot of intriguing and obscure aspects of cancer pathogenesis (i.e., cancer cell dormancy, chemoresistance, local and distant relapses). The complex pathophysiology of CSCs and its important direct and indirect implications in molecular and cellular biology of cancer, at present, render this topic particularly interesting for Chemists, Biochemists, Pharmacologists, Biologists, Geneticists who are studying different aspect of experimental oncology. Moreover, considering the enormity of the clinical implications related to CSCs and/or to "cancer cells like stem cell," a growing number of researchers should modify and/or adapt its field of study in consideration of this relatively new topic.

At last, the identification of a molecular phenotype for these modified stem cells, associated to an accurate definition of their typical derangement in cell differentiation and metabolism, can represent a fundamental advance in terms of early diagnosis and selective therapy of cancer. At last but not least, the knowledge of pathogenetic mechanisms at the basis of CSCs can enlarge and ameliorate the therapeutic applications of the normal adult stem cells (i.e., regenerative medicine, tissue engineering, biotechnology applications) by reducing the risk of a deranged, uncontrolled, and thereby potentially tumorigenic stem cell differentiation.

A critical and continuous updating to the different pathophysiological aspects of this CSC may certainly help the development of a research, not only limited to cancer but also really useful and harmless for patients, by stimulating potential clinical applications in terms of diagnosis and above all of therapy.

Rome, Italy

Roberto Scatena
Alvaro Mordente
Bruno Giardina

Contents

1 **Cancer Stem Cells: A Revisitation of the "Anaplasia" Concept** 1
   Roberto Scatena

2 **Stem Cells and Cancer Stem Cells: New Insights** 17
   Toru Kondo

3 **Molecular Biology of Cancer Stem Cells** 33
   Oswaldo Keith Okamoto

4 **Biomarkers of Cancer Stem Cells** 45
   Jun Dou and Ning Gu

5 **Cancer Stem Cells and the Microenvironment** 69
   Alfonso Colombatti, Carla Danussi, Eliana Pivetta, and Paola Spessotto

6 **Leukemia Stem Cells** 85
   Steven W. Lane and David A. Williams

7 **Cancer Stem Cells and the Central Nervous System** 105
   Serdar Korur, Maria Maddalena Lino, and Adrian Merlo

8 **Cancer Stem Cells and Glioblastoma Multiforme: Pathophysiological and Clinical Aspects** 123
   Akio Soeda, Mark E. Shaffrey, and Deric M. Park

9 **Breast Cancer Stem Cells** 141
   Nuria Rodríguez Salas, Enrique González González, and Carlos Gamallo Amat

10 **Colon Cancer Stem Cells** 155
   Ugo Testa

11	**Liver Tumor-Initiating Cells/Cancer Stem Cells: Past Studies, Current Status, and Future Perspectives** 181
	Kwan Ho Tang, Stephanie Ma, and Xin-Yuan Guan

12	**Pancreatic Cancer Stem Cells** 197
	Erica N. Proctor and Diane M. Simeone

13	**Cancer Stem Cells and Renal Carcinoma** 211
	Benedetta Bussolati and Giovanni Camussi

14	**Cancer Stem Cells: Proteomic Approaches for New Potential Diagnostic and Prognostic Biomarkers** 221
	Patrizia Bottoni, Bruno Giardina, and Roberto Scatena

15	**Cancer Stem Cells: An Innovative Therapeutic Approach** 239
	Roberto Scatena, Patrizia Bottoni, Alessandro Pontoglio, Salvatore Scarà, and Bruno Giardina

16	**Cancer Stem Cell and ATP-Binding Cassette: Which Role in Chemoresistance?** 267
	Andrea Silvestrini, Elisabetta Meucci, Giuseppe Ettore Martorana, Bruno Giardina, and Alvaro Mordente

17	**Stem Cells and Cancer Stem Cells: Biological and Clinical Interrelationships** 289
	Cinzia Bagalà and Carlo Barone

18	**Immunomodulatory Functions of Cancer Stem Cells** 301
	Tobias Schatton, Jennifer Y. Lin, and Markus H. Frank

Index 333

Contributors

Carlos Gamallo Amat Pathology Department, Medical School, Autónoma University, Madrid, Spain

Cinzia Bagalà Division of Medical Oncology, Department of Internal Medicine, Catholic University, Largo A. Gemelli 8, 00168 Rome, Italy
cinziabagala@libero.it

Carlo Barone Division of Medical Oncology, Department of Internal Medicine, Catholic University, Largo A. Gemelli 8, 00168 Rome, Italy
carlobarone@rm.unicatt.it

Patrizia Bottoni Department of Laboratory Medicine, Catholic University, Largo A. Gemelli 8, 00168 Rome, Italy
patrizia.bottoni@rm.unicatt.it

Benedetta Bussolati Renal and Vascular Physiopathology Laboratory, Department of Internal Medicine, Molecular Biotechnology Centre and Research Centre for Molecular Medicine, University of Torino, Cso Dogliotti 14, 10126 Torino, Italy
benedetta.bussolati@unito.it

Giovanni Camussi Renal and Vascular Physiopathology Laboratory, Department of Internal Medicine, Molecular Biotechnology Centre and Research Centre for Molecular Medicine, University of Torino, Cso Dogliotti 14, 10126 Torino, Italy

Alfonso Colombatti Division of Experimental Oncology 2, National Cancer Institute IRCCS-CRO, Via Franco Gallini 2, 33081 Aviano, Italy
acolombatti@cro.it

Carla Danussi Division of Experimental Oncology 2, National Cancer Institute IRCCS-CRO, Via Franco Gallini 2, 33081 Aviano, Italy

Jun Dou Department of Pathogenic Biology and Immunology, Medical School, Southeast University, Nanjing 210009, China
njdoujun@yahoo.com.cn

Markus H. Frank Transplantation Research Center, Children's Hospital Boston and Brigham and Women's Hospital, Harvard Medical School, 300 Longwood Avenue, Boston, MA 02115, USA

Department of Dermatology, Brigham and Women's Hospital, Harvard Medical School, 77 Avenue Louis Pasteur, Boston, MA 02115, USA

Bruno Giardina Department of Laboratory Medicine, Catholic University, Largo A. Gemelli 8, 00168 Rome, Italy
bgiardina@rm.unicatt.it

Enrique González González Surgery Department, Hospital del Henares, Madrid, Spain

Ning Gu School of Biological Science and Medical Engineering, Southeast University, Nanjing 210096, China
guning@seu.edu.cn

Xin-Yuan Guan Department of Clinical Oncology, Li Ka Shing Faculty of Medicine, Queen Mary Hospital, The University of Hong Kong, Pok Fu Lam, Hong Kong
xyguan@hkucc.hku.hk

Toru Kondo Laboratory for Cell Lineage Modulation, RIKEN Center for Developmental Biology, 2-2-3 Minatojima-Minamimachi, Chuo-ku, Kobe, Hyogo 650-0047, Japan

Department of Stem Cell Biology, Ehime University Proteo-Medicine Research Center, Shitsukawa, To-on, Ehime 791-0295, Japan
tkondo@m.ehime-u.ac.j

Serdar Korur Laboratory of Molecular Neuro-Oncology, University Hospital Basel, Buchserstrasse 26, Bern CH-3006, Basel, Switzerland
sedar.korur@unibas.ch

Steven W. Lane Division of Immonology, Queenland Institute of Medical Research, Brisbane, Australia
steven.lane@gimr.edu.au

Jennifer Y. Lin Department of Dermatology, Brigham and Women's Hospital, Harvard Medical School, 77 Avenue Louis Pasteur, Boston, MA 02115, USA

Maria Maddalena Lino Laboratory of Molecular Neuro-Oncology, University Hospital Basel, Buchserstrasse 26, Bern CH-3006, Basel, Switzerland

Stephanie Ma Department of Pathology, Li Ka Shing Faculty of Medicine, Queen Mary Hospital, The University of Hong Kong, Pok Fu Lam, Hong Kong
stephanie.ma@gmail.com

Contributors   xi

Giuseppe Ettore Martorana Institute of Biochemistry and Clinical Biochemistry, Catholic University, School of Medicine, Largo F. Vito, 1, 00168 Rome, Italy

Adrian Merlo Laboratory of Molecular Neuro-Oncology,
University Hospital Basel, Buchserstrasse 26, Bern CH-3006, Basel, Switzerland
adrian.merlo@gmx.ch

Elisabetta Meucci Institute of Biochemistry and Clinical Biochemistry, Catholic University, School of Medicine, Largo F. Vito, 1, 00168 Rome, Italy

Alvaro Mordente Institute of Biochemistry and Clinical Biochemistry, Catholic University, School of Medicine, Largo F. Vito 1, 00168 Rome, Italy
alvaro.mordente@rm.unicatt.it

Oswaldo Keith Okamoto Centro de Estudos do Genoma Humano, Departamento de Genética e Biologia Evolutiva, Instituto de Biociências, Universidade de São Paulo, CEP 05508-090, São Paulo – SP, Brazil
keith.okamoto@usp.br

Deric M. Park Department of Neurological Surgery, University of Virginia, 800212 Charlottesville, VA 22908, USA
dmp3j@virginia.edu

Eliana Pivetta Division of Experimental Oncology 2, National Cancer Institute IRCCS-CRO, Via Franco Gallini 2, 33081 Aviano, Italy

Alessandro Pontoglio Department of Laboratory Medicine, Catholic University, Largo A. Gemelli 8, 00168 Rome, Italy
espeedy@libero.it

Erica N. Proctor Departments of Surgery and Molecular and Integrative Physiology, University of Michigan Medical Center, 1500 E Medical Center Drive, TC 2210B, Ann Arbor, MI 48109, USA
eproctor@med.umich.edu

Nuria Rodríguez Salas Medical Oncology Unit, Hospital Universitario Infanta Leonor, C/ Gran Vía del Este n° 80, 28031 Madrid, Spain
nuria.rodriguez@salud.madrid.org

Salvatore Scarà Department of Laboratory Medicine, Catholic University, Largo A. Gemelli 8, 00168 Rome, Italy

Roberto Scatena Department of Laboratory Medicine, Catholic University, Largo A. Gemelli 8, 00168 Rome, Italy
r.scatena@rm.unicatt.it

Tobias Schatton Transplantation Research Center, Children's Hospital Boston and Brigham and Women's Hospital, Harvard Medical School,
300 Longwood Avenue, Boston, MA 02115, USA
tobias.schatton@tch.harvard.edu

Mark E. Shaffrey Department of Neurological Surgery, University of Virginia, 800212 Charlottesville, VA 22908, USA

Andrea Silvestrini Institute of Biochemistry and Clinical Biochemistry, Catholic University, School of Medicine, Largo F. Vito, 1, 00168 Rome, Italy

Diane M. Simeone Departments of Surgery and Molecular and Integrative Physiology, University of Michigan Medical Center, 1500 E Medical Center Drive, TC 2210B, Ann Arbor, MI 48109, USA
simeone@med.umich.edu

Akio Soeda Department of Neurological Surgery, University of Virginia, 800212 Charlottesville, VA 22908, USA

Paola Spessotto Division of Experimental Oncology 2, National Cancer Institute IRCCS-CRO, Via Franco Gallini 2, 33081 Aviano, Italy

Kwan Ho Tang Department of Pathology, Li Ka Shing Faculty of Medicine, Queen Mary Hospital, The University of Hong Kong, Pok Fu Lam, Hong Kong

Ugo Testa Department of Hematology, Oncology and Molecular Medicine, Istituto Superiore di Sanità, Viale Regina Elena 299, 00161 Rome, Italy
ugo.testa@iss.it

David A. Williams Division of Hematology/Oncology, Children's Hospital Boston, Department of Pediatrics, Harvard Medical School, Boston, MA, USA

Department of Pediatrics Oncology, Dana-Farber Cancer Institute, Harvard Stem Cell Institute, Boston, MA, USA

Chapter 1
Cancer Stem Cells: A Revisitation of the "Anaplasia" Concept

Roberto Scatena

Introduction

Cancer stem cells (CSCs) or, as defined by other authors, tumor-maintaining cells or cancer stem-like cells represent one of the most interesting topics of cancer pathophysiology studied in the last decade.

The American Association for Cancer Research Stem Cell Workshop defined a cancer stem cell as a cell within the tumor that possesses the capacity to self-renew and, in doing so, gives rise to the heterogeneous lineages that comprise the tumor (Clarke et al. 2006). This intriguing subpopulation of cancer cells should permit to justify some lethal clinical aspects of cancer, above all recidivism and radio/chemoresistance. Moreover, CSCs may represent a real new and more selective approach in cancer treatment. These innovative clinical potentials originate from an important revision of cancer molecular biology, with the clonal model of tumor evolution passing to a hierarchical model.

Specifically, the term "CSCs" describes a representative subpopulation of cancer cells with peculiar molecular aspects that resemble some of those typical of normal stem cells. In fact, these cells are capable of self-renewal (i.e., replenishing the repertoire of identical cancer cells), differentiation (i.e., creating heterogeneous progeny that differentiate into more mature cells), and show extraordinary proliferative potential (Stricker and Kumar 2010). Importantly, this particular subpopulation of tumor cells seems to show other similarities to normal stem cell physiology, including the following:

- They appear to be primarily in a more quiescent or dormant cell-cycle state
- Long-lived cells typically give rise to short-lived, more differentiated cells

R. Scatena (✉)
Department of Laboratory Medicine, Catholic University,
Largo A. Gemelli 8, 00168 Rome, Italy
e-mail: r.scatena@rm.unicatt.it

- They are highly influenced by signals from their microenvironment
- They are characterized by specific surface markers and/or signal transduction pathways that are also important in stem cell biology
- They express high levels of ABC transporters and DNA repair mechanisms, which, together with their low proliferation index, give these cells a particular resistance to classical radiotherapeutic and chemotherapeutic protocols (Visvader 2011; Wang and Dick 2008).

On the whole, these peculiar biological properties contribute to the possibility that CSCs are responsible for cancer recurrence, metastatic dissemination, and chemoresistance (Zhou et al. 2009). As a result, these intriguing cells seem to play an important role in the pathophysiology of cancer, with dramatic clinical implications in terms of prognosis and therapy. In this sense, it may be more appropriate to call them "tumor-maintaining," "tumor-sustaining," or "tumor-propagating" cells.

Interestingly, in the same way, cancer stem-like cells seem to introduce a modification to the definition of the term "anaplasia," which derives from the term Greek ἀνα-πλάσσω, meaning to mold, to shape, or to model again. In fact, classically, it implies a dedifferentiation or, better, a loss of the structural and functional peculiarities of normal cells, which lose the morphological and functional features of the original cell, either partially or totally (Stricker and Kumar 2010). This peculiar reversion and/or lack of differentiation are considered hallmarks of malignant neoplasms (tumors). This term also includes a derangement of the normal cytoarchitecture of the tissue/organ from which the tumor originates and sometimes, an increased proliferative potential.

Generally, to define anaplasia, a number of morphologic changes are required (Stricker and Kumar 2010), including the following:

(a) *Pleomorphism.* The cells and the nuclei characteristically display considerable variations in size and shape.
(b) *Abnormal nuclear morphology.* Nuclei are typically hyperchromatic and disproportionately large; nuclear shape is extremely variable, and chromatin is often coarsely clumped and distributed along the nuclear membrane. Large nucleoli are usually present.
(c) *Mitoses.* Anaplastic cells usually show large numbers of mitoses; moreover, unusual mitotic figures (tripolar, quadripolar, or multipolar spindles) are often present. These gross perturbations of the mitotic apparatus could also be responsible for the formation of tumor giant cells, some possessing only a single huge polymorphic nucleus and others having two or more nuclei.
(d) *Loss of polarity.* In addition to cytological abnormalities, the orientation of anaplastic cells is markedly deranged, indicating a complex derangement of cell–cell and cell–matrix interactions. These alterations cause sheets or large masses of tumor cells to grow in an anarchic, disorganized fashion.
(e) *Stromal alterations.* The structural and functional perturbations of cancer cells derange cell–cell and cell–matrix interactions that could have a causative role in the classic tumor cell–matrix disorganization. This occurrence, in turn, from a morphological point of view, may cause large areas of ischemic necrosis in

tumor masses, while, from a functional standpoint, this architectural disorder could have a role on the induction of the Warburg effect.

For many years, these morphological features have been associated with a simple dedifferentiation process, fitting well with the classic, clonal evolution of cancer.

It is now known, however, that cancer may arise from stem cells or progenitor cells in different tissues. In these tumors, failure of differentiation and/or abnormal differentiation, rather than dedifferentiation of specialized cells, accounts for the undifferentiated neoplastic cell. In fact, according to hierarchical model, instead of a neoplastic cell, it would be more appropriate to discuss about heterogeneous populations of tumor cells, which consist of both essentially differentiated cells with no or poor mitotic potential and rarer cells that function as a tumor reservoir by sustaining malignant growth. This mixed pathogenesis has important biological, pathological, and thereby clinical implications that push to reevaluate the morphological criteria of anaplasia.

Background

Are CSCs really progenitor/stem cells and the actual cells of origin in cancer? The answer is becoming more complex as more data is accumulating.

Virchow first suggested that some tumors could arise from embryonic cells (1855). Generally, however, the modern concept of cancer cells as cells that show or acquire some of the fundamental characteristics of normal stem cells (i.e., self-renewal, multipotency, and proliferation potential) was initially postulated by Pierce and Speers (1988) and more recently confirmed by Bonnet and Dick (1997), who, by adopting some clusters of differentiation as CSC biomarkers, elegantly showed that a single leukemic cell was able to transmit systemic disease when transplanted into a mouse. A decade following the initial prospective isolation of leukemic stem cells, Al-Hajj et al. (2003) showed that human breast cancers also seem to adhere to the hierarchical or CSC model.

Thereafter, similar stem cell-like cells were discovered in various solid tumors, including melanoma (Quintana et al. 2008), colon (O'Brien et al. 2007), prostate (Collins et al. 2005), liver (Sell and Leffert 2008), pancreas (Li et al. 2007), and brain tumors (Singh et al. 2003).

Specifically, Bonnet and Dick (1997), in acute myeloid leukemia, showed that only a small subset of CD34+CD38− cells harbored serial leukemic transplantation potential, whereas the bulk of leukemic cells did not show this capability. Thereby, just a defined subset of leukemic cells is responsible for maintaining the disease. Other evidence seems to confirm that few, but not all, cancers are organized in a hierarchical manner (Bonnet and Dick 1997; Reya et al. 2001). Moreover, a number of caveats of the CSC model were evident early that limited a general acceptance of the CSC concept and the hierarchical organization of cancer (Visvader and Lindeman 2008).

It is essential to appreciate that the field of CSC research is a work in progress. Specifically, as recently reviewed by Clevers (2011), the meaning of CSC is undergoing a profound re-evaluation in its main postulates. In reality, additional data give a more mature vision of the CSC concept and, at the same time, mitigate an overly enthusiastic approach to its potential clinical applications. These new data, moreover, reply efficaciously to criticism about the existence of CSCs and their pathophysiological role in cancer (Gupta et al. 2009; Maenhaut et al. 2010).

CSC Peculiarities

CSC Plasticity

Importantly, the most intriguing and new evidence about this subpopulation of CSCs seems to be their plasticity (Rapp et al. 2008; Leder et al. 2010). This term introduces a dynamic concept in the CSC definition, with fundamental biological and clinical implications.

For example, Roesch et al. (2010) isolated different melanoma subpopulations of tumor cells, using the H3K4 demethylase JARID1B as a biomarker. Using this technique, the authors characterized a small subpopulation of slow-cycling melanoma cells that cycle with doubling times of >4 weeks within the rapidly proliferating main population. These isolated JARID1B-positive melanoma cells give rise to highly proliferative progeny. Moreover, knockdown of JARID1B leads to an initial acceleration of tumor growth followed by exhaustion, which seems to suggest that the JARID1B-positive subpopulation is essential for maintaining tumor growth. Importantly, the expression of JARID1B was dynamically regulated and did not follow the typical hierarchical CSC model because JARID1B-negative cells can become positive, and even single melanoma cells, irrespective of selection, are tumorigenic. These results seem to suggest a new understanding of melanoma heterogeneity, with tumor maintenance as a dynamic process mediated by a temporarily and dynamically distinct subpopulation of cancer stem-like cells. These data pushed the authors to conclude that at least some stem-like cells from solid tumors may actually not be static entities, but rather tumor cells that may transiently acquire some stemness properties, depending on the tumor context (microenvironment, physical and chemical milieu). Moreover, analogous to normal stem cells, the epithelial–mesenchymal transition (EMT) seems to be a key developmental program that can induce not only the acquisition of mesenchymal traits but also the expression of functional and phenotypic stem cell markers, confirming previous studies (Mani et al. 2008).

At this point, it is already evident that the morphological concept of anaplasia is not static, but now extends to an extremely complex and dynamic, molecular pathophysiological disorder.

Strong evidence about this new complexity originates from the research of Anderson et al. (2011) and Notta et al. (2011). These authors, by adopting a Ph$^+$ acute lymphoblastic leukemia (ALL) xenograft model, carried out a combined genetic and functional study of the genomic diversity of functionally defined tumor-initiating cells derived from a diagnostic patient sample. The results clearly showed that multiple tumor clones coexist in the diagnostic patient sample and that these clones undergo divergent evolution from the diagnostic clone, supporting a branching model of tumor progression. Specifically, these genetically diverse subclones seem to be related through a complex evolutionary process and vary in their xenograft growth properties and leukemia-initiating cell frequency. Importantly, this intratumoral heterogeneity seems to promote clonal evolution by increasing the number of selectable traits under any given stress. This selective pressure could contribute to the genetic diversification that is probably important for tumor survival and evolution, which also affects outcomes in terms of clinical aggressiveness.

In practical terms, the evidence that, at diagnosis, genetically distinct subclones already possess variably aggressive growth properties points to the need to develop effective therapies to eradicate all intratumoral genetic subclones, to prevent further evolution and recurrence. In this sense, the ability to segregate even minor subclones in xenografts could be a useful tool for the preclinical development of new therapeutic strategies, but in reality, this ability will likely significantly complicate a true radical therapeutic approach.

From a pathophysiological point of view, the isolation of individual genetic subclones in xenografts could provide an opportunity to study the functional genetic evolution of subclones present in diagnostic samples. Moreover, because gene silencing and other epigenetic events may contribute to tumor progression, a genome-wide methylation analysis of individual subclones would be an interesting undertaking. In fact, this evolution by branching, stressing subclonal complexity, underscores the importance of gaining a better molecular understanding of each subclone. Most important, this research has shown that outgrowth of subclones in serial xenografts can only be sustained by leukemia-initiating cells, establishing that genetic diversity occurs in this functionally important cell type, as well. Moreover, in the opinion of the authors, the discoveries that specific genetic events influence leukemia-initiating cell frequency, and genetically distinct leukemia-initiating cells evolve through a complex evolutionary process, indicate that a close connection must exist between genetic and functional heterogeneity.

All that brings together the classical clonal evolution and the hierarchical model related to CSC. This unifying vision allows consideration of the leukemia stem cell not as a static entity, but as a cell able to evolve genetically in response to the selective pressure of tumor microenvironments. As tumors evolve, the frequency of leukemia stem cells can increase and eventually progress at different grades of differentiation until they lose the characteristics of a CSC.

From a clinical point of view, the isolation of CSCs should be interpreted with considerable care in tumors composed of genetically diverse subclones, as fractionation of CSC and non-CSC populations could segregate genetically distinct subclones with variable tumor-initiating cell capacity, different epigenetic/developmental programs, and possibly different phenotypic peculiarities. Finally, these findings indicate that more commonalities may exist between clonal evolution and CSC models of cancer than previously thought, and in the future, a unification of these concepts will likely be realized.

Moreover, data from the Anderson and Dick groups confirm a re-evaluation of a Darwinian model for cancer propagating cells and resultant clonal architecture. According to this revisitation, cells with self-renewing properties have varying genotypes that provide the units of selection in the evolutionary diversification and progression of cancer. Moreover, data have shown that sequential and concurrent genotypic variation in propagating cells occur in ALL and are likely to do so in other cancers, providing a rich substrate for disease progression.

Importantly, it is likely that genetic diversity of these new cancer stem-like cells may be associated with both frequency variation and diversity of functional properties, for example, differentiation status, niche occupancy, quiescence and drug or irradiation sensitivity. This picture may help to explain some of the criticisms related to the CSC hypothesis (Visvader and Lindeman 2008; Rosen and Jordan 2009; Greaves 2010).

In summary, plasticity and related genomic diversity in cancer varies in extent with stage of disease (Park et al. 2010; Anderson et al. 2011) and probably with time, but this diversity also varies according to space, depending on the local microenvironments, chemical and physical conditions of each cell, effects of intraclonal competition, and intrinsic genetic instability. In fact, in metastasis or recurrences, for example, data seem to indicate a continued diversification of propagating cells with a prevalence of dominant or therapy-resistant subclones (Scatena et al. 2008; Liu et al. 2009).

In this situation, a CSC-targeted therapy, directed at mutant molecules, may have limited efficacy if the targets themselves are not initiating lesions, but secondary mutations segregated into subclones. In other terms, this genetic and functional variation of cancer-propagating cells may represent a significant roadblock to effective, specific therapy (Scatena et al. 2011). CSCs plasticity thereby seems to reconcile clonal and hierarchical models, but it significantly complicates the pathophysiology of CSCs.

An additional new aspect of CSCs that also indirectly confirms to the concept of plasticity comes from the observation of Visvader (2011), who stressed that the cell of origin of cancer, i.e., the normal cell that acquires the first cancer-promoting mutation, is not necessarily related to the CSCs, the cellular subset that uniquely sustains malignant growth. In other words, the cell-of-origin and CSC concepts refer to cancer-initiating cells and cancer-propagating cells, which should be considered distinct.

Thereby, a stem cell might sustain the first oncogenic hit, but subsequent alterations required for the genesis of a real CSC can occur in descendent cells. For example, in chronic myeloid leukemia (CML), the hematopoietic stem cell (HMS) is the cell of origin in the more indolent phase of the disease, but in patients with CML blast crisis, granulocyte–macrophage progenitors acquire self-renewal capacity through a β-catenin mutation and emerge as the probable CSCs (Jamieson et al. 2004).

Interestingly, the stemness of CSC was indirectly validated by Janic et al. (2010) who showed that a number of genes typically involved in germline programming in fruit flies were also involved in the formation of glioblastoma. The authors found that inactivation of these germ cell genes can suppress tumor growth. Importantly, some of these genes have a related human counterpart known to be abnormally expressed in certain cancers and not only in glioblastoma.

Further strong evidence of CSC plasticity and/or stemness comes from the observations of Wang et al. (2010) and Ricci-Vitiani et al. (2010), which show that, in addition to recruiting vessels from the outside, glioblastomas may induce vessel formation by differentiating its tumor cells into cancer endothelial-like cells. Specifically, some cancer cells in the immediate environment of the nascent vessel are co-opted for this purpose. The co-opted cells are thought to retain most of their tumor-cell characteristics, while acquiring a limited number of endothelial-cell features. In fact, both authors showed independently that a subset of endothelial cells lining tumor vessels carry genetic abnormalities (i.e., monosomy of Cep 10 or polysomy of Tel19 and LSI22) found in the tumor cells themselves. Moreover, a comparable proportion of a cell population expressing endothelial cell markers and a population of neighboring tumor cells harbored three or more copies of either the *EGFR* gene or other parts of chromosome 7. Such cell populations also shared a mutated version of the oncogene *p53*. Another indicator of the tumor origin of some tumor vessel endothelial cells is that, as well as expressing characteristic endothelial cell markers, such as von Willebrand factor and VE-cadherin, they expressed the nonendothelial tumor marker GFAP. Moreover, the glioblastoma cell population that could differentiate into endothelial cells and form blood vessels in vitro was enriched in cells expressing the tumor stem cell marker CD133. Further, Wang et al. (2010) showed that a clone of cells derived from a single tumor cell, which expressed CD133 but not VE-cadherin, was multipotent in vitro, and these cells may differentiate into both neural cells and endothelial cells.

Interestingly, Ricci-Vitiani et al. (2010), on the basis of this evidence, hypothesized some clinical applications. In fact, studies examining exposure to the clinical antiangiogenesis agent bevacizumab (Calabrese et al. 2007) or to a γ-secretase inhibitor (Gilbertson and Rich 2007) utilizing knockdown shRNA have demonstrated that blocking VEGF or silencing *VEGFR2* inhibits the maturation of tumor endothelial progenitors into endothelium, but not the differentiation of CD133+ cells into endothelial progenitors, whereas γ-secretase inhibition or *NOTCH1* silencing blocks the transition into endothelial progenitors. These data may provide new perspectives on the mechanisms of failure of antiangiogenesis inhibitors currently in use.

In conclusion, such data demonstrate that lineage plasticity and the capacity to generate tumor vasculature of putative CSCs within glioblastoma are strong findings that provide new insight into the biology of gliomas and, above all, into the definition of cancer stemness.

These findings further confirm the pathophysiological role of CSCs in cancer. In fact, the expression of these multipotency factors, normally limited to early developmental stages, may inappropriately contribute "to specify and characterize" CSCs that can divide and differentiate into heterogeneous cell types. Importantly, from a therapeutic point of view, the direct and/or indirect drug-induced loss or inhibition of these stem cell program genes might prevent the formation of CSCs or lead to their death, thereby facilitating the prevention or cure of cancer. These observations clearly established that cancer cells, during their evolution, might acquire some stem cell peculiarities that are fundamental for the resultant course of disease.

If, on the one hand, this cancer stemness stresses the difference between stem cells and CSCs, which may better be defined as cancer "stem-like" cells, on the other hand, it induces the study of the physiology and pathophysiology of stem cells, allowing a better understanding of the molecular mechanisms that extend these new functional conditions of cancer cell, with dramatic clinical implications. Again, intriguingly, the term "anaplasia" does not seem to contain this new armament of powerful functional capabilities that, until now, have not been characterized by a peculiar morphological picture.

CSC Biomarkers

The revival of CSCs originated from the possibility to isolate these cells by adopting hypothetical, somewhat specific markers (i.e., the original research of Dick (2008) on the CD34+/CD34− fraction from AML). Afterward, other various biomarkers have been discovered that show the peculiarity to be more present in cancer cells with stemness properties, such as the following:

(a) Other cell surface proteins (CD 133, IL-3r, EpCAM, CXC chemokine receptor type 4 (CXCR-4) also known as fusin or CD184)
(b) Peculiar signaling pathways generally related to self-renewal mechanisms (Hedgehog, Notch, Wnt/β-catenin, BM1, BMI, Pten)
(c) Structural and/or functional components of the stem cell niche
(d) Various detoxifying mechanisms (ABC transporters, aldehyde dehydrogenase ALDH)
(e) Telomerase and pathways related to cellular senescence
(f) Oncogenes and oncosuppressors (p16INK4 – Rb)
(g) Cell differentiation-inducing pathways
(h) Various microRNAs

Each marker and its pathophysiological implications in cancer will be discussed in other sections; now it is important to outline that these structural molecules and/or functional pathways are not specific for CSCs but are present both in normal differentiated cells and stem cells. This could partially hamper potential clinical implications of these markers in diagnosis and, above all, therapy of cancer. In fact, recently developed drugs capable of modulating some of these functions and utilized in the preclinical phase have provided interesting results in terms of response to therapy but showed significant side effects (Von Hoff et al. 2009; Yauch et al. 2009).

As already cited, Dick (2008) adopted CD34+CD38− fractions to identify leukemic stem cells. Similarly, Al-Hajj et al. (2003) used the marker combination

CD24−/CD44+ in breast cancer. CD133 has been a widely used CSC marker, despite criticisms that it is also present in normal cells of different organs. From this original research, different authors have adopted several differentiation-clustering panels to characterize CSCs of various origins. However, as previously cited, CSCs may present other structural and functional characteristics that, at least partially, should permit identification (ALDH, Hedgehog, Notch, Wnt/β-catenin, BM1, BMI, telomerase and so on). It is important to reiterate, however, that these characteristics, although they prevail in CSCs, are not unique to this subpopulation of cancer cells. This difficulty to identify and isolate CSCs can impair research on the molecular pathophysiology of CSCs, in particular, and cancer, in general, with significant implications on the therapeutic index of drugs that could selectively target these tumor-maintaining cells. In fact, the possibility to recognize and selectively kill such cells could represent a real revolution in cancer treatment, with beneficial effects on the frequency of recidivism and metastasis. This therapeutic potential has caused an upsurge in research on different molecular aspects of this topic, and some new and old drugs have been rapidly produced to destroy these cells. Some of these molecules are already in the clinical phase, with conflicting results. In reality, actual CSC biomarkers are not specific and are present in normal stem cells, as well as in normal cells from different organs and tissues, a fact that is too often disregarded.

To further complicate the matter, the molecular mechanisms at the basis of CSC are really complex and above all, not static, but highly dynamic. This means that phenotypic and functional characteristics of these cells can vary by minimal influences of microenvironments, rendering their identification and analysis problematic. Just as an example to better understand the serious, but disregarded, aspect of the dynamic plasticity of CSCs, the dissimilar biomarker profiles of human colon CSCs from two different European and American biotechnology companies that produce various CSCs for research purposes are presented below:

- USA company positive markers of human colon CSCs : Vimentin, Variable S100, CEA, Galactosyl Transferase II, CK-7, CK-20, Smooth Muscle Actin (polyp), Bcl2, Ki-67, P504S, Mucin (MUC-1 and MUC-3)
- European company positive markers of human colon CSCs: CD133, CD44, CD34, CD 10SSEA3/4, Oct4, Tumorigenicity (<1,000 cells), Alkaline Phosphatase, Aldehyde Dehydrogenase, Telomerase, Sox2, cKit, Lin28

It is evident that genetic, proteomic, cellular and functional studies of these two groups of CSCs could give different results, with serious consequences in terms of translational research and thereby on pharmacotoxicological implications.

All these facts stress that the present fundamental task, not only from a pharmacological point of view, is the accurate identification/targeting of these CSCs. Such attempts must consider that these cells are tumor stem-like cells with only some aspects typical of physiological stem cells. This sharing of certain structural and functional characteristics not only should permit more selective therapeutic targeting but also may expose normal stem cells to iatrogenic insult, with potentially dangerous side effects.

Identification and Isolation of CSCs by Xenograft Assay

Another debated aspect of CSC validation is related to xenograft assay validity. Xenotransplantation of sorted cancer cells into immunodeficient mice is the choice method to identify CSCs. The transplanted cancer cell should be able to regenerate the original neoplasia. The frequency of cells able to regenerate tumor in the host depends also on the level of mouse immunocompromise, belittling in such a way the concept of CSCs is rare subpopulation of cancer cells (Quintana et al. 2008). Moreover, the frequency of CSCs can be dramatically improved if the species barrier is avoided. On the other hand, in some mouse leukemia models, CSC isolation by tumor cell transplantation has not been obtained. These data are ambiguous, as these models significantly limit the pathogenic role of the microenvironment that, in other different cancer experimental models, seems to have a fundamental importance in driving tumor progression (LaBarge 2010; Allen and Louise Jones 2011). Further, isolation by xenotransplantation could significantly impair morph-functional studies on CSCs because all fundamental niche functions are abruptly modified, with unavoidable alteration of proteome and genome expression of the original CSCs. Importantly, xenotransplantation attests that these cancer stem-like cells may survive and proliferate independently by otherwise fundamental interactions with adhesion molecule and growth factors. This seems to indicate that potential anticancer drugs targeting niche interactions would be, or would become, easily ineffective. Thereby, the interesting experimental results reported by Liu et al. (2011), which show that enforced expression of miR-34a in bulk or purified CD44(+) prostate cancer stem-like cells may inhibit clonogenic expansion, tumor regeneration, and metastasis by directly repressing CD44, should all be validated by in vivo studies. Similarly, the attractive data of Sodir et al. (2011), which showed that short-term systemic Myc inhibition in the (SV40)-driven pancreatic islet mouse tumor model is sufficient to trigger tumor regression by collapse of the tumor microenvironment, with concomitant death of endothelial cells, attenuation of inflammatory cells, vascular collapse, and hypoxia, need to be confirmed with more prolonged studies. In fact, it is fundamental to verify if such plastic and highly adaptable cancer stem-like cells can overcome this molecular stress signaling.

Existence of Distinctive CSCs Biomarkers?

The defined, so-called peculiarities of CSC, in terms of cluster of differentiations, signal transduction pathways, ATP-binding cassette transporters (ABC transporters), and so on, are not specific. It is evident that only one intriguing aspect is truly distinctive, i.e., its genetic, functional and phenotypic plasticity (Woodward and Sulman 2008; Scatena et al. 2011). The extreme adaptability of these cells to minimal variations of the environment recalls, in the opinion of some authors, Darwin's evolutionary theory, with its classic branching pattern of evolution that is based on natural selection. However, considering the high rate of this cellular evolution/

adaptation, it is probably in some ways more complex because it contains a further important factor, i.e., the mutator phenotype of cancer cells (Bristow and Hill 2008; Brégeon and Doetsch 2011).

This definition originates from the well-known observation that malignancies are characterized by a high rate of mutations. Normal human cells replicate their DNA with exceptional accuracy. It has been estimated that approximately one error occurs during DNA replication for each 10^9–10^{10} nucleotides polymerized. Typically, malignant cells exhibit genetic instability, which causes multiple chromosomal abnormalities and thousands of alterations in the nucleotide sequence of nuclear DNA that tend to progressively accumulate. Pathogenic mechanisms, which accelerate this process, may be favored carcinogenic pathways. Mutator mutations are, in fact, mutations in genetic stability genes that increase the mutation rate, speeding up the accumulation of oncogenic mutations. The mutator hypothesis states that mutator mutations play a critical role in carcinogenesis (Beckman 2010).

Importantly, this mutator phenotype can be not only the starting point for tumor development but also might promote the emergence of a more aggressively growing tumor, frequently characterized by the appearance of poorly differentiated cells with some typical properties of a more embryonic phenotype. Moreover, during the tumor course, considerable biochemical heterogeneity becomes manifest in the growing tumor and its metastases.

Thereby, the loss of genetic stability is expected to increase the rate of growth-promoting or survival-promoting mutations that could drive tumor growth. Importantly, genetic instability may also increase the rate of deleterious mutations that could kill cells before they develop into tumors. Understanding how these factors balance out will ultimately be the key to understanding tumor development via genome destabilization. Moreover, understanding this balance may also have clinical implications for cancer diagnosis, prognosis, and therapy. If deleterious, genome-destabilizing mutations with their phenotypic counterparts are found in the population of developing cancer cells, these targets may provide opportunities for more efficacious diagnostic and therapeutic procedures (Barbie et al. 2008).

Specifically, the unscheduled alterations caused by genetic instability may be either temporary or permanent within the genome. These genetic changes are generally categorized into two major sites of instability, at the chromosomal level and at the nucleotide level (Perera and Bapat 2007).

At the chromosomal level, for example, telomere attrition has been correlated with genome instability. The shortest telomeres, in fact, can cause telomere fusions and genomic rearrangement. Thus, telomere-related carcinogenesis may involve induction of senescence by shortened telomeres, followed by primary genomic instability, leading to acquisition of mutations in cells. Some mutations may provide a proliferative advantage. The induced cell proliferation may induce further telomere shortening. Telomeres that are shortened below their stability threshold can induce breakage-fusion-bridge (BFB) cycles, formation of dicentric or ring chromosomes, and so on (Raynaud et al. 2008).

Instability at the nucleotide level occurs because of faulty DNA repair pathways, such as base excision repair and nucleotide excision repair, and includes instability of microsatellite repeat sequences (MSI) caused by defects in the mismatch repair pathway. The second form of instability, chromosomal instability (CIN), defines the existence of an accelerated rate of chromosomal alterations, which result in gains or losses of whole chromosomes, as well as inversions, deletions, duplications, and translocations of large chromosomal segments. Aneuploidy, which refers to an abnormal karyotype, is a hallmark of many cancer cells and is thought to develop as a result of CIN. To date, several pathways and processes have been implicated in CIN including the following: (1) pathways involved in telomere and centromere stability, (2) cell cycle checkpoint pathways and kinases, (3) pathways regulating diverse proteins via posttranslational modifications, (4) sister chromatid cohesion and chromosome segregation, and v. centrosome duplication.

Valeri et al. (2010) and Tili et al. (2011) have proposed a new, fascinating cause of genetic instability. These authors showed that miR-155 might significantly downregulate the core MMR proteins hMSH2, hMSH6, and hMLH1, inducing a mutator phenotype and MSI. Moreover, Tili et al. (2011) showed that miR-155 enhances the mutation rate by simultaneously targeting different genes that suppress mutations and even can reduce the efficiency of DNA safeguard mechanisms by targeting cell-cycle regulators, such as WEE1. In conclusion, by simultaneously targeting tumor suppressor genes and inducing a mutator phenotype, miR-155 could allow the selection of gene alterations required for tumor development and progression.

Genetic instability in cancer may also depend on abnormal protein synthesis because of the following: (1) lapses in RNA polymerase (RNAP) fidelity, generating aberrant transcripts that are translated into erroneous proteins; (2) lapses in ribosome fidelity, caused by exposure to a genotoxic agent; and (3) modification of RNA molecules that could induce the production of erroneous proteins during translation because of their potentially altered codon–anticodon pairing during tRNA selection. This transcriptional mutagenesis, which alters proteins and possibly changes the physiology of the cell, could be crucial for cancer stem origin because, as opposed to the DNA replication-dependent production of erroneous proteins, the lapses hit quiescent or slowly replicating cells (Brégeon and Doetsch 2011).

For completeness, it could be useful to stress that derangement of cellular metabolism could also have a role in genetic instability of cancer cells, in general, and CSC, in particular. In fact, in an experimental model of radiation-induced genomic instability (Dayal et al. 2009), mitochondrial dysfunction of complex II caused increased steady-state levels of hydrogen peroxide, which increased mutation frequency and induced gene amplification. These results seem to indicate that mitochondrial ROS could have a role in inducing genetic instability. These data, when applied to the intriguing metabolism of CSC, open an interesting field of research.

Finally, it is useful to cite the work of Conway et al. (2009), who showed that CSC generation is associated with the acquisition of nonclonal genomic rearrangements not found in the original population. This study was carried out in a transplantation model of testicular germ cell tumor, created by transplanting murine embryonic germ cells into the testis of the adult severe combined immunodeficient mouse model. Interestingly, pretreatment of EGCs with a potent inhibitor of self-renewal, retinoic acid, prevented tumor formation and the emergence of genetically unstable CSCs. Moreover, microarray analysis revealed that EGCs and first- and second-generation CSCs were highly similar. Further, approximately 1,000 differentially expressed transcripts could be identified that corresponded to alterations in oncogenes and genes associated with motility and development. In the opinion of the authors, these data suggest that activation of oncogenic pathways in a cellular background of genetic instability, coupled with an inherent ability to self-renew, is involved in the acquisition of metastatic behavior in the CSC population of tumors derived from pluripotent cells.

Conclusions

The evidence that cancer cells may assume some functional characteristics of stem cells is substantially modifying cancer research. In fact, CSCs not only have led to the consideration that cancer is caused by a morphologically heterogeneous population of malignant cells but also have focused the attention of researchers on a particular subpopulation of cancer cells with intriguing, yet too often disregarded, functional, and consequently clinical, implications.

The pathophysiology of these particular malignant cells is progressively becoming more complex with the advances in the understanding of their various biological properties, from a simple vision of stem cells that acquire a malignant phenotype, maintaining some of their typical characteristics (i.e., self-renewal, differentiation, proliferation potential), to a model of a neoplastic cell with extraordinary genomic plasticity that permits adaptation, also by assuming some functions of stem cells, to the minimal modifications of the microenvironment to satisfy their primordial need, i.e., proliferation.

The original definition of CSC pointed to the research on stem cells, which, across their long lives, may easily undergo and accumulate mutations that cause neoplasia. This pathogenesis may perfectly adhere to the hierarchical model of cancer proliferation. Moreover, this definition of CSC permits the adoption of some typical biomarkers of stem cells, to selectively target "transformed" stem cells.

This targeting of various subpopulations of isolated CSCs has produced innovative, but debated, results. Most important, the possibility of targeting the cells responsible for recidivism and/or metastasis has induced a series of pharmacological studies on potential anti-CSCs drugs. Considering the peculiarity of these biomarkers (clusters of differentiation, signal transduction pathways including Hedgehog, WNT, TK), some preclinical and clinical studies have shown interesting results, but the real therapeutic index should be evaluated, considering, above all, the partial selectivity of these biomarkers for CSCs.

It is probably time to update the definition of CSCs. It could be sufficient to stress, as already adopted from some authors concerning "cancer-maintaining cells" or "cancer stem-like cells," the differences between these cells may be not only phenotypic and functional but also origin. Moreover, the frequently adopted definition of "tumor-initiating cell," as recently reviewed by Visvader (2011), should be limited to that stem, progenitor, or terminally differentiated cell that presents the first mutative hit leading to cancer. This cell could be different from, or subsequently become, the cancer "stem-like" cell.

Finally, it is beyond doubt that CSCs have stimulated attention toward some aspects of the pathophysiology of cancer, which, until recently, have been neglected, specifically:

- It is clear that metabolism of these cells, which can be considered dormant or with a low proliferation index, should be different from that of classical highly proliferating cancer cells, justifying a re-evaluation of the Warburg effect (Scatena et al. 2010), which could mean that all cancer cell metabolism should be revisited according to this functional heterogeneity of cancer cells. Could metabolic drugs, capable of inhibiting the cancer "stem-like cell" and inducing cell differentiation toward more specialized and less multipotent cancer cells, be developed?
- What is the role of the epigenome in maintaining the genetic program induced by selection pressure and/or genetic instability? Could epigenetic drugs, capable of deranging the mechanisms that permit the cancer cell to acquire its high and dramatic genetic plasticity, be developed?
- Could it be possible to pharmacologically target the molecular mechanisms at the basis of this pathogenetically relevant genetic plasticity of cancer "like-stem" cells?

In conclusion, the advances in knowledge on CSCs are confirming that the clonal and hierarchical models of cancer growth coexist, at least at some points, during neoplastic evolution.

Moreover, the complex molecular pathophysiology of the cancer cell, in general, and the CSC, in particular, should be considered when discussing the anaplastic cell.

References

Al-Hajj M, Wicha MS, Benito-Hernandez A et al. (2003) Prospective identification of tumorigenic breast cancer cells. Proc Natl Acad Sci USA 100:3983–88.

Allen M, Louise Jones J (2011). Jekyll and Hyde: the role of the microenvironment on the progression of cancer. J Pathol. 223: 162–76.

Anderson K, Lutz C, van Delft FW et al (2011). Genetic variegation of clonal architecture and propagating cells in leukaemia. Nature 469: 356–61.

Barbie DA, Hahn WC, Pelman DS (2008). Destabilization of cancer genome. In: Devita, Hellman & Rosenberg's Cancer: Principles & Practice of Oncology 8th Ed. DeVita VT; Lawrence TS.; Rosenberg SA (Eds). Lippincott Williams & Wilkins. Philadelphia, PA, USA.

Beckman RA (2010) Efficiency of carcinogenesis: is the mutator phenotype inevitable? Semin Cancer Biol. 20: 340–52.

Bonnet D, Dick JE (1997) Human acute myeloid leukemia is organized as a hierarchy that originates from a primitive hematopoietic cell. Nat Med 3: 730–7.

Brégeon D, Doetsch PW (2011). Transcriptional mutagenesis: causes and involvement in tumour development. Nat Rev Cancer 11: 218–27.

Bristow RG, Hill RP (2008). Hypoxia and metabolism. Hypoxia, DNA repair and genetic instability. Nat Rev Cancer 8: 180–92.

Calabrese C, Poppleton H, Kocak M et al (2007). A perivascular niche for brain tumor stem cells. Cancer Cell 11: 69–82.
Clarke MF, Dick JE, Dirks PB et al. (2006) Cancer stem cells – perspectives on current status and future directions: AACR Workshop on cancer stem cells. Cancer Res.66: 9339–9344.
Clevers H (2011). The cancer stem cell: premises, promises and challenges. Nat Med. 17: 313–9.
Collins AT, Berry PA, Hyde C (2005). Prospective identification of tumorigenic prostate cancer stem cells. Cancer Res. 65: 10946–51.
Conway AE, Lindgren A, Galic Z et al (2009). A self-renewal program controls the expansion of genetically unstable cancer stem cells in pluripotent stem cell-derived tumors. Stem Cells. 27: 18–28.
Dayal D, Martin SM, Owens KM, et al. (2009). Mitochondrial complex II dysfunction can contribute significantly to genomic instability after exposure to ionizing radiation. Radiat Res. 172: 737–45.
Dick JE (2008) Stem cell concepts renew cancer research. Blood 112: 4793–807.
Gilbertson RJ and Rich JN (2007). Making a tumour's bed: glioblastoma stem cells and the vascular niche. Nature Rev. Cancer 7: 733–736.
Greaves M (2010). Cancer stem cells: back to Darwin? Semin Cancer Biol. 20: 65–70.
Gupta PB, Chaffer CL, Weinberg RA (2009). Cancer stem cells: mirage or reality? Nat Med. 15: 1010–2.
Jamieson CH, Ailles LE, Dylla SJ et al (2004). Granulocyte-macrophage progenitors as candidate leukemic stem cells in blast-crisis CML. N Engl J Med. 351: 657–67.
Janic A, Mendizabal L, Llamazares S et al (2010) Ectopic expression of germline genes drives malignant brain tumor growth in Drosophila. Science. 330: 1824–7.
LaBarge MA (2010). The difficulty of targeting cancer stem cell niches. Clin Cancer Res. 16: 3121–9.
Leder K, Holland EC, Michor F (2010). The therapeutic implications of plasticity of the cancer stem cell phenotype. PLoS One. 5: e14366.
Li C, Heidt DG, Dalerba P et al (2007). Identification of pancreatic cancer stem cells. Cancer Res. 67: 1030–7.
Liu W, Laitinen S, Khan S et al (2009). Copy number analysis indicates monoclonal origin of lethal metastatic prostate cancer. Nat Med. 15: 559–65.
Liu C, Kelnar K, Liu B et al (2011). The microRNA miR-34a inhibits prostate cancer stem cells and metastasis by directly repressing CD44. Nat Med. 17: 211–5.
Maenhaut C, Dumont J E, Roger P Pand van Staveren W C G (2010). Cancer stem cells: a reality, a myth, a fuzzy concept or a misnomer? An analysis. Carcinogenesis 31: 149–158.
Mani SA, Guo W, Liao MJ et al (2008). The epithelial-mesenchymal transition generates cells with properties of stem cells. Cell. 133: 704–15.
Notta F, Mullighan CG, Wang JC et al (2011). Evolution of human BCR-ABL1 lymphoblastic leukaemia-initiating cells. Nature 469: 362–7.
O'Brien CA, Pollett A, Gallinger S, Dick JE (2007). A human colon cancer cell capable of initiating tumour growth in immunodeficient mice. Nature 445: 106–10.
Park SY, et al (2010). Cellular and genetic diversity in the progression of in situ human breast carcinomas to an invasive phenotype. J Clin Invest.120. 636–44.
Perera S, Bapat B (2007). Genetic Instability in Cancer. Atlas Genet Cytogenet Oncol Haematol. January 2007. URL: http://AtlasGeneticsOncology.org/Deep/GenetInstabilityCancerID20056.html.
Pierce GB, Speers WC (1988) Tumors as caricatures of the process of tissue renewal: prospects for therapy by directing differentiation. Cancer Res 48: 1996–2004.
Quintana E, Shackleton M, Sabel MS et al (2008) Efficient tumour formation by single human melanoma cells. Nature 456: 593–8.
Rapp UR, Ceteci F, Schreck R (2008). Oncogene-induced plasticity and cancer stem cells. Cell Cycle. 7: 45–51.
Raynaud CM, Sabatier L, Philipot O et al (2008). Telomere length, telomeric proteins and genomic instability during the multistep carcinogenic process. Crit Rev Oncol Hematol. 66: 99–117.

Reya T Morrison SJ, Clarke MF, Weissman IL (2001) Stem cells, cancer, and cancer stem cells. Nature 414: 105–11.

Ricci-Vitiani L, Pallini R, Biffoni M et al (2010). Tumour vascularization via endothelial differentiation of glioblastoma stem-like cells. Nature 468: 824–8.

Roesch A, Fukunaga-Kalabis M, Schmidt EC et al (2010). A temporarily distinct subpopulation of slow-cycling melanoma cells is required for continuous tumor growth. Cell 141: 583–94.

Rosen JM, Jordan CT (2009) The increasing complexity of the cancer stem cell paradigm. Science 324: 1670–3.

Scatena R, Bottoni P, Giardina B (2008). Modulation of cancer cell line differentiation: A neglected proteomic analysis with potential implications in pathophysiology, diagnosis, prognosis, and therapy of cancer. Proteomics Clin Appl. 2: 229–37.

Scatena R, Bottoni P, Pontoglio A, Giardina B (2010). Revisiting the Warburg effect in cancer cells with proteomics. The emergence of new approaches to diagnosis, prognosis and therapy. Proteomics Clin Appl. 4: 143–58.

Scatena R, Bottoni P, Pontoglio A, Giardina B (2011). Cancer stem cells: the development of new cancer therapeutics. Expert Opin Biol Ther. 11: 875–92.

Sell S, Leffert HL (2008). Liver cancer stem cells. J Clin Oncol. 26: 2800–5.

Singh SK, Clarke ID, Terasaki M (2003). Identification of a cancer stem cell in human brain tumors. Cancer Res. 63: 5821–8.

Sodir NM, Swigart LB, Karnezis AN et al (2011). Endogenous Myc maintains the tumor microenvironment. Genes Dev. 25: 907–16.

Stricker TP, Kumar V. Neoplasia (2010) In: Robbins and Cotran Pathologic Basis of Disease 8th Ed. Kumar V, Abbas AK, Fausto N, Aster JC (Eds) Saunders, Philadelphia.

Tili E, Michaille JJ, Wernicke D (2011) . Mutator activity induced by microRNA-155 (miR-155) links inflammation and cancer. Proc Natl Acad Sci USA. 108: 4908–13.

Valeri N, Gasparini P, Fabbri M (2010). Modulation of mismatch repair and genomic stability by miR-155. Proc Natl Acad Sci USA. 107: 6982–7.

Visvader JE and Lindeman GJ (2008).Cancer stem cells in solid tumours: accumulating evidence and unresolved questions. Nature Rev. Cancer 8: 755–768.

Visvader JE (2011). Cells of origin in cancer. Nature. 469: 314–22.

Von Hoff DD, LoRusso PM, Rudin CM et al (2009). Inhibition of the hedgehog pathway in advanced basal-cell carcinoma. N Engl J Med. 361: 1164–72.

Yauch RL, Dijkgraaf GJ, Alicke B et al (2009) Smoothened mutation confers resistance to a Hedgehog pathway inhibitor in medulloblastoma. Science 326: 572–4.

Wang JCY, Dick JE. Cancer Stem Cells. (2008) In: Devita, Hellman & Rosenberg's Cancer: Principles & Practice of Oncology 8th Ed. DeVita VT; Lawrence TS.; Rosenberg SA (Eds). Lippincott Williams & Wilkins. Philadelphia, PA, USA, 135–143.

Wang R, Chadalavada K, Wilshire J et al (2010) Glioblastoma stem-like cells give rise to tumour endothelium. Nature. 468: 829–33.

Woodward WA, Sulman EP (2008). Cancer stem cells: markers or biomarkers? Cancer Metastasis Rev. 27: 459–70.

Zhou BB, Zhang H, Damelin M et al (2009). Tumour-initiating cells: challenges and opportunities for anticancer drug discovery. Nat Rev Drug Discov. 8: 806–23.

Chapter 2
Stem Cells and Cancer Stem Cells: New Insights

Toru Kondo

Prologue to Cancer Stem Cell Research

Although the concept of the cancer stem cell (CSC) was advocated more than several decades ahead, it was not accepted widely due to the lack of a direct proof method. However, recent progresses in the stem cell biology and developmental biology revealed that cancers contain the hierarchy similar to normal tissues and that only CSCs in tumors have a strong self-renewal capability and are malignant (Fig. 2.1) (Reya et al. 2001). It is thought that the existence ratio of CSCs is several percent or less in tumors and cancer cell lines and the other cells (non-CSCs) are either cancer precursor cells, which have limited proliferation ability, or nondividing cancer cells. Together these findings suggest that characterization of CSCs is essential for the curable cancer therapy.

Definition of CSCs

CSCs were initially defined by their extensive self-renewal capacity, tumorigenicity, and multipotentiality. As a number of oncogenes, including *inhibitor of differentiation* (*Id*), *hairy and enhancer of splits* (*Hes*) and *Notch*, are expressed in CSCs as well as tissue-specific stem cells (TSCs) and block cell differentiation, it remains uncertain as to whether CSCs actually give rise to multilineage cells. Further evidence also exists suggesting that cancer cells co-express a number of lineage-specific

---

T. Kondo (✉)
Laboratory for Cell Lineage Modulation, RIKEN Center for Developmental Biology,
2-2-3 Minatojima-Minamimachi, Chuo-ku, Kobe, Hyogo 650-0047, Japan

Department of Stem Cell Biology, Ehime University Proteo-Medicine Research Center,
Shitsukawa, To-on, Ehime 791-0295, Japan
e-mail: tkondo@m.ehime-u.ac.jp

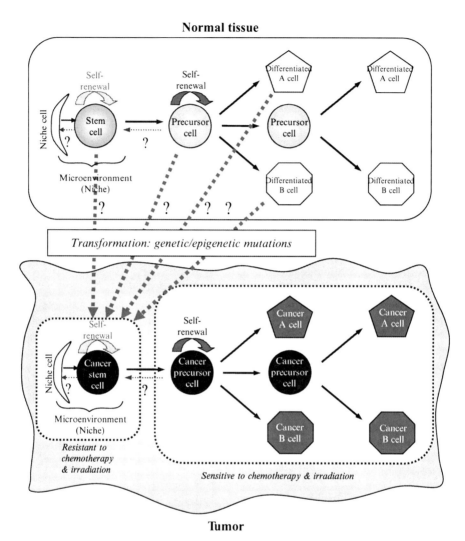

Fig. 2.1 Similarity between normal tissue and tumor. Tumors as well as normal tissues are likely to consist of small number of stem cells that have self-renewal capability and multipotentiality, precursor cells that have limited proliferative potency, and differentiated cells. CSCs are thought to be transformed from TSCs, precursor cells and/or differentiated cells by genetic/epigenetic mutations. Moreover, CSCs exist in special microenvironment "niche" and seem to keep their resistance to a variety of anti-cancer treatment methods

markers, each of which is exclusively expressed in normal differentiated cells, such as neurofilaments in neurons, glial fibrillary acidic protein in astrocytes and galactocerebrocide in oligodendrocytes, raising the question of whether such lineage-marker positive cells are in fact differentiated cells. Seen against this light then the obvious definition that can be applied to CSCs might be their unlimited self-renewal, expression of TSC markers, and tumorigenicity.

Cell-of-Origin of CSCs

Cancers have traditionally been thought to arise from either differentiated cells or their proliferating precursor cells, which have acquired oncogenic mutations. Since stem cells have been discovered in adult tissues, however, it has been suggested that TSCs might be a principal target of such mutations (Fig. 2.1). This speculation is supported by a number of different findings: First, it is likely that cancers arise from epithelia, which are in contact with the external environment and contain a wide variety of TSCs. Second, many cancers have been immunolabeled for TSC markers and for differentiation markers. Third, while TSCs survive and continue to proliferate throughout life, differentiated cells do not, suggesting that TSCs are more susceptible to accumulating oncogenic mutations. Finally, stem cells and precursor cells, which are transformed with oncogenic genes, have been shown to as developing cancer in vivo. Together, these findings suggest that either TSCs or amplifying precursor cells can be seen as the origin of malignant tumors.

Characteristics of CSCs

Resistance to Chemotherapy

A number of anti-cancer drugs have been successful in eliminating cancers; however, some cancer cells survive and the cancer recurs, indicating that the surviving cells are not only resistant to such anti-cancer drugs but are also malignant (Gottesman et al. 2002; Szakacs et al. 2006). It has been shown that glutathione and its related enzyme apparatus, topoisomerase II, O6-methylguanine-DNA-methyltransferase, dihydrofolate reductase, metallothioneins, and various ATP-binding cassette (ABC) transporters, such as the protein encoded by the multidrug resistant gene (MDR), the multidrug resistant protein (MRP), and the breast cancer resistant protein (BCRP1), contribute to such drug resistance in cancers. It is crucial to investigate relationship between CSCs and these factors.

Resistance to Irradiation

Irradiation is one of the most effective therapies for malignant tumors; however, a small population of cancerous cells tends to survive and cause tumor recurrence, suggesting that CSCs are radioresistant. Recently, Bao et al. (2006) have revealed that CD133-positive glioblastoma CSCs are much more resistant to irradiation than CD133-negative cells.

Invasion/Metastatic Activity

One characteristic of malignant tumor cells is their ability to invade and disseminate into normal tissue and to metastasize into other tissues. Some of the infiltrating cancer cells cannot be removed by surgical operation and causes recurrence, suggesting that CSCs retain high invasion activity. In fact, it has demonstrated that CD133-positive cancer cells highly express CD44 and chemokine receptor CXCR4, both of which mediate cell migration (Hermann et al. 2007; Liu et al. 2006).

Niche for CSCs

The number of TSCs is precisely regulated by both intrinsic mechanism and extracellular signals derived from specialized microenvironment "niche." For example, it was demonstrated that niche provides a limited number of physical anchoring sites, including beta1-integrin and N-cadherin, for TSCs and secretes both growth factors and anti-growth factors, including Wnt, FGF, hedgehog (Hh), bone morphogenic proteins, and Notch (Li and Neaves 2006; Moore and Lemischka 2006). Hypoxia is also shown to be essential for the maintenance of stemness, tumorigenesis, and resistance to anti-cancer treatments, chemotherapy and irradiation (Das et al. 2008; Matsumoto et al. 2009). Moreover, it was shown that the ablation of such niche results in loss of TSCs. It seems likely that CSCs also need niche for tumorigenesis. Kaplan and his colleagues have elegantly demonstrated that bone marrow-derived progenitors form the pre-metastatic niche in the tumor-specific pre-metastatic sites before cancer cells arrive and that the ablation of the niche prevents tumor metastasis (Kaplan et al. 2005). However, since transplanted cancer cells form tumors in any area in vivo, CSCs might be independent of the niche regulation or have a capability to make a new niche by recruiting bone marrow stem cells and other component cells.

Preparation of CSCs

The following methods are commonly used to prepare CSCs from cancers and cancer cell lines using the common characteristics of TSCs, such as cell surface markers, side population (SP), aldehyde dehydrogenase activity (ALDH), and a floating sphere formation.

Cell Surface Markers

Dick and colleagues have been able to show that the acute myeloid leukemia (AML)-initiating cells are found in primitive $CD34^+$ and $CD38^-$ populations, in which hematopoietic stem cells are enriched (Bonnet and Dick 1997; Lapidot et al. 1994).

Al-Hajj et al. have successfully separated tumorigenic breast CSCs from mammary tumors and breast cancer cell lines as CD44+ CD24−/low Lineage− cells. As few as 100 CD44+ CD24−/low Lineage− cells formed tumors in NOD/SCID mice, while tens of thousands of other cancer cell populations did not (Al-Hajj et al. 2003; Ponti et al. 2005). Another study by Singh et al. reported their success in separating brain CSCs from human medulloblastoma and glioblastoma multiforme (GBM) using an anti-CD133 antibody that recognizes a variety of different stem cells. Here, as few as 100 CD133+ GBM cells, although not CD133− cells, formed tumors in NOD/SCID brain (Singh et al. 2004). It has also revealed that colon CSCs are enriched in a CD133+ population (O'brien et al. 2007; Ricci-Vitiani et al. 2007). This is in addition to prostate CSCs being found to be enriched in CD44+ Integrin alpha2 beta1hi CD133+ (Collins et al. 2005). Very recent studies have shown that CD15, also known as stage-specific embryonic antigen 1 (SSEA1) or Lewis X (LeX), is a general CSC marker on GBM and medulloblastoma (Read et al. 2009; Son et al. 2009; Ward et al. 2009). It therefore seems likely that cell surface markers, such as CD133, are useful in separating CSCs from many types of tumors.

Side Population

It was revealed that cancer cells, as well as many kinds of normal stem cells, express a number of ABC transporters. BCRP1, for example, excludes the fluorescent dye Hoechst 33342, identifying a SP (Goodell et al. 1996), which is enriched for the various types of TSCs, although some research has shown that TSCs exist in both SP and non-SP and that SP cells do not express stem cell markers (Mitsutake et al. 2007; Morita et al. 2006). A number of research groups have found that some established cancer cell lines, which have been maintained in culture for decades, and tumors, such as AML, neuroblastoma, nasopharyngeal carcinoma, and ovarian cancer, contain a small SP. These studies have demonstrated that SP cells – but not non-SP cells – self-renew in culture, are resistant to anti-cancer drugs including Mitoxantrone, and form tumors when transplanted in vivo (Haraguchi et al. 2006; Hirschmann-Jax et al. 2004; Kondo et al. 2004; Patrawala et al. 2005; Ponti et al. 2005; Szotek et al. 2006). However, since many cancer cell lines do not contain any SP fraction and non-SP cells in some cancer cell lines likely generate SP fraction during culture, it is needed to evaluate whether SP is a general method to prepare CSCs.

Aldehyde Dehydrogenase Activity

ALDH is another detoxifying enzyme oxidizing intracellular aldehydes to carboxylic acids and blocking alkylating agents. Since it has been shown that ALDH increases in TSCs (Jones et al. 1995; Cai et al. 2004), it is now possible to identify and purify many types of TSCs, including hematopoietic stem cells and neural stem cells (NSCs), using fluorescent substrates of this enzyme and flow cytometry. There is increasing evidence that many types of CSCs strongly express ALDH and can be purified from tumors and cancer cell lines (Ginestier et al. 2007; Korkaya et al. 2008; Pearce et al. 2005).

Sphere Formation Assay

An increasing evidence points to the fact that CSCs as well as TSCs, such as NSCs and mammary gland stem cells, can form floating aggregates (tumor spheres) and be enriched in the spheres when cultured in serum-free medium with proper mitogens, such as bFGF and EGF (Fig. 2.2c) (Haraguchi et al. 2006; Hirschmann-Jax et al. 2004; Kondo et al. 2004; Ponti et al. 2005). Although many CSC researchers use sphere formation methods to concentrate their CSCs in culture, monolayer culture method might be better used to characterize CSCs as monolayer-cultured CSCs can be expanded as a homogenous population (Pollard et al. 2009).

Signaling Pathways Involved in CSC Maintenance

Since genetic alterations cause TSCs, amplifying precursors, or differentiated cells to transform to CSCs, it is important to classify the relationship between genetic alterations and tumor phenotype and malignancy.

p53 Pathway

It is well known that the loss of p53 function promotes the accelerated cell proliferation and malignant transformation (Toledo and Wahl 2006). Indeed, it was shown that over 65% of human glioma contains TP53 gene deletion and mutation (Kleihues and Ohgaki 1999). Moreover, additional evidences also indicated that other p53 signaling factors, including Murin-double-minute 2 (MDM2), which binds to, destabilizes, and inactivates p53, and chromodomain helicase DNA-binding domain 5 (Chd5), which regulates cell proliferation, cellular senescence, apoptosis, and tumorigenesis, are mutated in malignant glioma (Bagchi et al. 2007; Kleihues and Ohgaki 1999; Reifenberger et al. 1993; Toledo and Wahl 2006) In total, it was revealed that about 90% of human GBM have mutations in p53 signaling pathway (Cancer Genome Atlas Research Network 2008; Parsons et al. 2008). Although the effector molecule of p53 pathway is the p21 cyclin-dependent kinase (cdk) inhibitor that regulates progression of cells through the G1 cell-cycle phase, it has not been demonstrated that p21 gene itself is an oncogenic target in human cancers.

Rb Pathway

Retinoblastoma (Rb) is another essential tumor suppressor protein that regulates the G1 checkpoint (Classon and Harlow 2002). Hypophosphorylated form of Rb sequesters E2F transcription factor and arrest cells at the G1 checkpoint. Once Rb is hyperphosphorylated by cyclin D and cdk4/6 complex, phosphorylated Rb releases E2F, E2F induces the expression of cell cycle regulators, and then the cells enter S phase. In contrast, p16/Ink4a cdk inhibitor binds to cdk4/6, prevents the complex formation of cdk4/6 and cyclin D, and maintains Rb hypophosphorylation. Mutations in Rb pathway have been frequently identified in many types of malignant tumors. For example, mutations in Rb signaling pathway, including cdk4 amplification and p16/Ink4a deletion, was found in about 80% of GBM (Cancer Genome Atlas Research Network 2008; Parsons et al. 2008; Schmidt et al. 1994).

Activation of Receptor Tyrosine Kinase Pathway

Signaling pathways (Ras/Raf/MAPK and PTEN/AKT pathways) of Receptor Tyrosine Kinases (RTKs) including PDGFR, EGFR, FGFR, and IGFR, many of which play a role for the maintenance of TSCs and amplifying precursors, are frequently mutated in tumors (Schubbert et al. 2007). For instance, activation of RTK pathway was found in about 90% of GBM (Cancer Genome Atlas Research Network 2008; Parsons et al. 2008). In particular, it has been shown that small GTP protein Ras, one of essential oncogenes, and its negative regulator, type1 Neurofibromas gene (NF1), are mutated in many kinds of human cancers and that phosphatase tensin homolog (PTEN), which inhibits function of phosphoinositol tri-phosphate kinase (PI3K) that activates Akt, is frequently inactivated in malignant tumors (Duerr et al. 1998).

Notch Signaling Pathway

Notch receptors are involved in a number of biological functions, including cell proliferation, differentiation, survival, and tumorigenesis (Radtke and Raj 2003). There are four known mammalian Notch receptors, Notch 1–4, and five ligands, Delta-like-ligand (Dll) 1, 3, and 4, and Jagged 1 and 2 in mammals. Following the activation, Notch is cleaved in its extracellular region by metalloproteases and in its intracellular region by presenilins (PS), releasing the Notch intracellular domain (NICD) from the plasma membrane. The NICD then translocates into the nucleus, associates with the CSL transcription factor CBF1/RBP-Jk, and activates a number of target genes, including the hairy and enhancer-of-split (Hes) genes

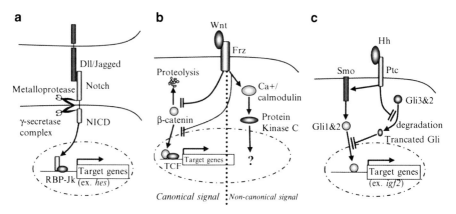

Fig. 2.2 Notch, Wnt, Hh signaling pathways are involved in CSC maintenance. Notch (**a**), Wnt/Frz (**b**), or Hh/Ptc/Smo (**c**) signaling pathway activates a number of genes, which regulate cell proliferation and cell fates. The constitutive activation of any of these pathways leads to abnormal development and tumorigenesis

(Fig. 2.2a). It has been shown that the inactivation of Notch signaling leads to serious developmental defects: Jagged1, Notch1, Notch2, and PS1and 2 knockout mice are all embryonically or perinatally lethal (Krebs et al. 2000; Swiatek et al. 1994; Xue et al. 1999). There is accumulating evidence that Notch activation not only maintains the multipotentiality of NSCs but is also involved in tumorigenesis. Depletion of Notch1, Dll1, or Jagged1 by RNAi was shown to block proliferation of glioma cells in vivo and in vitro (Purow et al. 2005). Together, these findings suggest that Notch signaling is involved in tumorigenesis, as well as in normal development.

Wnt Signaling Pathway

The Wnt family of secreted proteins coordinates diverse developmental processes, including cell proliferation and fate decisions (Logan and Nusse 2004; Moon et al. 2004; Reya and Clevers 2005). In mammals, there are 20 Wnt members, 10 Wnt receptors (called Frizzled, Frz), and 5 soluble forms of Frz, which are natural inhibitors of Wnt signaling. Once Frz is activated, β-catenin, which is a central player in canonical Wnt signaling, accumulates in the nucleus and induces the expression of Wnt target genes, including *c-myc* and *cyclin D1*, by associating with LEF/TCF transcription factors (Fig. 2.2b). The noncanonical Wnt signaling pathway activates calcium/calmodulin-dependent protein kinase and protein kinase C, although the molecular details are still uncertain (Logan and Nusse 2004; Moon et al. 2004; Reya and Clevers 2005).

Wnt signaling is also crucial for CNS development. Wnt1 and 3a, Frz5 and β-catenin, for example, are expressed in the ventricular and subventricular zones (VZ/SVZ) in the developing brain (Chenn and Walsh 2002; Ikeya et al. 1999; Lee et al. 2000). Inactivation of Wnt1, Wnt3a, or β-catenin causes developmental brain defects (McMahon and Bradley 1990; Reya and Clevers 2005). Moreover, overexpression of a stabilized form of β-catenin in neural precursor cells caused a hyperplasia of lateral ventricles (Chenn and Walsh 2002). Some factors in the Wnt signaling pathway, including β-catenin and axin1 (an inhibitor in the pathway), are mutated in medulloblastomas (Dahmen et al. 2001; Zurawel et al. 1998). Thus these findings suggest that hyper-activation of Wnt signaling may promote brain tumorigenesis.

Hedgehog Signaling Pathway

Hh signaling is also involved in proliferation, development, and tumorigenesis (Pasca di Magliano and Hebrok 2003; Ruiz i Altaba et al. 2002a, b). In mammals, there are three Hh members, Sonic, Desert, and Indian, all of which are secreted proteins. When Sonic Hh (Shh), for example, binds to the Patched1 (Ptc1) transmembrane receptor, another transmembrane protein, Smoothened (Smo), which is normally restrained by Ptc, is relieved and activates the zinc-finger transcription factor Gli. Activated Gli accumulates in the nucleus and induces the expression of target genes, including *wnt, insulin-growth factor 2 (igf2)*, and *pdgf receptor α* (Fig. 2.2c). There are three Gli transcription factors in mammals. Gli1 and 2 function as activators of Shh signaling, whereas the cleaved form of either Gli2 or Gli3 antagonizes the Shh-Gli1/2 signaling pathway. The Shh signaling pathway is essential for CNS development: Shh, Ptc, Gli2, or Gli3 knockout mice die before birth with severe defects in the brain, although Gli1 knockout mice develop normally (Ding et al. 1998; Matise et al. 1998; Palma and Ruiz i Altaba 2004; Park et al. 2000). Conditional inactivation of Smo blocks NSC proliferation in vivo and in vitro (Machold et al. 2003). Together with the finding that Glis, Ptc1, and Smo are all expressed in the VZ/SVZ, these observations suggest that Shh signaling may be essential for the maintenance of NSCs.

Ectopic activation of Hh signaling in CNS is likely to lead to brain tumor formation (Pasca di Magliano and Hebrok 2003; Ruiz i Altaba et al. 2002a, b). For example, Gli1 is highly activated in many brain cancers, including medulloblastoma, glioblastoma, and primitive neuroectodermal tumors, some of which also have mutations in Ptc1 (Goodrich et al. 1997). It was shown that overexpression of Gli1 in the developing tadpole CNS gives rise to brain tumors (Dahmane et al. 2001). Moreover, cyclopamine, which is a specific inhibitor of Smo, blocks the growth of several primary gliomas, medulloblastomas, and glioma cell lines (Berman et al. 2002; Dahmane et al. 2001). Taken together, these findings suggest that Hh signaling plays an important role in brain tumorigenesis.

CSC Models

In Vivo Models

Using a combination of transgenic mice and a retrovirus system, some groups have demonstrated that TSCs and differentiating cells form tumors in vivo. For instance, Holland and his colleagues infected transgenic mice that expressed the avian leukosis virus (ALV) receptor under the regulation of either a *nestin* enhancer or a *gfap* promoter, with recombinant ALVs encoding oncogenic genes, such as platelet-derived growth factor (PDGF) receptor beta, or activated Akt, or activated Ras, and found GBM had developed in the brain (Dai et al. 2001; Uhrbom et al. 2002). De Pinho and colleagues overexpressed a constitutively active form of epidermal growth factor (EGF) receptor in either NSCs or astrocytes from Ink4a/Arf$^{-/-}$ mice, transplanted them into the brain, and found that the cells formed high-grade gliomas (Bachoo et al. 2002). Thus, these findings suggest that NSCs and astrocytes are cells of origin for brain tumors. However, since tumors would be, in theory, generated from one transformed cell, these tumor models, in which many transformed cells are generated or injected at the same time, may not provide an answer to whether NSCs and astrocytes are *bona fide* cells of origin for malignant glioma.

In Vitro Models

It still remains controversial whether CSCs arise from TSCs, committed precursor cells, or differentiated cells. In addition, the relationship between cell of origin for CSCs and genetic alterations have not yet been elucidated, although a number of oncogenes and tumor suppressor genes have been well characterized in tumorigenesis. Using cell lineage markers and new methods including Fluorescence-activated cell sorting, it is possible to purify the cells. We can then overexpress oncogenes or knock down tumor-suppressor genes in the cells, examine the relationship between cell of origin for tumors and genetic alterations and find therapeutic targets (Fig. 2.3). Indeed, it has been demonstrated that overexpression of exogenous oncogenes can induce hematopoietic stem/progenitor cells to transform into leukemic stem cells (Cozzio et al. 2003; Huntly et al. 2004; Krivtsov et al. 2006). We and others also succeeded in generating glioma stem cells by overexpressing glioma-related oncogenes in neural lineage cells and in finding therapeutic targets by comparing gene expression profile of induced CSC models with that of human tumor spheres (Hide et al. 2009; Hide et al. 2011; Ligon et al. 2007). Thus these data suggest that, using similar methods, we might generate any CSCs from TSCs, amplifying precursor cells and/or differentiated cells, characterize them, and identify targets for curable therapy.

Fig. 2.3 Strategy for identifying factors specific to CSCs. Purified TSCs, committed precursor cells, and differentiated cells that are transfected with various types of oncogenes and/or siRNA/shRNA for tumor suppressor genes, transform into CSCs that are capable of self-renewal, positive for TSC markers and show malignancy. By comparing gene expression profiles of such induced CSCs with that of human CSC-enriched population (tumor spheres and TSC marker-positive cells), novel CSC markers and therapeutic targets would be identified

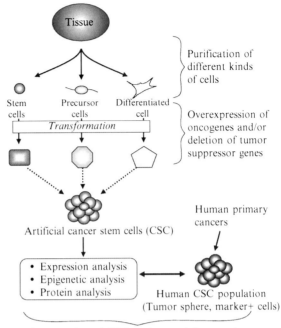

Conclusion

A number of new stem cell markers and techniques have been utilized to identify and purify CSCs during last several years. However, it is not yet known whether or not such CSCs consist of homogenous population, as CD133$^-$ and non-SP cells as well as CD133$^+$ and SP cells contain tumorigenic cells. Therefore it is still essential to establish experimental strategies, including the single cell analysis, to identify bona fide CSCs and to characterize them, leading to the discovery of novel therapeutic targets and methods.

Conflict of Interest

None declared.

Acknowledgments I apologize to authors whose works were not referenced due to limitations of space. I thank Hazuki Hiraga for critical reading of the manuscript. TK was supported by RIKEN internal funds.

References

Al-Hajj M, Wicha MS, Benito-Hernandez A et al (2003) Prospective identification of tumorigenic breast cancer cells. Proc Natl Acad Sci USA 100:3983–3988

Bachoo RM, Maher EA, Ligon KL et al (2002) Epidermal growth factor receptor and Ink4a/Arf: convergent mechanisms governing terminal differentiation and transformation along the neural stem cell to astrocyte axis. Cancer Cell 1:269–277

Bagchi A, Papazoglu C, Wu Y et al (2007) CHD5 is a tumor suppressor at human 1p36. Cell 128:459–475

Bao S, Wu Q, McLendon RE et al (2006) Glioma stem cells promote radioresistance by preferential activation of the DNA damage response. Nature 444:756–760

Berman DM, Karhadkar SS, Hallahan AR et al (2002) Medulloblastoma growth inhibition by hedgehog pathway blockade. Science 297:1559–1561

Bonnet D, Dick JE (1997) Human acute myeloid leukemia is organized as a hierarchy that originates from a primitive hematopoietic cell. Nat Med 3:730–737

Cai J, Cheng A, Luo Y et al (2004) Membrane properties of rat embryonic multipotent neural stem cells. J Neurochem 88:212–226

Cancer Genome Atlas Research Network (2008) Comprehensive genomic characterization defines human glioblastoma genes and core pathways. Nature 455:1061–1068

Chenn A, Walsh CA (2002) Regulation of cerebral cortical size by control of cell cycle exit in neural precursors. Science 297:365–369

Classon M, Harlow E (2002) The retinoblastoma tumour suppressor in development and cancer. Nat Rev Cancer 2:910–917

Collins AT, Berry PA, Hyde C et al (2005) Prospective identification of tumorigenic prostate cancer stem cells. Cancer Res 65:10946–10951

Cozzio A, Passegué E, Ayton PM et al (2003) Similar MLL-associated leukemias arising from self-renewing stem cells and short-lived myeloid progenitors. Genes Dev 17:3029–3035

Dahmen RP, Koch A, Denkhaus D et al (2001) Deletions of AXIN1, a component of the WNT/wingless pathway, in sporadic medulloblastomas. Cancer Res 61:7039–7043

Dahmane N, Sanchez P, Gitton Y et al (2001) The Sonic Hedgehog-Gli pathway regulates dorsal brain growth and tumorigenesis. Development 128:5201–5212

Dai C, Celestino JC, Okada Y et al (2001) PDGF autocrine stimulation dedifferentiates cultured astrocytes and induces oligodendrogliomas and oligoastrocytomas from neural progenitors and astrocytes in vivo. Genes Dev 15:1913–1925

Das B, Tsuchida R, Malkin D et al (2008) Hypoxia enhances tumor stemness by increasing the invasive and tumorigenic side population fraction. Stem Cells 26:1818–1830

Ding Q, Motoyama J, Gasca S et al (1998) Diminished Sonic hedgehog signaling and lack of floor plate differentiation in Gli2 mutant mice. Development 125:2533–2543

Duerr EM, Rollbrocker B, Hayashi Y et al (1998) PTEN mutations in gliomas and glioneuronal tumors. Oncogene 16:2259–2264

Ginestier C, Hur MH, Charafe-Jauffret E et al (2007) ALDH1 is a marker of normal and malignant human mammary stem cells and a predictor of poor clinical outcome. Cell Stem Cell 1:555–567

Goodell MA, Brose K, Paradis G et al (1996) Isolation and functional properties of murine hematopoietic stem cells that are replicating in vivo. J Exp Med 183:1797–1806

Goodrich LV, Milenkovic L, Higgins KM et al (1997) Altered neural cell fates and medulloblastoma in mouse patched mutants. Science 277:1109–1113

Gottesman MM, Fojo T, Bates SE (2002) Multidrug resistance in cancer: role of ATP-dependent transporters. Nat Rev Cancer 2:48–58

Haraguchi N, Utsunomiya T, Inoue H et al (2006) Characterization of a side population of cancer cells from human gastrointestinal system. Stem Cell 24:506–513

Hermann PC, Huber SL, Herrler T et al (2007) Distinct populations of cancer stem cells determine tumor growth and metastatic activity in human pancreatic cancer. Cell Stem Cell 1:313–323

Hide T, Takezaki T, Nakatani Y et al (2009) Sox11 prevents tumorigenesis of glioma-initiating cells by inducing neuronal differentiation. Cancer Res. 69:7953–7959

Hide T, Takezaki T, Nakatani Y et al (2011) Combination of a ptgs2 inhibitor and an epidermal growth factor receptor-signaling inhibitor prevents tumorigenesis of oligodendrocyte lineage-derived glioma-initiating cells. Stem Cells 29:590–599

Hirschmann-Jax C, Foster AE, Wulf GG et al (2004) A distinct "side population" of cells with high drug efflux capacity in human tumor cells. Proc Natl Acad Sci USA 101:14228–14233

Huntly BJ, Shigematsu H, Deguchi K et al (2004) MOZ-TIF2, but not BCR-ABL, confers properties of leukemic stem cells to committed murine hematopoietic progenitors. Cancer Cell 6:587–596

Ikeya M, Lee SM, Johnson JE et al (1999) Wnt signalling required for expansion of neural crest and CNS progenitors. Nature 389:966–970

Jones RJ, Barber JP, Vala MS et al (1995) Assessment of aldehyde dehydrogenase in viable cells. Blood 85:2742–2746

Kaplan RN, Riba RD, Zacharoulis S et al (2005) VEGFR1-positive haematopoietic bone marrow progenitors initiate the pre-metastatic niche. Nature 438:820–827

Kleihues, P, Ohgaki H (1999) Primary and secondary glioblastoma: from concept to clinical diagnosis. Neuro-Oncol 1:44–51

Kondo T, Setoguchi T, Taga T (2004) Persistence of a small subpopulation of cancer stem-like cells in the C6 glioma cell line. Proc Natl Acad Sci USA 101:781–786

Korkaya H, Paulson A, Iovino F et al (2008) HER2 regulates the mammary stem/progenitor cell population driving tumorigenesis and invasion. Oncogene 27:6120–6130

Krebs LT, Xue Y, Norton CR et al (2000) Notch signaling is essential for vascular morphogenesis in mice. Genes Dev 14:1343–1352

Krivtsov AV, Twomey D, Feng Z et al (2006) Transformation from committed progenitor to leukaemia stem cell initiated by MLL-AF9. Nature 442:324–331

Lapidot T, Sirard C, Vormoor J et al (1994) A cell initiating human acute myeloid leukaemia after transplantation into SCID mice. Nature 367:645–648

Lee SMK, Tole S, Grove E et al (2000) A local Wnt-3a signal is required for development of the mammalian hippocampus. Development 197:457–467

Li L, Neaves WB (2006) Normal stem cells and cancer stem cells: The niche matters. Cancer Res 66:4553–4557

Ligon KL, Huillard E, Mehta S et al (2007) Olig2-regulated lineage-restricted pathway controls replication competence in neural stem cells and malignant glioma. Neuron 53:503–517

Liu G, Yuan X, Zeng Z et al (2006) Analysis of gene expression and chemoresistance of CD133+ cancer stem cells in glioblastoma. Mol Cancer 5:67–78

Logan CY, Nusse R (2004) The Wnt signaling pathway in development and disease. Annu Rev Cell Dev Biol 20:781–810

Machold R, Hayashi S, Rutlin M et al (2003) Sonic hedgehog is required for progenitor cell maintenance in telencephalic stem cell niches. Neuron 39:937–950

Matise MP, Epstein DJ, Park HL et al (1998) Gli2 is required for induction of floor plate and adjacent cells, but not most ventral neurons in the mouse central nervous system. Development 125:2759–2770

Matsumoto K, Arao T, Tanaka K et al (2009) mTOR signal and hypoxia inducible factor-1 alpha regulate CD133 expression in cancer cells. Cancer Res 69:7160–7164

McMahon AP, Bradley A (1990) The Wnt-1 (int-1) proto-oncogene is required for development of a large region of the mouse brain. Cell 62:1073–1085

Mitsutake N, Iwao A, Nagai K et al (2007) Characterization of side population in thyroid cancer cell lines: cancer stem-like cells are enriched partly but not exclusively. Endocrinology 148:1797–1803

Moon RT, Kohn AD, De Ferrari GV et al (2004) WNT and beta-catenin signalling: diseases and therapies. Nat Rev Genet 5:691–701

Moore KA, Lemischka IR (2006) Stem cells and their niches. Science 311:1880–1885

Morita Y, Ema H, Yamazaki S et al (2006) Non-side-population hematopoietic stem cells in mouse bone marrow. Blood 108:2850–2856

O'brien CA, Pollett A, Gallinger S et al (2007) A human colon cancer cell capable of initiating tumour growth in immunodeficient mice. Nature 445:106–110

Palma V, Ruiz i Altaba A (2004) Hedgehog-GLI signaling regulates the behavior of cells with stem cell properties in the developing neocortex. Development 131:337–345

Park HL, Bai C, Platt KA et al (2000) Mouse Gli1 mutants are viable but have defects in SHH signaling in combination with a Gli2 mutation. Development 127:1593–1605

Parsons DW, Jones S, Zhang X et al (2008) An integrated genomic analysis of human glioblastoma multiforme. Science 321:1807–1812

Pasca di Magliano M, Hebrok M (2003) Hedgehog signalling in cancer formation and maintenance. Nat Rev Cancer 3:903–911

Patrawala L, Calhoun T, Schneider-Broussard R et al (2005) Side population is enriched in tumorigenic, stem-like cancer cells, whereas ABCG2+ and ABCG2- cancer cells are similarly tumorigenic. Cancer Res 65:6207–6219

Pearce DJ, Taussig D, Simpson C et al (2005) Characterization of cells with a high aldehyde dehydrogenase activity from cord blood and acute myeloid leukemia samples. Stem Cells 23:752–760

Ponti D, Costa A, Zaffaroni N et al (2005) Isolation and in vitro propagation of tumorigenic breast cancer cells with stem/progenitor cell properties. Cancer Res 65:5506–5511

Pollard SM, Yoshikawa K, Clarke ID et al (2009) Glioma stem cell lines expanded in adherent culture have tumor-specific phenotypes and are suitable for chemical and genetic screens. Cell Stem Cell 4:568–580

Radtke F, Raj K (2003) The role of Notch in tumorigenesis: oncogene or tumour suppressor? Nat Rev Cancer 3:756–767

Purow BW, Haque RM, Noel MW et al (2005) Expression of Notch-1 and its ligands, Delta-like-1 and Jagged-1, is critical for glioma cell survival and proliferation. Cancer Res 65:2353–2363

Read TA, Fogarty MP, Markant SL et al (2009) Identification of CD15 as a marker for tumor-propagating cells in a mouse model of medulloblastoma. Cancer Cell 15:135–147

Reifenberger G, Liu L, Ichimura K et al (1993) Amplification and overexpression of the MDM2 gene in a subset of human malignant gliomas without p53 mutations. Cancer Res 53:2736–2739

Reya T, Clevers H (2005) Wnt signalling in stem cells and cancer. Nature 434:843–850

Reya T, Morrison SJ, Clarke MF et al (2001) Stem cells, cancer, and cancer stem cells. Nature,414: 105–111

Ricci-Vitiani L, Lombardi DG, Pilozzi E et al (2007) Identification and expansion of human colon-cancer-initiating cells. Nature 445:111–115

Ruiz i Altaba A, Palma V, Dahmane N (2002a) Hedgehog-Gli signalling and the growth of the brain. Nat Rev Neurosci 3:24–33

Ruiz i Altaba A, Sanchez P, Dahmane N (2002b) Gli and hedgehog in cancer: tumours, embryos and stem cells. Nat Rev Cancer 2:361–372

Schmidt EE, Ichimura K, Reifenberger G et al (1994) CDKN2 (p16/MTS1) gene deletion or CDK4 amplification occurs in the majority of glioblastomas. Cancer Res 54:6321–6324

Schubbert S, Shannon K, Bollag G (2007) Hyperactive Ras in developmental disorders and cancer. Nat Rev Cancer 7:295–308

Singh SK, Hawkins C, Clarke ID et al (2004) Identification of human brain tumour initiating cells. Nature 432:396–401

Son MJ, Woolard K, Nam DH et al (2009) SSEA-1 is an enrichment marker for tumor-initiating cells in human glioblastoma. Cell Stem Cell 4:440–452

Swiatek PJ, Lindsell CE, del Amo FF et al (1994) Notch1 is essential for postimplantation development in mice. Genes Dev 8:707–719

Szakacs G, Paterson JK, Ludwig JA et al (2006) Targeting multidrug resistance in cancer. Nat Rev Drug Discov 5:219–234

Szotek PP, Pieretti-Vanmarcke R, Masiakos PT et al (2006) Ovarian cancer side population defines cells with stem cell-like characteristics and Mullerian Inhibiting Substance responsiveness. Proc Natl Acad Sci USA 103:11154–11159

Toledo F, Wahl GM (2006) Regulating the p53 pathway: in vitro hypotheses, in vivo veritas. Nat Rev Cancer 6:909–923

Uhrbom L, Dai C, Celestino JC et al (2002) Ink4a-Arf loss cooperates with KRas activation in astrocytes and neural progenitors to generate glioblastomas of various morphologies depending on activated Akt. Cancer Res 62:5551–5558

Ward RJ, Lee L, Graham K et al (2009) Multipotent CD15+ cancer stem cells in patched-1-deficient mouse medulloblastoma. Cancer Res 69:4682–4690

Xue Y, Gao X, Lindsell CE et al (1999) Embryonic lethality and vascular defects in mice lacking the Notch ligand Jagged1. Hum Mol Genet 8:723–730

Zurawel RH, Chiappa SA, Allen C et al (1998) Sporadic medulloblastomas contain oncogenic beta-catenin mutations. Cancer Res 58:896–899

Chapter 3
Molecular Biology of Cancer Stem Cells

Oswaldo Keith Okamoto

Introduction

Cancer Stem Cells and Disease Progression

Tumors are comprised by a heterogeneous cell population with subsets of cells displaying distinct tumorigenic capabilities. In some types of cancer, only a few cells with stem cell properties have been reported capable of initiating tumors in vivo, supporting the so-called cancer stem cell (CSC) model of tumor development.

At the molecular level, CSC display distinctive patterns of gene expression that correlates with poor clinical prognosis. For instance, an increased expression of genes from the Bcl-2 family and from the ATP-binding cassette (ABC) superfamily has been reported in CSC. Flow cytometry analyses have confirmed increased resistance to apoptosis and enhanced ability to efflux drugs in neuroblastoma, glioblastoma, breast, and lung stem cells (Hirschmann-Jax et al. 2004; Hadnagy et al. 2006; Jørgensen and Holyoake 2007). Furthermore, functional studies have confirmed that CSCs are more resistant to treatment with classical chemotherapy agents such as daunorubicin, temozolomide, carboplatin, and taxol (Costello et al. 2000; Liu et al. 2006a).

Likewise, recent studies with both CD133+ glioblastoma cells and CD44+/CD24− breast cancer cells have demonstrated that these cell populations exhibit a lower sensitivity to radiation than the remainder of the respective tumor cells, most likely due to the combined effects of an exacerbated expression of antiapoptotic,

O.K. Okamoto (✉)
Centro de Estudos do Genoma Humano, Departamento de Genética e Biologia Evolutiva,
Instituto de Biociências, Universidade de São Paulo, CEP 05508-090, São Paulo – SP, Brazil
e-mail: keith.okamoto@usp.br

drug resistance, DNA damage checkpoint, and DNA repair genes (Liu et al. 2006b; Phillips et al. 2006). These mechanisms allowing CSC to become more resistant to chemotherapy and radiotherapy may explain events of tumor relapse after conventional therapies that are observed in the clinics for some cancer patients.

In addition to the ability of developing new tumors and the enhanced resistance to radiation and drugs, other intrinsic properties of CSC include infiltration into surrounding tissues and migration to distant sites, facilitating tumor metastasis. Therefore, CSC seems to be directly implicated in tumor development, response to therapy, and disease progression, which makes them interesting targets for new forms of therapy.

Applied Stem Cell Molecular Biology

Although the genetic and epigenetic events resulting in CSC are not completely elucidated, there are evidences supporting the involvement of alterations in genes controlling stem cell pluripotency, self-renewal, and senescence. The identification of such molecular alterations in CSC seems highly appealing for therapeutic purposes. Yet, CSCs are still somewhat poorly characterized at the molecular level. For instance, the identification of specific CSC antigens suitable for therapeutic purposes is still limited. Most CSC markers reported so far are also expressed in normal adult stem cells, such as CD34 for myeloid leukemia and lung adenocarcinoma, CD105 for bone sarcoma, CD133 for brain and colon tumors, CD20 for metastatic melanomas, and CD44 for breast, pancreatic, and prostate tumors. The lack of targets restricted to CSC urges molecular profiling studies of CSC and their normal counterparts aiming at the identification of new biomarkers for diagnosis and development of smart drugs. The ultimate goal, in terms of therapeutics, would be to devise ways of specifically targeting CSC while avoiding harming normal cells.

However, since CSC are typically minor cellular constituents of tumors, such low abundance, in addition to purity issues in cell sorting protocols, poses several technical challenges for the study of CSC molecular biology. Some studies have suggested the use of established human tumor cell lines as tools for CSC characterization, since some of them have been shown to be comprised by subsets of more tumorigenic stem-like cells (Qiang et al. 2009).

Alternatively, the search for CSC targets may benefit from the knowledge of common molecular players regulating stem cell biology and cancer development. The development of innovative approaches for diagnosis and targeted therapy of cancer may gain from a deep understanding of the mechanisms controlling critical stem cell properties such as self-renewal, pluripotency, and longevity, and how deregulation of these processes may contribute to neoplastic transformation. Ultimately, this knowledge could be useful for detection of precancerous lesions, improving prevention and early tumor diagnosis.

Some examples of genes and molecular pathways linking stem cell and cancer biology are discussed in the next sections.

"Stemness" in Tumor Cells

Ectopic Expression of Genes Determining Pluripotency

According to the CSC model of tumor development, due to a relative long half-life within the tissues, adult stem cells could suffer prolonged exposure to genotoxic stresses and therefore accumulate the initial mutations leading to cancer (Lobo et al. 2007). Indeed, most tumors seem to arise from a single cell until eventually become heterogeneous with anomalous cells displaying distinct phenotypes, somewhat resembling the normal process that originates the cellular constituents of the original tissue.

Transformation of mature cells may also occur due to aberrant expression of stemness genes, resulting in cell clones with a dedifferentiated phenotype and self-renewing capacity resembling stem cells. Recent experimental evidence supporting this proposal has been provided with the induction of adult somatic cells into pluripotent stem (iPS) cells through ectopic expression of four genes encoding the pluripotency factors Oct4 and Sox2, the transcription factor Klf4, and the oncoprotein c-Myc in mouse or human fibroblasts (Takahashi et al. 2007; Yu et al. 2007).

However, along with pluripotency comes the capability of generating teratomas. This tumorigenicity could be partly explained by the enforced expression of c-Myc, a well-known oncogene. However, attempt to suppress tumorigenicity of iPS cells by retrieving *c-Myc* expression resulted only in partial reduction of tumor formation and was not enough to fully block tumorigenesis (Nakagawa et al. 2008). More recently, ectopic expression of *Oct4* alone was reported sufficient to directly reprogram mouse neural stem cells to pluripotency, in part due to the fact that these stem cells already express *Sox2*, *c-Myc*, and *Klf4* in addition to other factors related to stem cell activity (Kim et al. 2009). Only after reprogramming were the cells capable of inducing teratomas in vivo, indicating that pluripotency and tumorigenesis share a similar gene expression program that is still not so obvious to dissect.

Furthermore, expression of the pluripotency gene *Oct4* is detected in embryonal carcinomas, seminomas, and also in somatic cancers such as gliomas, lung adenocarcinomas, and prostate cancer. Interestingly, increased Oct4 expression is verified in high-grade gliomas and in prostate cancers with high Gleason scores, suggesting correlation with tumor malignancy (Du et al. 2009; Ngan et al. 2008; Karoubi et al. 2009; Sotomayor et al. 2009). Re-expression of embryonic stem cell-related genes, including downstream targets of *Nanog*, *Oct4*, and *Sox2*, is also predominantly found in aggressive tumors and correlates with poor clinical outcome (Ben-Porath et al. 2008). Expression of both *Oct4* and *Nanog* pluripotency genes have been detected in tumor initiating cells isolated from fresh specimens of ovarian and oral squamous cell carcinomas (Chiou et al. 2008; Zhang et al. 2008). Established cell lines from glioma (C6), osteosarcoma (3AB-OS), lung carcinoma (3LL), and breast carcinoma (MCF7) also express Oct4 at high levels (Hu et al. 2008; Di Fiore et al. 2009). Oct4 silencing by RNA interference in rat C6 cells and human MCF7 cells inhibited proliferation and increased apoptosis, respectively, suggesting a functional relevance of *Oct4* in tumorigenesis.

Another pluripotency factor, LIN28, is known to be aberrantly expressed in cancer cells. LIN28 is an RNA-binding protein that, together with OCT4, NANOG, and SOX2, has been shown to induce pluripotency in mature cells like fibroblasts (Yu et al. 2007). Interestingly, LIN28 expression is detected in aggressive, poorly differentiated, tumor cells and is correlated with poor prognosis (Viswanathan et al. 2009). Some of the mechanisms by which LIN28 is ectopically expressed in cancer involve interaction with microRNAs, discussed further in this chapter.

Enhanced Self-Renewal Capacity

Under normal conditions, stem cells respond to signals coming from their niche and activate a complex molecular program in a concerted fashion, which defines their self-renewal or differentiation into more specialized cells. Along the differentiation pathway, the proliferation capacity of stem cells tends to decline as their degree of maturation increases. Mutations in genes comprising the self-renewal program may disrupt the control of these processes and lead to neoplastic transformation. The resulting effects of such mutations on stem cells may include increased sensitivity to self-renewal signals coming from their own niche or autonomous proliferation in the absence of external growth signals. Alternatively, mutations may turn down the differentiation of stem cells while sustaining their proliferation capacity.

In agreement with this notion, many genes known to be involved in the regulation of stem cell self-renewal are proto-oncogenes, tumor suppressors, or genes belonging to signaling pathways involved in cancer such as MEK/ERK, PI3K/AKT, WNT, NOTCH, IGF, and TGF, among others. Some of these pathways, for instance, control the G1–S checkpoint of the cell cycle which intersects with the growth (MEK/ERK), survival (PI3K/AKT), and death pathways. Mutations in genes belonging to these pathways are frequently observed in human cancers. For instance, some of the genes regulating hematopoietic stem cell self-renewal have been found to be aberrantly expressed or mutated in patients with hematological malignancies (Toren et al. 2005). Members of the growth arrest and DNA damage 45 family, GADD45-beta and GADD45-gamma, have been found down-regulated during quiescence abrogation of hematopoietic stem cells (Okamoto et al. 2007a). These ubiquitous nuclear proteins are activated during stress conditions and are involved in maintenance of genomic stability, DNA repair, suppression of cell growth through interaction with cell cycle proteins, and induction of apoptosis via activation of the JNK and p38 MAPK pathways. Down-regulation of GADD45-beta and GADD45-gamma during self-renewal may facilitate accumulation of somatic mutations in stem cells. Accordingly, transcriptional silencing of *GADD45*-gamma due to promoter hypermethylation has been reported in several tumor cell lines and this epigenetic inactivation correlated with increased susceptibility to genetic instability and tumorigenesis (Ying et al. 2005).

The involvement of NOTCH, Sonic Hedgehog (SHH), and WNT pathways in neurogenesis as well as in development of gliomas, as a result of gene mutations affecting these pathways, is another example (de Bont et al. 2008). In glioblastoma stem cells, an aberrant expression of *E2F2*, encoding a member of a family of transcription factors with well-known roles in regulation of cell proliferation and development, has been reported (Okamoto et al. 2007b). Both frequency and hyperexpression of *E2F2* were found to correlate with the degree of tumor malignancy. E2F2 regulates the expression of *Bmi1*, *MYB*, and *MELK*, which are involved in the control of stem cell proliferation and malign transformation (Godlewski et al. 2008; Nakano et al. 2008; Malaterre et al. 2008).

Altogether, these observations strongly support a potential link between deregulation of stem cell self-renewal and neoplastic transformation.

Overcoming Senescence

DNA defense and cell cycle check point systems responsible for minimizing somatic mutations must be particularly fine-tuned in stem cells to suppress transformation and prevent dissemination of detrimental mutations to their progeny cells. When neither defense nor repair systems are sufficient to avoid DNA damage and mutagenesis, mechanisms of cell senescence are activated suppressing cell cycle and activating cell death pathways, thus inhibiting cancer development. While the efficacy of stem cell senescence mechanisms contribute to the aging process through a decline in self-renewing stem cell pools, its bypass should therefore facilitate neoplastic transformation.

Under normal culture conditions, primary mesenchymal stem cells (MSC) become senescent after about 30 population doublings, displaying impaired differentiation capacity in vitro, albeit preserving normal karyotype and inability to form tumors in vivo (Kim et al. 2008). Spontaneous in vitro transformation of MSC may occur, however, when cells are forced to grow beyond the senescence phase, after which only a subset of few transformed cells eventually overcome a crisis growth phase and dominate the cell culture (Rubio et al. 2008). Genetic alterations favoring telomere maintenance are likely implicated in this transformation process since telomerase dysfunction is known to induce replicative senescence and apoptosis (Ju and Rudolph 2006). Indeed, ectopic expression of hTERT, the catalytic unit of the enzyme telomerase responsible for telomere elongation, prolong the in vitro life span of MSC (up to 275 population doublings) while preserving their differentiation capacity. Cells at such high passages still present normal karyotype and inability to form tumors in NOD-SCID mice (Huang et al. 2008), indicating that hTERT is an important determinant of stem cell longevity.

Ionizing radiation is long known to cause DNA damage. When normal MSC are exposed to ionizing radiation, there is an accelerated telomere shortening and an increased chromosomal instability, leading to neoplastic transformation evidenced by tumor formation in SCID mice (Christensen et al. 2008). An increased resistance to ionizing radiation is also attained by enforced expression of hTERT in MSC (Serakinci et al. 2007). Interestingly, increased telomerase expression is detected in radioresistant CSCs such as those from prostate tumors (Marian and Shay 2009), supporting the relevance of hTERT to the balance between senescence and longevity of normal and neoplastic stem cells.

Posttranscriptional Orchestration by MicroRNAs

Many aspects of the biology of stem cells, including maintenance of pluripotency, self-renewal, and differentiation, are controlled by the phenomenon of RNA interference involving a variety of small molecules of RNA. The mRNA of a target gene can be degraded through the action of small interfering RNAs (siRNAs). These 21–25 nucleotide long molecules result from the cleavage of double strand RNAs by the RNaseIII enzyme Dicer. In a similar mechanism, microRNAs (miRNA) are also produced from precursor RNAs, or pre-miRNA, which have a hairpin structure recognized and cleaved by the enzymes Drosha and Dicer. Besides degrading mRNA, miRNA can also silence gene expression by physically blocking the interaction of mRNA with ribosomes, preventing its translation.

In the posttranscriptional regulation, both siRNA and miRNA form a large ribonucleoprotein complex known as RISC (RNA-induced silencing complex), in which the interfering RNA is transformed into a single strand RNA molecule, whose antisense sequence may be paired with a complementary sequence in the mRNA. In general, the complementary base pairing produces a new structure of double-stranded RNA, which is then enzymatically cleaved.

The control of gene expression by RNA interference appears to be powerful and wide ranging. Over 700 types of miRNA have been identified so far in the human genome and their respective sequences indicate that each miRNA has the potential to inhibit hundreds of molecules of mRNA.

The let-7 was one of the first miRNA to have its expression correlated with inhibition of proliferation and self-renewal of embryonic stem cells. One of the let-7 targets is the transcript of the *Hmga2* (high mobility group A2) gene, which encodes a chromatin protein that increases the activity of certain transcription factors. In embryonic stem cells, Hmga2 inhibits the expression of p16INK4a and Arf, two classical inhibitors of the cell cycle involved in senescence. This inhibitory effect of let-7 on self-renewal can be reversed by the expression of LIN28, a protein highly expressed in embryonic stem cells that blocks the cleavage of pre-let-7 and the consequent production of its mature form. LIN28 helps rescue pluripotency and inhibits neural commitment of stem cells mediated by let-7. During differentiation, other highly expressed miRNA such as miR-125a and miR-125b inhibit LIN28 translation and its repression effect on let-7. There are many other miRNAs reported to be involved in the regulation of embryonic stem cell self-renewal (e.g., miR-371, miR-372, miR-373, miR-200C, miR-368, miR-154) and differentiation (e.g., miR-301, miR-374, miR-21, miR-29) (Mallanna and Rizzino 2010).

Regulation of stemness genes by microRNAs may involve epigenetic mechanisms. One example is the inhibition of miR-21 by REST (Repressor element 1 silencing transcription factor), a transcriptional repressor that recruits multiple chromatin-modifying enzymes. Expression of *Nanog, Oct4,* and *Sox2* genes are silenced by miR-21, but REST remove this silencing by epigenetically suppressing miR-21, thus keeping ESC pluripotency. Oct4 expression may also be epigenetically repressed through the action of DNA methyltransferases such as DNMT1. The miR-290-295 cassette inhibits Oct4 expression by indirectly activating DNMT1.

Small RNAs are also important in controlling the biology of adult stem cells. The miR-128 and miR-181 are highly expressed in hematopoietic stem cells, helping to maintain their undifferentiated state. The miR-221, miR-222, and miR-223 induce the differentiation of hematopoietic progenitors while blockade of differentiation is regulated by miR-16, miR-103, and miR-107, among others. Inhibition of stem cell differentiation may occur indirectly, by silencing genes involved in self-renewal. This is the case of *Bmi-1* silencing by miR-128. Another example is the effect of miR-16, which has the antiapoptotic gene *Bcl-2* as one of its targets. The absence of miR-16 expression due to a deletion in chromosome 13 is found in patients with chronic lymphocytic leukemia, indicating that the miR-16 has a tumor suppressor activity (Navarro and Lieberman 2010).

Actually, many of these stem cell-related microRNAs exhibit a differential expression in cancer cells. Changes in the expression pattern of miRNAs affect stem cell fate and disruption of this mechanism may have a contribution in the development of cancer. The interaction of some miRNAs with other factors regulating stem cell biology is illustrated in Fig. 3.1. The manipulation of miRNAs has become an important platform for molecular studies of different pathological processes. In cancer, miRNAs are being explored as diagnostic markers of malign tumors, as well as therapeutic tools (Sarkar et al. 2010).

Perspectives

One fundamental issue in cancer therapeutics is the elucidation of the molecular mechanism of the disease. This knowledge should guide the identification of suitable molecular targets, a critical step for the therapeutic success of drugs such as those based on the action of monoclonal antibodies and small molecules. Typically, the desired characteristics of a therapeutic target include hyper expression in tumor cells, low or absent expression in normal cells, functional relevance to cancer, biochemical accessibility, widespread distribution in tumors, and be a molecular trait representative of a given tumor type or category.

Although not trivial, the search for molecular targets falling into this profile has been facilitated with the advent of genomic technologies, including further improvements in DNA sequencing. For instance, new generation of DNA sequencing machines allow faster and affordable sequencing of entire genomes. This technology is being used to sequence the genome of cancer cells and normal counterparts from the same individuals in order to identify somatic mutations associated with a particular malignancy.

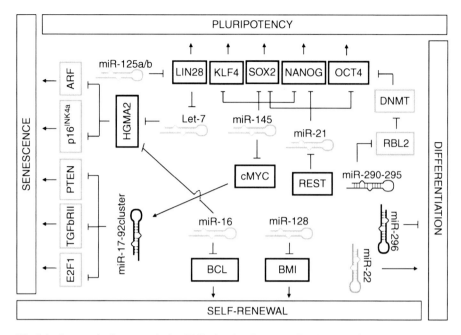

Fig. 3.1 A network of genes and microRNAs involved in stem cell and cancer biology. Deregulation of critical genes and pathways controlling typical stem cell properties may have a cumulative contribution toward malignant transformation and tumor development from cancer stem cells. Several genes regulating stem cell pluripotency are overexpressed in tumors. Likewise, classic oncogenes and tumor supressors have been shown to regulate stem cell self-renewal under nonpathological conditions. Expression of some of these stemness genes is posttranscriptionally regulated by microRNAs. Differential expression of these microRNAs has also been reported in human cancers. Color code: *bold black* = hyper-expressed in tumors; *grey* = hypo-expressed in tumors

Another important aspect that deserves attention in therapeutic development is the cellular bases of cancer. It could help refine drug delivery and enhance the efficiency of a targeting strategy. In theory, the efficacy of a molecular therapy is expected to be higher if the targeted molecule is present on cells with fundamental relevance in cancer physiopathology.

The CSC model of tumorigenesis combines these two aspects of cancer biology, bringing a new paradigm to cancer research and therapeutic development. Current technologies are allowing detailed genome-wide studies of neoplastic and non-neoplastic stem cell counterparts aiming at identifying mutations, chromosomal aberrations, and epigenetic alterations likely involved in CSC properties as well as possible association with disease progression and clinical outcome. For instance, cytogenetic screening and epigenetic analysis of highly pure cancer cell populations should enable the identification of chromosomal aberrations that may contribute to the tumor-initiation cell phenotype. Exon re-sequencing of key genes displaying differential expression in cancer is another example of strategy that could be performed in attempt to narrow down the screening of new mutations affecting both stem cell properties and tumor initiation capacity.

Based on this knowledge, future development of molecular therapeutic approaches with selective targeting of CSC can be envisioned and they should be of great value to cancer management. From the diagnostic perspective, it could devise more sensitive methods to detect the early formation and spread of tumors, allowing therapeutic interventions at initial disease stages when the chances of improving clinical outcome are higher. Likewise, new molecular targeted treatments focusing on CSC eradication have the potential to restrain tumor growth, invasion, and metastasis more effectively than currently available treatments.

After discussing a few aspects of CSC, it becomes evident that studies about the molecular biology of CSC are likely to impact both basic and translational cancer research fields. In addition to academia, such critical studies are of great interest of the biotechnological and pharmaceutical sectors, where they should catalyze the development of a new generation of drugs for cancer therapy.

References

Ben-Porath I, Thomson MW, Carey VJ, et al. An embryonic stem cell-like gene expression signature in poorly differentiated aggressive human tumors. *Nat. Genet.* 40(5), 499–507 (2008).

Costello RT, Mallet F, Gaugler B et al. Human acute myeloid leukemia CD34+/CD38progenitor cells have decreased sensitivity to chemotherapy and Fas-induced apoptosis, reduced immunogenicity, and impaired dendritic cell transformation capacities. *Cancer Res.* 60, 4403–4411 (2000).

Chiou SH, Yu CC, Huang CY, et al. Positive correlations of Oct-4 and Nanog in oral cancer stem-like cells and high-grade oral squamous cell carcinoma. *Clin. Cancer Res.* 14(13), 4085–4095 (2008).

Christensen R, Alsner J, Brandt Sorensen F, Dagnaes-Hansen F, Kolvraa S, Serakinci N. Transformation of human mesenchymal stem cells in radiation carcinogenesis: long-term effect of ionizing radiation. *Regen. Med.* 3(6), 849–861 (2008).

de Bont JM, Packer RJ, Michiels EM, den Boer ML, Pieters R. Biological background of pediatric medulloblastoma and ependymoma: a review from a translational research perspective. *Neuro Oncol.* 10(6), 1040–1060 (2008).

Di Fiore R, Santulli A, Ferrante RD, et al. Identification and expansion of human osteosarcoma-cancer-stem cells by long-term 3-aminobenzamide treatment. *J. Cell Physiol.* 219(2), 301–313 (2009).

Du Z, Jia D, Liu S, Wang F, Li G, Zhang Y, Cao X, Ling EA, Hao A. Oct4 is expressed in human gliomas and promotes colony formation in glioma cells. *Glia.* 57(7), 724–733 (2009).

Godlewski J, Nowicki MO, Bronisz A, et al. Targeting of the Bmi-1 oncogene/stem cell renewal factor by microRNA-128 inhibits glioma proliferation and self-renewal. *Cancer Res.* 68(22), 9125–9130 (2008).

Hadnagy A, Gaboury L, Beaulieu R, Balicki D. SP analysis may be used to identify cancer stem cell populations. *Exp. Cell Res.* 312, 3701–3710 (2006).

Hirschmann-Jax C, Foster AE, Wulf GG et al. A distinct "side population" of cells with high drug efflux capacity in human tumor cells. *Proc. Natl. Acad. Sci. USA.* 101, 14228–14233 (2004).

Hu T, Liu S, Breiter DR, Wang F, Tang Y, Sun S. Octamer 4 small interfering RNA results in cancer stem cell-like cell apoptosis. *Cancer Res.* 68(16), 6533–6540 (2008).

Huang G, Zheng Q, Sun J, et al. Stabilization of cellular properties and differentiation multipotential of human mesenchymal stem cells transduced with hTERT gene in a long-term culture. *J. Cell Biochem.* 103(4), 1256–1269 (2008).

Jørgensen HG, Holyoake TL. Characterization of cancer stem cells in chronic myeloid leukaemia. *Biochem. Soc. Trans.* 35(Pt 5), 1347–1351 (2007).

Ju Z, Rudolph KL. Telomeres and telomerase in stem cells during aging and disease. *Genome Dyn*.1, 84–103 (2006).

Karoubi G, Gugger M, Schmid R, Dutly A. OCT4 expression in human non-small cell lung cancer: implications for therapeutic intervention. Interact. *Cardiovasc. Thorac. Surg.* 8(4):393–7 (2009).

Kim J, Kang JW, Park JH, et al. Biological characterization of long-term cultured human mesenchymal stem cells. *Arch. Pharm. Res.* 32(1), 117–126, (2008).

Kim JB, Sebastiano V, Wu G, et al. Oct4-induced pluripotency in adult neural stem cells. *Cell.* 136(3), 411–419 (2009).

Liu G, Black KL, Yu JS. Sensitization of malignant glioma to chemotherapy through dendritic cell vaccination. *Expert. Rev. Vaccines* 5, 233–247 (2006a).

Liu G, Yuan X, Zeng Z et al. Analysis of gene expression and chemoresistance of CD133+ cancer stem cells in glioblastoma. *Mol. Cancer.* 2, 5–67 (2006b).

Lobo NA, Shimono Y, Qian D, Clarke MF. The biology of cancer stem cells. *Annu. Rev. Cell Dev. Biol.* 23, 675–99 (2007).

Malaterre J, Mantamadiotis T, Dworkin S, et al. c-Myb is required for neural progenitor cell proliferation and maintenance of the neural stem cell niche in adult brain. *Stem Cells*. 26(1), 173–181 (2008).

Mallanna SK, Rizzino A. Emerging roles of microRNAs in the control of embryonic stem cells and the generation of induced pluripotent stem cells. Dev Biol. 344(1):16–25 (2010).

Marian CO, Shay JW. Prostate tumor-initiating cells: A new target for telomerase inhibition therapy? *Biochim. Biophys. Acta.* 1792(4), 289–96 (2009).

Nakagawa M, Koyanagi M, Tanabe K, et al. Generation of induced pluripotent stem cells without Myc from mouse and human fibroblasts. *Nat. Biotechnol.* 26(1), 101–106 (2008).

Nakano I, Masterman-Smith M, Saigusa K, et al. Maternal embryonic leucine zipper kinase is a key regulator of the proliferation of malignant brain tumors, including brain tumor stem cells. *J. Neurosci. Res.* 86(1), 48–60 (2008).

Navarro F, Lieberman J. Small RNAs guide hematopoietic cell differentiation and function. J Immunol. 184(11), 5939–47 (2010).

Ngan KW, Jung SM, Lee LY, Chuang WY, Yeh CJ, Hsieh YY. Immunohistochemical expression of OCT4 in primary central nervous system germ cell tumours. *J. Clin. Neurosci.* 15(2), 149–152. (2008).

Okamoto OK, Carvalho AC, Marti LC, Vêncio RZ, Moreira-Filho CA. Common molecular pathways involved in human CD133+/CD34+ progenitor cell expansion and cancer. *Cancer Cell Int*. 8, 7–11 (2007a).

Okamoto OK, Oba-Shinjo SM, Lopes L, Nagahashi Marie SK. Expression of HOXC9 and E2F2 are up-regulated in CD133(+) cells isolated from human astrocytomas and associate with transformation of human astrocytes. *Biochim. Biophys. Acta.* 1769(7-8), 437–442 (2007b).

Phillips TM, McBride WH, Pajonk F. The response of CD24(-/low)/CD44+ breast cancer – initiating cells to radiation. *J. Natl. Cancer Inst.* 98, 1777–1785 (2006).

Qiang L, Yang Y, Ma YJ, et al. Isolation and characterization of cancer stem like cells in human glioblastoma cell lines. Cancer Lett. 28;279(1), 13–21. (2009)

Rubio D, Garcia S, Paz MF, et al. Molecular characterization of spontaneous mesenchymal stem cell transformation. *PLoS ONE*. 3(1), e1398 (2008).

Sarkar FH, Li Y, Wang Z, Kong D, Ali S. Implication of microRNAs in drug resistance for designing novel cancer therapy. Drug Resist Updat. 13(3), 57–66 (2010).

Serakinci N, Christensen R, Graakjaer J, et al. Ectopically hTERT expressing adult human mesenchymal stem cells are less radiosensitive than their telomerase negative counterpart. *Exp. Cell Res.* 313(5), 1056–1067 (2007).

Sotomayor P, Godoy A, Smith GJ, Huss WJ. Oct4A is expressed by a subpopulation of prostate neuroendocrine cells. *Prostate.* 69(4), 401–410 (2009).

Takahashi K, Tanabe K, Ohnuki M, et al. Induction of pluripotent stem cells from adult human fibroblasts by defined factors. *Cell.* 131(5), 861–872 (2007).

Toren A, Bielorai B, Jacob-Hirsch J, *et al.* CD133-positive hematopoietic stem cell "stemness" genes contain many genes mutated or abnormally expressed in leukemia. *Stem Cells.* 23(8), 1142–53 (2005).

Viswanathan SR, Powers JT, Einhorn W, et al. Lin28 promotes transformation and is associated with advanced human malignancies. Nat Genet. 41(7), 843–8. (2009).

Ying J, Srivastava G, Hsieh WS, *et al.* The stress-responsive gene GADD45G is a functional tumor suppressor, with its response to environmental stresses frequently disrupted epigenetically in multiple tumors. *Clin. Cancer Res.* 11, 6442–6449 (2005).

Yu J, Vodyanik MA, Smuga-Otto K, *et al.* Induced pluripotent stem cell lines derived from human somatic cells. *Science.* 318(5858), 1917–1920 (2007).

Zhang S, Balch C, Chan MW, *et al.* Identification and characterization of ovarian cancer-initiating cells from primary human tumors. *Cancer Res.* 68(11), 4311–4320 (2008).

Chapter 4
Biomarkers of Cancer Stem Cells

Jun Dou and Ning Gu

Introduction

A hypothesis of cancer stem cells (CSCs) originally formulated for hematologic malignancies and extended to solid tumors is receiving increasing interest in cancer researchers who now gradually change their classical view on tumors. The hypothesis of CSCs also called tumor stem cells (TSCs) or tumor-initiating cells (TICs) is a population of rare tumor cells bearing stem cell properties and this rare cells are responsible for the initiating and maintaining the tumor tissues, allowing the tumor cell propagation, colonizing distant sites, having resistant to standard chemotherapeutic drugs, and the inimical conditions of the tumor microenvironment. Investigation of CSCs has been conducted using primary patient tumor samples, cancer cell lines, and xenograft animal models. Each method has its usefulness and limitations; for example, stable cancer cell lines are simple to identify cancer cell characteristic except have been selected to grow in culture, whereas patient samples are the gold standard, however, they are difficult to obtain regularly (Stephen and Antonio 2010).

Recent rapid progress in CSC research has encountered increasing challenges in which identifying them is hotly debated topics. Additional challenges are presented by such factors as limited number of CSCs in tumor tissues, technical difficulties in keeping CSCs in any culture, and their unusually strong drug resistance. Nevertheless, the existence of CSCs, a subpopulation of tumor cells with stem-like characteristics, has significant implications in clinical therapy (Al-Hajj et al. 2003; Pannuti et al. 2010). Currently, CSC markers must be clearly defined for each tissue, and clarifying

---

J. Dou (✉)
Department of Pathogenic Biology and Immunology, Medical School,
Southeast University, Nanjing 210009, China
e-mail: njdoujun@yahoo.com.cn

N. Gu
School of Biological Science & Medical Engineering, Southeast University,
Nanjing 210096, China
e-mail: guning@seu.edu.cn

cellular and signaling functions of CSCs is key to conduct better identification and diagnosis based on CSC biomarkers and eventually targeting to CSCs, which will undoubtedly result in improved prevention and treatment of many types of CSCs (Stephen and Antonio 2010; Jun and Ning 2010).

Since CSCs possess the potential to give rise to more mature nonstem cell cancer that present the phenotypically diverse progeny through a process of epigenetic change, differentiation or partial differentiation and ultimately form functionally diverse sets of nontumorigenic cancer cells, thus, there are many different types of cells in a tumor in which some are cancerous and others are infiltrating normal cells that are thought to support the growth of the cancer cells (Amitava and Jose 2010; Neethan et al. 2007). A crucial question in CSC hypothesis is which cells can be transformed to form tumors? To date, it is unclear why some tumor cells are more or less tumorigenic than others and the scientists have not been able to distinguish the characteristics of CSCs from the characteristics of stem cells because the CSCs are similar to normal stem cells, and molecular mechanisms regulating the process of CSC differentiation are not completely understood (Amitava and Jose 2010). Despite existence of difficulties and challenges in identification and isolation of CSCs, such as obtaining CSCs in sufficient quantities and maintaining their undifferentiated state, accumulating evidence indicates that the existence of CSCs in many different kinds of malignancies, including leukemia, multiple myeloma, glioblastoma, brain tumors, pancreatic cancer, gastric cancer, colon cancer, hepatocellular cancer, prostate cancer, lung cancer, head/neck cancer, melanoma, breast cancer, ovarian cancer, etc. The questions we should currently resolve are how we can identify and analyze CSCs? and what agents are being designed to kill this chemotherapy-refractory CSCs? Thus, the isolation and characterization of CSCs represent a revolutionary approach in cancer research with considerable therapeutic implications. In the chapter, we look at how researchers succeeded in identification and isolation of CSCs and critically discuss the methods for identification of CSCs based on the proposed biomarkers of CSCs as well as outlook future tasks in the field.

Biomarkers in CSCs

CSC markers are expressed in the different cancers with the different patterns seen for the different histological types and degrees of differentiation. These markers are necessary to isolate CSCs and analyze their biological characteristics in order to use the markers to target them efficiently for therapeutic purposes.

CD Molecules

CD133

CD133 molecule (a transmembrane pentaspan protein) is considered a universal marker of normal hematopoietic stem cells and organ-specific stem cells (Miraglia et al. 1997), and it has been proposed as a surface marker of CSCs in solid primary tumors such as medulloblastomas and glioblastomas (Kusumbe et al. 2009) and subsequently of CSCs in a growing number of cancers of epithelial tissues. Other cancers had similar observations [epithelial ovarian CSCs (Suetsugu et al. 2006), hepatocellular carcinoma (HCC) (Baba et al. 2009; Yao et al. 2009), pancreatic cancer (Hermann et al. 2007; Moriyama et al. 2010), gastric cancer (Ishigami et al. 2010), human cutaneous melanoma (Sharma et al. 2010), mouse melanoma (Dou et al. 2007), and colon CSCs (O'Brien et al. 2007)]. In particular, O'Brien et al. showed that human colon CSCs within the CD133$^+$ population were able to maintain themselves, to differentiate, and to re-establish tumor heterogeneity upon a serial transplantation in non-obese diabetic/severe combined immunodeficiency (NOD/SCID) mice. In their study, subcutaneous injection of colon cancer CD133$^+$ cells readily reproduced the original tumor in NOD/SCID mice (Ricci-Vitiani et al. 2007; Mizrak et al. 2008). The similar reports showed that the isolated primary tumor cells from 13 surgically resected colon tumor specimens were cultured in serum-free CSC-selective conditions and showed that the CD133$^+$ tumor cells gave rise to long-term tumor spheroid that were CD133$^+$ cells and were able to self-renew and differentiate into adherent epithelial lineages and recapitulate the phenotype of the original tumor. The spheroid cells were more resistant to the chemotherapeutic irinotecan than that of the differentiated progeny (Fang et al. 2010). Also, the CD133 expression in colorectal cancer is associated with some features attributable to stemness including enhanced colony formation and cell motility, and there is plasticity of CD133 expression (Elsaba et al. 2010).

However, CD133 is controversially discussed as putative marker for CSCs in epithelial tumors including colorectal carcinomas, and the precise contribution of CD133$^+$ CSCs in mediating colon cancer metastasis has remained controversial. In generated knockin lacZ reporter mouse (CD133lacZ/+), the expression of lacZ was driven by the endogenous CD133 promoters. Using this model and immunostaining, researchers discovered that CD133 expression in the colon is not restricted to stem cells; on the contrary, CD133 was ubiquitously expressed on differentiated colonic epithelium in both adult mice and humans. Both CD133$^+$ and CD133$^-$ metastatic tumor subpopulations formed colonosphere in vitro cultures and were capable of long-term tumorigenesis in a NOD/SCID serial xenotransplantation model (Shmelkov et al. 2008; Dittfeld et al. 2010). Furthermore, CD133 expressive variation in stem cells and CSCs were not limited to colon tissues. HSC, neural stem cells, glioblastoma, and their corresponding CSCs also have been reported with conflicting findings in the literature. For instance, the neural stem cell marker CD133$^+$ is proposed as identifying cells within glioblastoma that can initiate neurosphere growth and tumor formation; nevertheless, instances of CD133$^-$ cells exhibit similar properties. Some PTEN-deficient glioblastoma tumors generate a series of CD133$^+$ and CD133$^-$ self-renewing CSC types and show that both CD133$^+$ and CD133$^-$ cells could constitute a lineage hierarchy, and that the capacities for self-renewal and tumor initiation in glioblastoma need not be restricted to CD133$^+$ population (Chen et al. 2010a).

The function and the mechanisms regulating CD133 expression remain unknown. In light of this inconsistency in the research findings, one explanation may be hidden in the potential difference between the presence of mRNA and the CD133 protein in epithelial cells or CD133 expression on stem cells may vary between species (mouse vs. humans). Alternatively, this inconsistency may be due to the antibody affinity and different glycosylation and/or splice variants of CD133. The half-life of the beta-galactosidase relative to CD133 may also affect the readout in the knock in situation. The utilization of destabilized forms of lacZ or GFP is to more accurately determine expression patterns (Mark et al. 2008). In addition, in the previous studies, the detection of CD133 was done using commercially available antibodies, which may not recognize the full gamut of CD133 expression pattern. The antibody from the different commercial companies may also identify the different epitopes. The use of such commercial antibodies whose epitope and specificity have never been thoroughly investigated could be one of reasons that inconsistent findings were yielded in those experiments of the previous studies.

Nonetheless, there is increasing evidence that has indicated that the CD133 molecule is a specific marker (uniquely or in part) in isolation of CSCs that include prostate cancer (CD44$^+$/$\alpha_2\beta_1^{hi}$/CD133$^+$) (Kasper 2005), murine melanoma (CD133$^+$/CD44$^+$/CD24$^+$) (Dean et al. 2005; Kimberly et al. 2009), childhood acute lymphoblastic leukemia (CD133$^+$/CD19$^-$/CD38$^-$) (Cox et al. 2009), ameloblastic tumors (CD133$^+$/Bmi-1/ABCG2) (Kumamoto and Ohki 2010), HCC (CD133$^+$/CD44$^+$) (Zhu et al. 2010), ovarian cancer (Curley et al. 2009), lung carcinoma (Eramo et al. 2008), etc. If CD133 expression is elevated, it may serve as a predictive marker of a distant recurrence and a poor survival after preoperative chemoradiotherapy in the residual rectal cancer (Yasuda et al. 2009). These data suggest that the CSCs are heterogeneous in their CD133 expression and considerable overlap exists between different organ stem cells and CSCs in their repertoire of gene expression (Goodell et al. 1996). Thus, the identification of CD133$^+$ cells may thus be a potentially powerful tool for investigating the tumorigenic process. Caution, however, should be exercised when using the expression of CD133 as the primary means to identify CSCs. This is due to the fact that the CD133 molecule may change during a culture process and in any particular organ, such as the brain in which only CSCs express CD133 (Zhou et al. 2009).

CD44

CD44 is a multifunctional protein involved in cell adhesion, motility, proliferation, drug resistance, and cell survival (Marhaba and Zoller 2004; Afify et al. 2009) and has been implicated in lymphocyte homing, wound healing, and cell migration, as well as cancer cell growth and metastasis (Ponta et al. 2003; Ishimoto et al. 2009). It is a primary receptor for hyaluronan (HA), a major component of the extracellular matrix (ECM) where their interactions play a critical role in cell signaling in cancer. The standard CD44 (CD44s) molecule is an 85- to 90-kDa transmembrane glycoprotein containing 10 standard exons, whereas tissue-specific splice variants (CD44v1-10) contain the standard set and combinations of the 10 variable exons. HA has been shown to be enriched in the stem cell niche and is also likely to play an integral role in the behavior of CD44 in CSCs (Stephen and Antonio 2010). Recently, CD44 has been detected as a cell surface marker in CSCs of several solid tumors (Miletti-González et al. 2005) including prostate cancer (Hao et al. 2010), head and neck cancer (Prince et al. 2007), glioblastoma (Xu et al. 2010), and gastric cancer (Takaishi et al. 2009). The CD44$^+$ gastric cancer cells showed increased resistance for chemotherapy- or radiation-induced cell death. The data support the existence of gastric CSCs that represent a possible therapeutic target for the tumor and the underlying mechanisms for the emergence of CD44$^+$ CSCs during tumorigenesis. The CSC tumorigenesis may involved in CD44$^+$ slow-cycling tumor cell expansion that is triggered by cooperative actions of Wnt and prostaglandin E2 in gastric cancer (Takaishi et al. 2009). CD44 molecule may also be detected as one of CSC markers such as breast cancer (CD44$^+$/CD24$^{-/low}$/Lin) (Al-Hajj et al. 2003), colon carcinoma (EpCAM^{hi}/CD44$^+$) (Dalerba et al. 2007), colorectal cancer (CD44$^+$/CD24$^+$) (Yeung et al. 2010), prostate cancer CD44$^+\alpha_2\beta_1^{hi}$ CD133$^+$ (Collins et al. 2005), pancreas cancer (CD44$^+$/CD24$^+$/ESA$^+$) (Li et al. 2010), murine melanoma (CD133$^+$/CD44$^+$/CD24$^+$) (Dou et al. 2007), HCC (CD133$^+$/CD44$^+$) (Kumamoto and Ohki 2010), gastrointestinal stromal tumors (CD44$^+$/CD24$^+$ Kit^{low}) (Bardsley et al. 2010), ovarian cancer (CD44$^+$/CD117$^+$ or CD133$^+$/CD117$^+$) (Zhang et al. 2008; Liu et al. 2010b), etc. To validate the existence of CSCs, 100 dissociated nonadherent spheroid cells, which were derived from disaggregated ovarian serous adenocarcinomas and cultured in serum-free growth conditions, were injected into female athymic BALB/c nude mice and the cells generated full recapitulation of the original tumor, whereas >10^5 unselected cells (cultured in common growth conditions) remained nontumorigenic in mice. To identify the CSC cell surface phenotype, spheroid immunostaining showed significant up-regulation of the HA receptor CD44 and stem cell factor receptor CD117 (c-kit), a tyrosine kinase oncoprotein. Similar to sphere-forming CSCs, inoculation of only 100 CD44$^+$CD117$^+$ cells could also serially propagate their original tumors, whereas 10^5 CD44$^-$CD117$^-$ cells remained nontumorigenic in athymic BALB/c nude mice. These findings provide a rational explanation for the observation that epithelial ovarian cancers derive from a subpopulation of CD44$^+$CD117$^+$ cells representing an ovarian cancers development, progression, metastasis, and recurrence (Liu et al. 2010). The invasive CD44$^+$ prostate cells had increased expression of Nanog, BMI1, and SHH, as well as a genetic signature similar to stem cells. Interactions between CD44 and the ECM glycosaminoglycan HA have been tied to pathways closely related to epithelial-to-mesenchymal transition (EMT), cancer, and "stemness" in head and neck, breast, and ovarian cancer cells (Klarmann et al. 2009). The EMT is involved in a differentiation process crucial to normal development and has been implicated in conferring metastatic ability on carcinomas. For instance, following induction of EMT in human breast cancer and related cell lines, these cells display the CD44$^{(high)}$/CD24$^{(low)}$ phenotype and increase the ability of cells to form mammospheres (Turner and Kohandel 2010). Consistent with this observation, CD44 promotes tumor cell resistance to reactive oxygen species-induced and cytotoxic agent-induced stress by attenuating activation of the Hippo signaling pathway and CD44 antagonists potently inhibit glioma growth in preclinical mouse models (Xu et al. 2010). An another report, however, has indicated that the positivity of

CD44 staining in 25 HCC specimens was significantly lower than in viral hepatitis specimens but the positive rate of CD133 in HCC was similar to viral hepatitis specimens (Lingala et al. 2010). Combined, these data demonstrate that the CD44 molecule is at least one characteristic of CSCs across tissues and that CD44 target therapy could be effective in CSCs.

CD24

CD24 is a small (27 amino acid single-chain protein), highly glycosylated cell surface molecule that is linked to the membrane through a glycosylphosphatidylinositol (GPI) anchor. Expression of CD24 in adult nonmalignant tissue is limited to B cells, granulocytes, and the stratum corneum. Early results show that the increased proliferation, cell adhesion, and migration when CD24$^-$ cell lines are made to express the CD24 protein (Aigner et al. 1997). CD24 is overexpressed in many human carcinomas and its expression is linked to bad prognosis, such as tumor migration and invasion. Recently, CD24 has been implicated in playing a part downstream of the developmental hedgehog pathway that is often active in CSCs (Pirruccello and Lebien 1986). In the ovarian study, a series of cancer cell clones were isolated from ovarian tumor specimens of a patient and identified a subpopulation enriched for ovarian CSCs defined by CD24 phenotype. These CD24$^+$ cell clones were heterogeneous in growth rate, cell cycle distribution, and expression profile of genes and proteins. The experiments in vitro demonstrated CD24$^+$ cell clones possessed stem cell-like characteristics of remaining quiescence and more chemoresistant compared with CD24$^-$ cells, as well as a specific capacity for self-renewal and differentiation. Injection of 5×10^3 CD24$^+$ cells was able to form tumor xenografts in nude mice, whereas equal number of CD24$^-$ cells remained nontumorigenic. CD24$^+$ cells expressed higher mRNA levels of some "stemness" genes, including Nestin, β-catenin, Bmi-1, Oct4, Oct3/4, Notch1, and Notch4. These data suggest human ovarian tumor cells are organized as a hierarchy and CD24 demarcates an ovarian cancer-initiating cell population (Gao et al. 2010). Liu and his colleagues detected the side population (SP) fraction in BxPc-3, CFPAC-1, MIA PaCa-2, PANC-1, and SW1990 pancreatic cancer cell lines by fluorescence activated cell sorting (FACS) analysis and showed that the SP cells contained more CD44$^+$, CD24$^+$, and CD133$^+$ cells than the non-SP cells. Since SP cells exhibited increased tumorigenetic ability in BALB/C nude mice and increased chemoresistance following in vitro exposure to gemcitabine. These data suggest that SP cells in the pancreatic cancer cell lines possess the property of CSCs that higher expressions of CD44, CD24, and CD133 molecules and that the CD24 molecule may be one of biomarkers in CSCs (Yao et al. 2010). Similar reports in CSCs include CD44$^+$/CD24$^+$ colorectal cancer (Yeung et al. 2010), CD44$^+$/CD24$^+$/ESA$^+$ pancreas cancer (Li et al. 2010), CD133$^+$/CD44$^+$/CD24$^+$ murine melanoma (Dou et al. 2007), CD44$^+$/CD24$^+$ Kit^{low} gastrointestinal stromal tumors (Zhang et al. 2008), CD173$^+$/CD174$^+$/CD44$^+$ breast carcinomas (Lin et al. 2010), etc.

However, lack or low expression of CD24 was also used to identify CSCs resulting in conflicting data on the usefulness of this marker (Kristiansen et al. 2010). Cancer cells expressing the cell surface marker CD44 but not CD24 (CD44$^+$/CD24$^{-/low}$) were the first described breast cancer CSCs (Al-Hajj et al. 2003). CD44$^+$/CD24$^{-/low}$ cells are generally enriched in basal subtype breast cancers as well as in cell lines that have undergone EMT. In contrast, luminal type breast cancers that express estrogen receptor-alpha (ERα) contain less than 1% CD44$^+$/CD24$^{-/low}$ cells. The study demonstrate enrichment of CD44$^+$/CD24$^-$ cells upon fractionated radiation of ERα$^+$ breast cancer cell lines MCF-7 and T47-D (Nakshatri 2010). In addition, CD44$^+$/CD24$^-$ prostate CSCs cells that were able to migrate through matrigel had suppressed CD24 expression. It is thus evident that these findings suggest that the presence or absence of CD24 on the cell surface has been used as a marker for putative CSCs.

CD138

Multiple myeloma (MM) is the leading cause of death in hematologic malignancies. Most patients eventually relapse and die as a consequence of their disease despite several novel agents improving therapeutic responses. Tumor regrowth following initial reductions in disease burden suggests that tumor cells capable of clonogenic growth are relatively drug resistant, and in several human cancers these functional properties have been attributed to CSCs (Matsui et al. 2004). CD 138 (syndecan-1) is expressed by MM cells from the majority of MM cell lines and patient specimens, but the self-renewing cells responsible for tumor initiation in immunodeficient mice phenotypically resemble memory B cells and are CD138$^-$. The human MM cell lines RPMI 8226 and NCI-H929 contain approximately 2–5% of total cells. These small subpopulations that lack CD138 expression have greater clonogenic potential in vitro than putative CD138$^+$ plasma cells. The D138$^-$ cells derived from clinical MM samples are similarly clonogenic both in vitro and in nonobese diabetic/severe combined immunodeficiency (NOD/SCID) mice, whereas CD138$^+$ cells are not. Thus, CSCs in MM have been well defined as CD138$^-$ B cells with the ability to replicate and subsequently differentiate into malignant CD138$^+$ plasma cells (Matsui et al. 2004).

Other CD Molecules

In addition to CD133, CD44, CD24, and CD138, CSCs have been defined populations in prostate cancer (CD147$^+$) (Hao et al. 2010), non-Hodgkin lymphoma (CD47$^+$) (Chao et al. 2010), HCC (CD90$^+$) (Lingala et al. 2010a), osteosarcoma (CD117$^+$) (Adhikari et al. 2010), acute myeloid leukemia [CD32$^+$ or CD25$^+$ or both (Saito et al. 2010) or CD34$^+$ CD38$^-$ (Natasha and Markus 2009)], MM (CD138$^-$ CD20$^+$/CD27$^+$) (Matsui et al. 2008), CD20$^+$ (classic Hodgkin lymphoma) (Oki and Younes 2010), etc. Stuelten and his colleagues hypothesized that the NCI60 tumor cell line panel that includes cell lines derived from hematopoietic malignancies and solid tumors including brain tumor, small- and non-small-cell lung cancer, central nervous system, colon, breast, ovarian, melanoma, and prostate cancer contains CSCs expressing putative CSC markers (CD15, CD24, CD44, CD133, CD166, CD326). The investigative results showed that the expression levels of individual markers varied widely across the 60 cell lines, and neither single marker expression nor simple combinations nor co-expression patterns correlated with the colony-formation capacity of cell lines and all investigated markers were expressed in cell lines of the NCI60 panel. These tumor cell lines display CSC markers in a complex pattern that relates to the tumor type (Stuelten et al. 2010). Clearly, more work is required to determine the complexity and tumor type specificity of marker in CSCs. Researchers will meet with more challenges for the application of cell sorting and other approaches to isolation of putative CSCs and whether these CD molecules are tissue dependent and a viable marker for identification and isolation.

ATP-Binding Cassette Transporters

Many putative stem cells have acquired the ability to withstand cytotoxic insults through either efficient enzyme-based detoxification systems or with their ability to rapidly export potentially harmful xenobiotics. The resistant tumor cells often over-express one of several ATP-binding cassette (ABC) transporters. To date, about 50 human ABC transporters have been identified in a variety of mammalian cells, which include multidrug resistance 1 (MDR1) (ABCB1 or P-glycoprotein), MRP1 (the multidrug resistance protein 1, ABCC1), ABCB5, and ABCG2/BCRP1 (breast cancer resistance protein 1), etc. These protein expressions are associated with MDR (Kim et al. 2002; Schinkel and Jonker 2003; Patrawala et al. 2005; Henriksen et al. 2005). Technically, ABC transporters act to enable a cancer to escape the cytotoxic effects of chemotherapy that kills most cells in a tumor but CSCs are believed to leave behind, which might be an important mechanism of resistance. Thus, the ABC drug transporters have been shown to protect CSCs from chemotherapeutic agents (Dean et al. 2005).

ABCG2

ABCG2 is a half-transporter, requiring dimerization to become functionally active. Unlike other ABC half-transporters, which are usually expressed in cellular membranes, ABCG2 localizes predominantly to the plasma membrane (Rocchi et al. 2000). The chemotherapy agents and natural substrates can be transported by ABCG2 transporters that are widely distributed in normal tissues and are highly expressed in a subpopulation of stem cells. Given that the ABCG2$^+$ subset of tumor cells is often enriched with cancer stem-like cell phenotypes, it is proposed that ABCG2 activity may enable cancer cells to regenerate postchemotherapy

(Schinkel and Jonker 2003). Because the SP cell phenotype both in human and mouse has also often been correlated with ABC expression, ABCG2 is responsible for Hoechst 33342 dye efflux pattern. Therefore, ABCG2 has been suggested as one of CSC markers, and the expression of ABCG2 has been analyzed in various cancer stem-like cells (Frank et al. 2005). For example, breast cancer SP cells that have been recently isolated from the MCF-7 and Cal-51 cell lines are found to possess ABCG2 transporter properties and may represent stem cell-like cancer cells. The level of ABCG2 mRNA and protein was also reported to be increased in purified MCF7 SP cells relative to non-SP cells, and the purified MCF7 SP cells had an increased ability to colonize the mouse mammary gland (Diah et al. 2001). The study from Christgen et al. indicated that the genuine nature of Cal-51 SP cells was unambiguously verified by showing the 30-fold increased ABCG2-expression in isolated Cal-51 SP cells, and by showing that Cal-51 SP cells generated heterologous non-SP cells, and the ABCG2⁻ expression declined dramatically. In contrast, non-SP cells failed to sustain proliferation (Christgen et al. 2007). A serial reports indicated that an elevated expression of ABCG2 has been observed in a number of putative CSCs from retinoblastoma (Seigel et al. 2005), lung cancer (Ho et al. 2007), human HCC cell lines (Zen et al. 2007), and pancreas cancer (Wang et al. 2009). Additionally, CD133⁺/ABCG2⁺, the widely identified CSC marker are co-expressed in melanoma and pancreatic carcinoma cell lines (Monzani et al. 2007; Olempska et al. 2007; Ding et al. 2010).

However, Patrawala's study demonstrated that the highly purified ABCG2⁺ cancer had very similar tumorigenicity to the ABCG2⁻ cancer cells, and that ABCG2⁻ cancer cells can also generate ABCG2⁺ cells. Furthermore, the ABCG2⁻ population preferentially expressed several "stemness" genes (Graf et al. 2002; Gou et al. 2007). A study by Zhang also reported that the ABCG2⁺ cells did not exhibit its obvious tumorigenic capability compared with the ABCG2⁻ cells in Balb/c null mice. On the proliferative capacity and clonal formative capacity in vitro, the ABCG2⁺ cells and the ABCG2⁻ cells shared similar characteristics, but a few of the SP cells with high expression of ABCG2 molecule had CSC-like characteristics in human ovarian A2780 cell line and in A549 lung cancer cells (Zhang et al. 2009; Su et al. 2010a). Together, these findings suggest that ABCG2 expression is a conserved feature of stem cells or cancer stem-like cells from a wide variety of sources. ABCG2 is an attractive candidate marker useful for identifying and isolating stem cells and CSCs.

ABCB5

ABCB5 is a chemoresistance mediator first identified and characterized in human skin and human malignant melanoma. Recently, the studies of Frank and Schatton indicated that ABCB5 was a novel molecular marker for a distinct subset of chemoresistant, stem cell phenotype-expressing tumor cells among melanoma bulk populations (Stuelten et al. 2010; Su et al. 2010a). In serial human-to-mouse xenotransplantation experiments, ABCB5⁺ melanoma cells were found to possess greater tumorigenic capacity than ABCB5⁻ bulk populations and re-establish clinical tumor heterogeneity. In vivo genetic lineage tracking demonstrated a specific capacity of ABCB5⁺ subpopulations for self-renewal and differentiation, because ABCB5⁺ cancer cells were able to generate both ABCB5⁺ and ABCB5⁻ progeny, whereas ABCB5⁻ tumor populations could only, exclusively to ABCB5⁻ cells and at lower rates. Recently, the studies indicated that a significant overexpression of ABCB5 was noted in tissues from lymph node and distant metastases compared with benign nevi from patients with melanoma, whereas none of the benign nevi of nonmelanoma patients demonstrated expression of ABCB5 (Schatton et al. 2008), and that ABCB5 blockade significantly reversed resistance of G3361 melanoma cells to doxorubicin. Therefore, ABCB5 is a novel molecular marker for a distinct subset of chemoresistant, stem cell phenotype-expressing tumor cells among melanoma bulk populations (Sharma et al. 2010). Together, ABCB5, including both ABCB 5α and ABCB 5β, is potentially a robust CSC biomarker in melanoma (Frank et al. 2005). More experiments, however, are still needed to verify these findings because the malignant CD34⁺ CD38⁻ stem cells were shown to express higher levels of ABC transporter genes, including ABCB1, ABCB4, and ABCB5 (Natasha and Markus 2009).

EpCAM

The epithelial cell adhesion molecule (EpCAM/CD326) was described 30 years ago as a dominant antigen in human colon carcinoma tissue (Chen et al. 2005). EpCAM is a homophilic, Ca^{2+}-independent adhesion molecule with an apparent molecular weight of EpCAM is a glycosylated, 30- to 40-kDa type I membrane protein of 314 amino acids, which is comprised of an extracellular domain with epidermal growth factor (EGF)- and thyroglobulin repeat-like domains, a single transmembrane domain, and a short 26-amino acid intracellular domain. EpCAM is expressed in a variety of human epithelial tissues, cancers, and progenitor and stem cells (Herlyn et al. 1979), thus it is one of the markers that identifies tumor cells with high tumorigenicity. Recent studies provide the evidence that the HCC growth and invasiveness was dictated by a subset of EpCAM⁺ cells (Münz et al. 2005). For instance, the sorted EpCAM⁺ subpopulation from HCC cell lines or HCC specimens identified (Kimura et al. 2010) by the fluorescence-activated cell sorting showed a greater colony formation rate than the sorted EpCAM⁻ subpopulation from the same cell lines or HCC specimens, and displayed hepatic CSC-like traits. Moreover, a smaller number of EpCAM⁺ cells (minimum 100) than EpCAM⁻ cells were capable of initiating highly invasive HCC in NOD/SCID mice. The bifurcated differentiation of EpCAM⁺ cell clones into both EpCAM⁺ and EpCAM⁻ cells was obvious both in vitro and in vivo, but EpCAM⁻ clones sustained their phenotype (Münz et al. 2005). More interestingly, the introduction of exogenous EpCAM into EpCAM⁺ clones, but not into EpCAM⁻ clones, markedly enhanced their tumor-forming ability. Therefore, these results suggest that the EpCAM⁺ cells are biologically quite different from the EpCAM⁻ cells in HCC cell lines or HCC specimens, and preferentially contains a highly tumorigenic cell population with the characteristics of CSCs. The study of Wang et al. indicated that the established characterization of a novel cell line (CSQT-2) with high metastatic activity derived from portal vein tumor thrombus of HCC also showed varied expression of CSC markers such as CD133, CD90, and EpCAM (Yamashita et al. 2009). Moreover, human embryo kidney (HEK) 293 cells expressing full-length EpCAM generated large tumors in 100% of animals, whereas only one out of eight injected mice developed a small tumor with control transfected HEK293 cells (Wang et al. 2010). The murine homolog of EpCAM, however, led to decreased growth, colony formation, and invasiveness of murine colorectal carcinoma cells, whereas overexpressed human EpCAM solely impaired invasiveness (Basak et al. 1998; Maetzel et al. 2009). Hence, there are marked differences between the species in the oncogenic potential and effects on invasiveness of EpCAM, which may depend on the different experimental system (Lugli et al. 2010). Although expression of human EpCAM is evidently associated with increased proliferation of CSCs, the effects of EpCAM expression on CSC metastatic activity and invasiveness seem to be more complex.

ALDH1

A high activity of aldehyde dehydrogenase-1 (ALDH1), the enzyme responsible for the oxidation of intracellular aldehydes, has been shown to be a marker for normal stem cells and CSCs in MM and leukemia patients with high capability of engraftment into NOD-SCID mice (Osta et al. 2004). In breast cancer, CSCs are identified by the cell-surface markers CD44$^+$/CD24$^-$/EpCAM$^+$ and/or possess ALDH1 enzyme activity. ALDH1-positive CSCs mediate metastasis and poor clinical outcome in inflammatory breast cancer (IBC). Charafe-Jauffret et al. showed that CSCs were isolated from SUM149 and MARY-X, an IBC cell line and primary xenograft and ALDH1 activity was analyzed, and invasion and metastasis of CSC populations were assessed by in vitro and mouse xenograft assays. The results indicated that both in vitro and xenograft assays, invasion and metastasis in IBC are mediated by a cellular component that displays ALDH1 activity. ALDH1 expression in IBC or breast cancer was an independent predictive factor for early metastasis and decreased survival in this patient population. The metastatic, aggressive behavior of IBC may be mediated by a CSC component that displays ALDH enzymatic activity (Ginestier et al. 2007; Charafe-Jauffret et al. 2010). Su and his colleagues investigated the stem cell-related function and clinical significance of the ALDH1A1 in bladder urothelial cell carcinoma. Stem cell or stem-like cancer cell characteristics of the ALDH1A1$^+$ cells were assessed by in vitro and in vivo approaches. They used immunohistochemistry assay to evaluate ALDH1A1 expression on 22 normal bladder tissues and 216 bladder tumor specimens of different stage and grade. The results indicated that ALDH1A1$^+$ cancer cells displayed higher in vitro tumorigenicity and generated xenograft tumors that resembled the histopathologic characteristics and heterogeneity of the parental cells, whereas isogenic ALDH1A1$^-$ cells did not have the effect in the same experiments.

Moreover, the ALDH1A1 expression was inversely associated with cancer-specific and overall survival of the patients. Therefore, ALDH1A1 may serve as a useful marker for identifying CSCs in bladder cancer patients and monitoring the progression of bladder tumor (Kawasaki et al. 2010). Furthermore, clusters of CD133+/ALDH^{high} cells were identified in HCC specimens and dysplastic tissues as well (Su et al. 2010a, b). ALDH1 positive CSCs may also be a source of rapidly dividing progeny cells having a biological aggressive phenotype in breast cancer, head and neck squamous cell cancer, neuroblastomas, and colorectal cancer cell lines (Ginestier et al. 2009; Lingala et al. 2010; Lugli et al. 2010; Chen et al. 2010b). Besides, only the presence of ALDH1 positive cells is associated with poor clinical outcome in breast cancer (Wesbuer et al. 2010) or with malignant transformation in ovarian cancer (Penumatsa et al. 2010).

CXCR4

The human chemokine system is currently known to include more than 40 chemokines and 18 chemokine receptors. Chemokine receptors are a family of seven transmembrane G protein-coupled cell surface receptors (GPCR) that are classified into four groups (CXC, CC, C, and CX3C) based on the position of the first two cysteines (Emmanuelle et al. 2000). CXCR4 is one of the best studied chemokine receptors and is a 352-amino acid rhodopsin-like GPCR that selectively binds the CXC chemokine stromal cell-derived factor 1 (SDF-1), also known as CXCL12 (Zlotnik and Yoshie 2000). CXCR4 is expressed on normal stem cells of various organs and tissues. Interestingly, when CXCR4 is expressed in a variety of cancers, its expression in adjacent normal tissue is minimal or absent, which may explain why some tumor cells express CXCR4 and why many researchers suggest that malignant cells may be derived from CXCR4-expressing normal stem cells (Fredriksson et al. 2003). A growing body of evidence now shows that CXCR4 has a role not only in cancer metastasis but also in regulating CSCs (Muller et al. 2001). A study of Chauchereau et al. showed that by culturing human prostate primary tumor cells onto human epithelial ECM, they successfully selected a new prostate cancer cell line, IGR-CaP1 cells, which harbor a tetraploid karyotype, high telomerase activity and mutated TP53, rapidly induced subcutaneous xenografts in nude mice. Moreover, IGR-CaP1 clones exhibit the original features of both basal prostate tissue and CSCs, which are reported to be prostate CSC markers that express high levels of CD44, CD133, and CXCR4 (Furusato et al. 2010). Since the interactions between the SDF-1-CXCR4 is a master regulator of trafficking of both normal stem cells and CSCs, CXCR4 is expressed on the surface of CSCs, as a result, the SDF-1-CXCR4 axis is also involved in directing their trafficking/metastasis to organs (e.g., lymph nodes, lungs, liver, and bones) that highly express SDF-1. If the metastasis of CSCs involve similar mechanisms, strategies aimed at modulating the SDF-1-CXCR4 axis could have important clinical applications in clinical hematology/oncology to inhibit metastasis of CSCs. Supporting this is experimental evidence that serum-free media in the presence of SDF-1 protected the breast cancer cells from apoptosis and CXCR4-low-expressing MCF-7 formed small tumor at inoculated site in SCID mice 8–9 weeks after inoculation while completely failed to metastasis into various organs, whereas CXCR4-high-expressing MDA-231 cells were most efficient in the formation of a large tumor and organ-metastasis within 3 weeks in SCID mice (Chauchereau et al. 2011). Up to date, CXCR4-expressing CSCs have been identified in breast cancer (Hwang-Verslues et al. 2009), HCC (Dewan et al. 2006), prostate cancer (Tomuleasa et al. 2010), melanoma (Hirbe et al. 2010), pancreatic cancer (Kucerova et al. 2010), acute myeloid leukemia (Mueller et al. 2010), neuroblastoma (113), etc. From a basic science perspective, a great deal remains to be learned about CXCR4 and its association with CSCs, and the role of CXCR4 in various CSCs has yet to gain widespread investigation.

Telomerase

Telomerase is expressed during early development and remains fully active in specific germline cells, but is undetectable in most normal somatic cells. High level of telomerase activity is detected in almost 90% of human tumors and immortalized cell lines. The telomere and telomerase system is critical for the biology of normal HSCs. Genetic instability associated with telomere dysfunction (i.e., short telomeres) is an early event in carcinogenesis, resulting in increased risk of myelodysplastic syndrome (MDS) and acute myeloid leukemia (AML). The length of telomeres can serve as a genetic damage marker and could be a potential clinical marker of neoplasia and CSCs (Konoplev et al. 2007; Gančarčíková et al. 2010; Brennan et al. 2010 and Wesbuer et al. 2010). Brennan and his colleagues demonstrated that clonotypic B cells can engraft and recapitulate disease in SCID mice, suggested that these cells serve as the MM CSCs that share functional features with normal stem cells such as drug resistance and self-renewal potential. Since telomerase activity is required for the maintenance of normal adult stem cells and is a common feature of nearly all human cancers, they examined the activity of the telomerase inhibitor imetelstat against MM CSC. Human MM CSC were isolated from cell lines and primary clinical specimens and treated with imetelstat that is a specific inhibitor of the reverse transcriptase activity of telomerase and resulted in a significant reduction in telomere length and the inhibition of clonogenic MM growth both in vitro and in vivo. The data suggest that telomerase activity serves as not only a novel biomarker in MM CSCs but also regulates the clonogenic growth of MM CSCs (Gančarčíková et al. 2010). In neuroblastoma cell lines CHLA-90 and SK-N-SH or prostate cancer cell line IGR-CaP1, high telomerase activity is one distinct CSC feature and in combination with stem cell markers like CD133, ALDH-1 and SP cells, which may be useable to investigate the impact of telomerase activity on CSC survival under therapy (Brennan et al. 2010). Therefore, an understanding of telomere dynamics and telomerase activity in normal and CSCs may provide additional insights into how tumors are initiated, and how they should be monitored and treated (Wesbuer et al. 2010).

SP Cells

SP cells usually represent only a small fraction of the whole cell population that is identified by efflux of Hoechst dye and are present in virtually all normal and malignant tissues (Shay and Wright 2010). SP cell properties have shown to possess some stem cell characteristics. The studies of the hematopoietic origin and some solid tumors have provided evidence that SP cells not only have been identified in cancer cell lines (e.g., neuroblastoma, Goodell et al. 1996), melanoma (Hirschmann-Jax et al. 2004), ovarian (Grichnik et al. 2006), and nasopharyngeal cancer cell lines (Szotek et al. 2006), but also have been used for identification of CSCs [e.g., hepatocellular cancer (Wang et al. 2007), glioma (Kondo et al. 2004; Chiba et al. 2006), myeloma (Dou et al. 2009a), melanoma (Dou et al. 2009b), prostate cancer (Collins et al. 2005a), murine mantle cell lymphoma (Vega et al. 2010), small-cell lung cancer (Salcido et al. 2010), and breast cancer (Nakanishi et al. 2010)]. Noteworthy, there has also been a heightened controversy over the expression of SP markers in tumor tissue samples compared with cell lines. Burker et al. demonstrated that the SP phenotype as a universal marker for stem cells should not be applied to gastrointestinal cancer cell lines (Burkert et al. 2008). They tested four gastrointestinal cancer cell lines (HT29, HGT101, Caco2, and HRA19a1.1) for detailed phenotypic and behavioral analyses of stem cell characteristics. Sorted SP and non-SP cells were similarly clonogenic in vitro and tumorigenic in vivo, and both displayed similar multipotential differentiation potential in vitro and in vivo. The similar result was acquired in the aggressive brain tumor glioblastoma multiforme (GBM) (Broadley et al. 2010).

Besides, Hoechst 33342 dye itself induces SP cell apoptosis and the SP cells isolated by such method have limited uses. For accurate assessment, SP cells must be isolated without Hoechst 33342 (Burkert et al. 2008).

Despite some limitations, SP cells isolated from tumors have proven to be an attractive alternative strategy to the study of CSCs, especially in cases where specific surface marker associations with normal stem cells of the organ of origin have not been identified (Jun et al. 2011). Since SP cells isolated from normal tissues are enriched in normal stem cells, the same population from tumors may also be enriched in CSCs. For example, Grichnik et al. isolated SP cells from human melanoma samples and showed that SP cells had overlapping properties that were common with normal stem cells and included smallness, possess the capacity to become larger cells, and have the greatest ability to expand in culture (Grichnik et al. 2006; Xu et al. 2007). Thus, the SP cells have been well documented as an enriched source of stem cells in specific settings and have remained a valid and promising tool, at least in part, for the identification, isolation, and characterization of stem cells, particularly when this approach is combined with other cell markers such as ABCG2 marker (Jun et al. 2011). A recent study showed that the human epidermal growth factor receptor 2 (HER2) expression was significantly correlated with the occurrence of SP cells and the SP cells from luminal-type MCF-7 cells with enforced expression of HER2, and displayed enrichment in MCF-7 cells capable of repopulating tumors in NOD/SCID mice. The results indicated SP cells in luminal-type breast cancer have

TIC properties, and are regulated by HER2 expression and signaling transduction, which may account for the poor responsiveness of HER2-positive breast cancer to chemotherapy, as well as their aggressiveness (Salcido et al. 2010). Thus, SP cells and HER2 may be novel specific targets for the effective treatment of CSCs.

Other Novel Biomarkers

DCAMKL-1

The putative stem cell marker doublecortin and CaM kinase-like-1 (DCAMKL-1), a microtubule-associated kinase expressed in postmitotic neurons and also was identified as a Gene Ontogeny-enriched transcript expressed in comparison with gastric epithelial progenitor and whole stomach libraries (Lin et al. 2000). May et al. demonstrated the expression patterns of the putative intestinal stem cell marker DCAMKL-1 in the pancreas of uninjured C57BL/6 mice compared with other pancreatic stem/progenitor cell markers. The data suggest that DCAMKL-1 is a novel putative stem/progenitor marker, can be used to isolate normal pancreatic stem/progenitors, and potentially regenerates pancreatic tissues. This may represent a novel tool for regenerative medicine and a target for antistem cell-based therapeutics in pancreatic cancer or pancreatic CSCs (May et al. 2010).

Podocalyxin

Podocalyxin is an integral plasma membrane cell-adhesion glycoprotein that is a marker of human pluripotent and multipotent stem cells and is also a marker of many types of cancers. The expression of podocalyxin is associated with an aggressive and poor-prognosis tumor phenotype. Podocalyxin protein isolated from embryonal carcinoma CSCs reveals peptide sequence of the glucose-3-transporter. Cell imaging studies confirm co-localization of podocalyxin and glucose-3-transporter and the interaction in vivo. The data demonstrate that the podocalyxin is expressed in embryonal carcinoma CSCs and also suggest a novel interaction of the glucose-3-transporter and the cell-adhesion protein podocalyxin that may function in part to regulate and maintain the cell surface expression of the glucose-3-transporter in pluripotent stem cells and in human CSC disease (Schopperle et al. 2010).

Piwil2

Piwil2, a member of AGO/PIWI family of proteins, has been reported to be expressed in precancerous stem cells (pCSCs), tumor cell lines, and various types of human cancers. Liu et al. examined for the expressions of piwil2 in archival formalin-fixed, paraffin-embedded breast cancer specimens at various developmental stages by tissue microarrays and immunohistochemical staining. The results indicated that the piwil2 was expressed in cytoplasm, nucleus, or both cytoplasm and nucleus in all of breast cancer tissue microarrays cores. The nucleus pattern was less observed in breast precancers, whereas all three patterns were observed in invasive and metastatic cancers. These findings demonstrate that the piwil2 has the potential to be used as a novel biomarker of CSCs (Liu et al. 2010a).

Nestin

Nestin belongs to class VI of the intermediate filaments and it is expressed primarily in mammalian nervous tissue during embryonic development. In adults, nestin occurs only in a small subset of cells and tissues. In various types of human solid tumors, as well as in the corresponding established cell lines, nestin expression together with the CD133 surface molecule has also been detected, such as brain CSCs and HCC CSCs, etc. (Krupkova et al. 2010; Yang et al. 2010; Burkert et al. 2010).

LRCs

Stem cells seem prudent to limit stem cell replications due to the error-prone nature of DNA synthesis. Nevertheless, due to this infrequently dividing nature, the stem cells in animals that incorporate DNA synthesis labels such as Bromodeoxyuridine (BrdU) tend to remain "labeled" for a longer time than transit amplifying cells whose more rapid cycling would quickly dilute the label BrdU below detection levels, whereas long-term label retaining cells (LRCs) divide actively during tissue development and remain quiescent at homeostasis. Therefore, the identification of LRCs is often used as a stem cell marker or cancer stem-like cells in the SP2/0 myeloma cell line (Kondo et al. 2004) and mammary stem cells, etc. (Leah et al. 2009; Fernandez-Gonzalez et al. 2010).

Outlook

The hypothesis of CSCs that represent malignant cell subsets in hierarchically organized tumors has also been gradually accepted by both basic and clinical scientists. Regardless of whether these CSCs come from TICs within heterogeneous tumor populations or from transformed stem cells or from progenitor cells, it is clear that CSCs have a role in the initial tumor formation. Understanding the biologic characteristic of CSCs is crucial to start with discovery of specific, sensitive, and reliable CSC biomarkers that can be useful for better identification and diagnosis of CSCs and development of novel therapeutic strategies aiming at thwarting the menacing power of CSCs (Stephen and Antonio 2010; Jun and Ning 2010).

References

Adhikari AS, Agarwal N, Wood BM et al (2010) CD117 and Stro-1 identify osteosarcoma tumor-initiating cells associated with metastasis and drug resistance. Cancer Res 70:4602–4612

Afify A, Purnell P, Nguyen L (2009) Role of CD44s and CD44v6 on human breast cancer cell adhesion, migration, and invasion. Exp Mol Pathol 86:95–100

Aigner S, Sthoeger ZM, Fogel M et al (1997) CD24, a mucin-type glycoprotein, is a ligand for P-selectin on human tumor cells. Blood 89:3385–3395

Al-Hajj M, Wicha MS, Benito-Hernandez A et al (2003) Morrison SJ, Clarke MF. Prospective identification of tumorigenic breast cancer cells. Proc Natl Acad Sci USA 100:3983–3988

Amitava E and Jose A C (2010) Cancer Stem Cells: A Stride Towards Cancer Cure? J Cell Physiol 225: 7–14

Baba T, Convery PA, Matsumura N et al (2009) Epigenetic regulation of CD133 and tumorigenicity of CD133⁺ ovarian cancer cells. Oncogene 28:209–218

Bardsley MR, Horváth VJ, Asuzu DT et al (2010) Kit^{low} stem cells cause resistance to Kit/platelet-derived growth factor alpha inhibitors in murine gastrointestinal stromal tumors. Gastroenterology 139:942–952

Basak S, Speicher D, Eck S et al (1998) Colorectal carcinoma invasion inhibition by CO17-1A/GA733 antigen and its murine homologue. J Natl Cancer Inst 90:691–697

Brennan SK, Wang Q, Tressler R et al (2010) Telomerase inhibition targets clonogenic multiple myeloma cells through telomere length-dependent and independent mechanisms. 5 pii: e12487

Broadley KW, Hunn MK, Farrand KJ et al (2010) Side Population is not Necessary or Sufficient for a Cancer Stem Cell Phenotype in Glioblastoma Multiforme. Stem Cells 2011;29:452–461

Burkert J, Otto WR, Wright NA (2008) Side populations of gastrointestinal cancers are not enriched in stem cells. J Pathol 214:564–573

Burkert J, Wright NA, Alison MR et al (2010) Stem cells and cancer: an intimate relationship. J Pathol 209:287–297

Chao MP, Alizadeh AA, Tang C et al (2010) Anti-CD47 antibody synergizes with rituximab to promote phagocytosis and eradicate non-Hodgkin lymphoma. Cell 142:699–713

Charafe-Jauffret E, Ginestier C, Iovino F et al (2010) Aldehyde dehydrogenase 1-positive cancer stem cells mediate metastasis and poor clinical outcome in inflammatory breast cancer. Clin Cancer Res 16:45–55

Chauchereau A, Al Nakouzi N, Gaudin C et al (2011) Stemness markers characterize IGR-CaP1, a new cell line derived from primary epithelial prostate cancer. Exp Cell Res 317:262–275

Chen KG, Szakács G, Annereau JP et al (2005) Principal expression of two mRNA isoforms (ABCB 5alpha and ABCB 5beta) of the ATP-binding cassette transporter gene ABCB 5 in melanoma cells and melanocytes. Pigment Cell Res 18:102–112

Chen R, Nishimura MC, Bumbaca SM et al (2010) A hierarchy of self-renewing tumor-initiating cell types in glioblastoma. Cancer Cell 17:362–375

Chen YC, Chang CJ, Hsu HS et al (2010) Inhibition of tumorigenicity and enhancement of radiochemosensitivity in head and neck squamous cell cancer-derived ALDH1-positive cells by knockdown of Bmi-1. Oral Oncol 46:158–65

Chiba T, Kita K, Zheng YW et al (2006) Side population purified from hepatocellular carcinoma cells harbors cancer stem cell-like properties. Hepatology 44:240–251

Christgen M, Ballmaier M, Bruchhardt H et al (2007) Identification of a distinct side population of cancer cells in the Cal-51 human breast carcinoma cell line. Mol Cell Biochem 306:201–212

Collins AT, Berry PA, Hyde C et al (2005) Prospective identification of tumorigenic prostate cancer stem cells. Cancer Res 65:10946–10951

Cox CV, Diamanti P, Evely RS et al (2009) Expression of CD133 on leukemia initiating cells in childhood ALL. Blood 113:3287–3296

Curley MD, Therrien VA, Cummings CL et al (2009) CD133 expression defines a tumor initiating cell population in primary human ovarian cancer. Stem Cells 12:2875–2883

Dalerba P, Dylla S J, Park I K et al (2007) Phenotypic characterization of human colorectal cancer stem cells. Proc Natl Acad Sci USA 104:10158–10163

Dean M, Fojo T, Bates S. (2005) Tumor stem cells and drug resistance. Nat Rev Cancer 5:275–284

Dewan MZ, Ahmed S, Iwasaki Y et al (2006) Stromal cell-derived factor-1 and CXCR4 receptor interaction in tumor growth and metastasis of breast cancer. Biomed Pharmacother 60:273–276

Diah SK, Smitherman PK, Aldridge J et al (2001) Resistance to mitoxantrone in multidrug-resistant MCF-7 breast cancer cells: evaluation of mitoxantrone transport and the role of multidrug resistance protein family proteins. Cancer Res 61:5461–5467

Ding X W, Wu JH, Jiang CP (2010) ABCG2: A potential marker of stem cells and novel target in stem cell and cancer therapy. Life Sciences 86:631–637

Dittfeld C, Dietrich A, Peickert S et al (2010) CD133 expression is not selective for tumor-initiating or radioresistant cell populations in the CRC cell line HCT-116. Radiother Oncol 94:375–383

Dou J, Li Y, Hu W et al (2009) Identification of tumor stem like cells in mouse myeloma cell lines. Cell Mol Biol 55 (Suppl): OL1151–1160

Dou J, Pan M, Wen P et al (2007) Isolation and identification of cancer stem like cells from murine melanoma cell lines. Cell Mol Immunol 4:467–472

Dou J, Wen P, Pan M et al (2009) Identification of tumor stem-like cells in mouse melanoma cell line by analysis characteristics of side population cells. Cell Bio Inter 33:807–815

Elsaba TM, Martinez-PomaresL, Robins AR et al (2010) The Stem Cell Marker CD133 Associates with Enhanced Colony Formation and Cell Motility in Colorectal Cancer. PLoS ONE 5: e10714

Emmanuelle C J, Christophe G and Daniel B (2000) Cancer stem cells: Just sign here! Cell Cycle. 229–30

Eramo A, Lotti F, Sette G et al (2008) Identification and expansion of the tumorigenic lung cancer stem cell population. Cell Death Differ 15:504–514

Fang DD, Kim YJ, Lee CN et al (2010) Expansion of CD133(+) colon cancer cultures retaining stem cell properties to enable cancer stem cell target discovery. Br J Cancer 102:1265–1275

Fernandez-Gonzalez R, Illa-Bochaca I, Shelton DN et al (2010) In situ analysis of cell populations: long-term label-retaining cells. Methods Mol Biol 621:1–28

Frank NY, Margaryan A, Huang Y et al (2005) ABCB5-mediated doxorubicin transport and chemoresistance in human malignant melanoma. Cancer Res 65:4320–4333

Fredriksson R, Lagerstrom MC, Lundin LG et al (2003) The G-protein-coupled receptors in the human genome form five main families. Phylogenetic analysis, paralogon groups, and fingerprints. Mol Pharmacol 63:1256–1272

Furusato B, Mohamed A, Uhlén M et al (2010) CXCR4 and cancer. Pathol Int 60:497–505

Gančarčíková M., Zemanová Z., Březinováet al (2010) The Role of Telomeres and Telomerase Complex in Haematological Neoplasia: The Length of Telomeres as a Marker of Carcinogenesis and Prognosis of Disease. Prague Medical Report 111:910–1105

Gao MQ, Choi YP, Kang S et al (2010) CD24+ cells from hierarchically organized ovarian cancer are enriched in cancer stem cells. Oncogene 29:2672–2680

Ginestier C, Hur MH, Charafe-Jauffret E et al (2007) ALDH1 is a marker of normal and malignant human mammary stem cells and a predictor of poor clinical outcome. Cell Stem Cell 1:555–567

Ginestier C, Wicinski J, Cervera N et al (2009) Retinoid signaling regulates breast cancer stem cell differentiation. Cell Cycle 8:3297–3302

Goodell MA, Brose K, Paradis G et al (1996) Isolation and functional properties of murine hematopoietic stem cells that are replicating in vivo. J Exp Med 183:1797–1806

Goodell MA, Brose K, Paradis G et al (1996) Isolation and functional properties of murine hematopoietic stem cells that are replicating in vivo. J Exp Med 183:1797–1806

Gou S, Liu T, Wang C et al (2007) Establishment of clonal colonyforming assay for propagation of pancreatic cancer cells with stem cell properties. Pancreas 34:429–435

Graf GA, Li WP, Gerard RD (2002) Coexpression of ATP-binding cassette proteins ABCG5 and ABCG8 permits their transport to the apical surface. J Clin Invest 110:659–669

Grichnik JM, Burch JA, Schulteis RD et al (2006) Melanoma, a tumor based on a mutant stem cell? J Invest Dermatol 126:142–153

Hao JL, Cozzi PJ, Khatri A et al (2010) CD147/EMMPRIN and CD44 are Potential Therapeutic Targets for Metastatic Prostate Cancer. Current Cancer Drug Targets 10:287–293

Hao JL, Cozzi PJ, Khatri A et al (2010) CD147/EMMPRIN and CD44 are potential therapeutic targets for metastatic prostate cancer. Curr Cancer Drug Targets 10:287–306

Henriksen U, Gether U, Litman T (2005). Effect of Walker A mutation (K86M) on oligomerization and surface targeting of the multidrug resistance transporter ABCG2. J Cell Sci 118:1417–1426

Herlyn D, Herlyn M, Steplewski Z et al (1979) Monoclonal antibodies in cell-mediated cytotoxicity against human melanoma and colorectal carcinoma. Eur J Immunol 9:657–659

Hermann PC, Huber SL, Herrler T et al (2007) Distinct populations of cancer stem cells determine tumor growth and metastatic activity in human pancreatic cancer. Cell Stem Cell 1:313–323

Hirbe AC, Morgan EA, Weilbaecher KN (2010) The CXCR4/SDF-1 chemokine axis: a potential therapeutic target for bone metastases? Curr Pharm Des 16:1284–1290

Hirschmann-Jax C, Foster AE, Wulf GG et al (2004). A distinct "side population" of cells with high drug efflux capacity in human tumor cells. Proc Natl Acad Sci USA 101: 14228–14233

Ho MM, Ng AV, Lam S, Hung JY (2007) Side population in human lung cancer cell lines and tumors is enriched with stem-like cancer cells. Cancer Res 67:4827–4833

Hwang-Verslues WW, Kuo WH, Chang PH et al (2009) Multiple lineages of human breast cancer stem/progenitor cells identified by profiling with stem cell markers. PLoS One 4:e8377

Ishigami S, Ueno S, Arigami T et al (2010) Prognostic impact of CD133 expression in gastric carcinoma. Anticancer Res 30:2453–2457

Ishimoto T, Oshima H, Oshima M (2009) CD44(+) slow-cycling tumor cell expansion is triggered by cooperative actions of Wnt and prostaglandin E(2) in gastric tumorigenesis. Cancer Sci 101:673–678

Jun D and Ning G (2010) Emerging strategies for the identification and targeting of cancer stem cells. Tumor Biol 31:243–253

Jun D, Chuilian J, Jing W et al (2011) Using ABCG2-molecule-expressing side population cells to identify cancer stem-like cells in a human ovarian cell line. Cell Biol Int 35:227–234

Kasper S. (2005) Exploring the origins of the normal prostate and prostate cancer stem cell. Stem Cell Rev 4:193–201

Kawasaki H, Ogura H, Arai Y et al (2010) Aggressive progression of breast cancer with microscopic pulmonary emboli possessing a stem cell-like phenotype independent of its origin. Pathol Int 60:228–234

Kim M, Turnquist H, Jackson J (2002) The multidrug resistance transporter ABCG2 (Breast Cancer Resistance Protein 1) Effluxes Hoechst 33342 and is overexpressed in hematopoietic stem cells. Clin Cancer Res 8:22–28

Kimberly EF, Paola R, Clodia O et al (2009) The cancer stem cell hypothesis. In: Bagley RG and Teicher BA (eds) Cancer drug discovery and development: stem cells and cancer. 1st edn. LLC: Humana Press Publishing

Kimura O, Takahashi T, Ishii N et al (2010) Characterization of the epithelial cell adhesion molecule (EpCAM)+ cell population in hepatocellular carcinoma cell lines. Cancer Sci 101:2145–2155

Klarmann GJ, Hurt EM, Mathews LA et al (2009) Invasive prostate cancer cells are tumor initiating cells that have a stem cell-like genomic signature. Clin Exp Metastasis 26:433–446

Kondo T, Setoguchi T, Taga T (2004) Persistence of a small subpopulation of cancer stem-like cells in the C6 glioma cell line. Proc Natl Acad Sci USA 101:781–786

Konoplev S, Rassidakis GZ, Estey E et al (2007) Overexpression of CXCR4 predicts adverse overall and event-free survival in patients with unmutated FLT3 acute myeloid leukemia with normal karyotype. Cancer 109:1152–1156

Kristiansen G, Machado E, Bretz N et al (2010) Molecular and clinical dissection of CD24 antibody specificity by a comprehensive comparative analysis. Lab Invest 90:1102–1116

Krupkova O Jr, Loja T, Zambo I et al (2010) Nestin expression in human tumors and tumor cell lines. Neoplasma 57:291–298

Kucerova L, Matuskova M, Hlubinova K et al (2010) Tumor cell behaviour modulation by mesenchymal stromal cells. Mol Cancer 9:129

Kumamoto H, Ohki K (2010) Detection of CD133, Bmi-1, and ABCG2 in ameloblastic tumors. J Oral Pathol Med 39:87–93

Kusumbe AP, Mali AM, Bapat SA. (2009) CD133-expressing stem cells associated with ovarian metastases establish an endothelial hierarchy and contribute to tumor vasculature. Stem Cells 27:498–508

Leah O, Benjamin T, Yibin K (2009) Cancer stem cells and metastasis: emerging themes and therapeutic implications. In: Bagley RG and Teicher BA, (eds) Cancer drug discovery and development: stem cells and cancer. 1rd edn. LLC: Humana Press Publishing

Li C, Heidt DG, Dalerba P et al (2010) Identification of pancreatic cancer stem cells. Cancer Res 67:1030–1037

Lin PT, Gleeson JG, Corbo JC et al (2000) DCAMKL1 encodes a protein kinase with homology to doublecortin that regulates microtubule polymerization. J Neurosci 20:9152–9161

Lin WM, Karsten U, Goletz S et al (2010) Co-expression of CD173 (H2) and CD174 (Lewis Y) with CD44 suggests that fucosylated histo-blood group antigens are markers of breast cancer-initiating cells. Virchows Arch 456:403–409

Lingala S, Cui YY, Chen X et al (2010) Immunohistochemical staining of cancer stem cell markers in hepatocellular carcinoma. Exp Mol Pathol 89:27–35

Liu JJ, Shen R, Chen L et al (2010) Piwil2 is expressed in various stages of breast cancers and has the potential to be used as a novel biomarker. Int J Clin Exp Pathol 3:328–337

Liu T, Cheng W, Lai D Huang et al (2010) Characterization of primary ovarian cancer cells in different culture systems. Oncol Rep 23:1277–1284

Lugli A, Iezzi G, Hostettler I et al (2010) Prognostic impact of the expression of putative cancer stem cell markers CD133, CD166, CD44s, EpCAM, and ALDH1 in colorectal cancer. Br J Cancer 103:382–390

Maetzel D, Denzel S, Mack B et al (2009) Nuclear signalling by tumour-associated antigen EpCAM. Nat Cell Biol 11:162–171

Marhaba R, Zoller M (2004) CD44 in cancer progression: adhesion, migration and growth regulation. J Mol Histol 35:211–231

Mark A, La B, Mina JB (2008) Is CD133 a marker of metastatic colon cancer stem cells? J Clin Invest 118:2021–2024

Matsui W, Huff CA, Wang Q et al (2004) Characterization of clonogenic multiple myeloma cells. Blood 103:2332–2336

Matsui W, Wang Q, Barber JP et al (2008) Clonogenic multiple myeloma progenitors, stem cell properties, and drug resistance. Cancer Res 68:190–197

May R, Sureban SM, Lightfoot SA et al (2010) Identification of a novel putative pancreatic stem/progenitor cell marker DCAMKL-1 in normal mouse pancreas. Am J Physiol Gastrointest Liver Physiol 299:G303–10

Miletti-González K E, Chen S, Muthukumaran N et al (2005) The CD44 receptor interacts with P Glycoprotein to promote cell migration and invasion in cancer. Cancer Res 65:6660–6667

Miraglia S, Godfrey W, Yin AH et al (1997) A novel five-transmembrane hematopoietic stem cell antigen: isolation, characterization, and molecular cloning. Blood 90:5013–5021

Mizrak D, Brittan M, Alison MR (2008) CD133: molecule of the moment. J Pathol 214:3–9

Monzani E, Facchetti F, Galmozzi E et al (2007) Melanoma contains CD133 and ABCG2 positive cells with enhanced tumourigenic potential. Eur J Cancer 43:935–946

Moriyama T, Ohuchida K, Mizumoto K et al (2010) Enhanced cell migration and invasion of CD133+ pancreatic cancer cells cocultured with pancreatic stromal cells. Cancer 116:3357–3368

Mueller MT, Hermann PC, Heeschen C (2010) Cancer stem cells as new therapeutic target to prevent tumour progression and metastasis. Front Biosci (Elite Ed) 2:602–613

Muller A, Homey B, Soto H et al (2001) Involvement of chemokine receptors in breast cancer metastasis. Nature 410:50–56

Münz M, Zeidler R, Gires O (2005) The tumour-associated antigen EpCAM upregulates the fatty acid binding protein E-FABP. Cancer Lett 225:151–157

Nakanishi T, Chumsri S, Khakpour N et al (2010) Side-population cells in luminal-type breast cancer have tumour-initiating cell properties, and are regulated by HER2 expression and signalling. Br J Cancer 102:815–826

Nakshatri H (2010) Radiation resistance in breast cancer: are CD44+/CD24-/proteosome low/ PKH26+ cells to blame? Breast Cancer Res 12:105

Natasha Y F, and Markus H F (2009) ABCB5 gene amplification in human leukemia cells. Leuk Res 33:1303–1305

Neethan A L, Yohei S, Dalong Q et al (2007) The Biology of Cancer Stem Cells. Annu Rev Cell Dev Biol 23:675–699

O'Brien CA, Pollett A, Gallinger S et al (2007) A human colon cancer cell capable of initiating tumour growth in immunodeficient mice. Nature 445:106–110

Oki Y, Younes A (2010) Does rituximab have a place in treating classic hodgkin lymphoma? Curr Hematol Malig Rep 5:135–139

Olempska M, Eisenach PA, Ammerpohl O et al (2007) Detection of tumor stem cell markers in pancreatic carcinoma cell lines. Hepato Pancre Dis Int 6:92–97

Osta WA, Chen Y, Mikhitarian K et al (2004) EpCAM is overexpressed in breast cancer and is a potential target for breast cancer gene therapy. Cancer Res 64:5818–5824

Pannuti A, Foreman K, Rizzo P et al (2010) Targeting Notch to target cancer stem cells. Clin Cancer Res. 16:3141–3152

Patrawala L, Calhoun T, Schneider-Broussard R et al (2005) Side population is enriched in tumorigenic, stem-like cancer cells, whereas ABCG2+ and ABCG2-cancer cells are similarly tumorigenic. Cancer Res 65:6207–6219

Penumatsa K, Edassery SL, Barua A et al (2010) Differential expression of aldehyde dehydrogenase 1A1 (ALDH1) in normal ovary and serous ovarian tumors. J Ovarian Res 3:28

Pirruccello SJ, LeBien TW (1986) The human B cell-associated antigen CD24 is a single chain sialoglycoprotein. J Immunol 136:3779–3784

Ponta H, Sherman L, Herrlich PA (2003) CD44: from adhesion molecules to signalling regulators. Nat Rev 4:33–45

Prince ME, Sivanandan R, Kaczorowski A et al (2007) Identification of a subpopulation of cells with cancer stem cell properties in head and neck squamous cell carcinoma. Proc Natl Acad Sci USA 104:973–978

Ricci-Vitiani L, Lombardi DG, Pilozzi E et al (2007) Identification and expansion of human coloncancer-initiating cells. Nature 445:111–115

Rocchi E, Khodjakov A, Volk EL et al (2000) The product of the ABC half-transporter gene ABCG2 (BCRP/MXR/ABCP) is expressed in the plasma membrane. Biochem Biophys Res Commun 271:42–46

Saito Y, Kitamura H, Hijikata A, et al (2010) Identification of therapeutic targets for quiescent, chemotherapy- resistant human leukemia stem cells. Sci Transl Med 2:17–19

Salcido CD, Larochelle A, Taylor BJ et al (2010) Molecular characterisation of side population cells with cancer stem cell-like characteristics in small-cell lung cancer. Br J Cancer 102:1636–1644

Schatton T, Murphy GF, Frank NY et al (2008) Identification of cells initiating human melanomas. Nature 451:345–349

Schinkel AH, Jonker JW (2003) Mammalian drug efflux transporters of the ATP binding cassette (ABC) family: an overview. Advanced Drug Delivery Reviews 55:3–29

Schopperle WM, Lee JM, Dewolf WC (2010) The human cancer and stem cell marker podocalyxin interacts with the glucose-3-transporter in malignant pluripotent stem cells. Biochem Biophys Res Commun 398:372–376

Seigel GM, Campbell LM, Narayan M et al (2005) Gonzalez-Fernandez F. Cancer stem cell characteristics in retinoblastoma. Molecular Vision 11:729–737

Sharma BK, Manglik V, Elias EG (2010) Immuno-expression of human melanoma stem cell markers in tissues at different stages of the disease. J Surg Res 163:e11–5

Shay JW, Wright WE (2010) Telomeres and telomerase in normal and cancer stem cells. FEBS Lett 584:3819–3825

Shmelkov JM, Butler AT, Hooper AH et al (2008) CD133 expression is not restricted to stem cells, and both CD133+ and CD133- metastatic colon cancer cells initiate tumors. J Clin Invest 118:2111–2120

Stephen B. K and Antonio J (2010) More than Markers: Biological Significance of Cancer Stem Cell-Defining Molecules. Mol Cancer Ther 9:2450–2457

Stuelten CH, Mertins SD, Busch JI et al (2010) Complex display of putative tumor stem cell markers in the NCI60 tumor cell line panel. Stem Cells 28:649–660

Su C, Picard P, Rathbone MP et al (2010) Guanosine-induced decrease in side population of lung cancer cells: lack of correlation with ABCG2 expression. J Biol Regul Homeost Agents 24:19–25

Su Y, Qiu Q, Zhang X et al (2010) Aldehyde dehydrogenase 1 A1-positive cell population is enriched in tumor-initiating cells and associated with progression of bladder cancer. Cancer Epidemiol Biomarkers Prev 19:327–337

Suetsugu A, Nagaki M, Aoki H et al (2006) Characterization of CD133+ hepatocellular carcinoma cells as cancer stem/progenitor cells. Biochem Biophys Res Commun 351:820–824

Szotek PP, Pieretti-Vanmarcke R, Masiakos PT et al (2006) Ovarian cancer side population defines cells with stem cell–like characteristics and Mullerian inhibiting substance responsiveness. Proc Natl Acad Sci USA 103:11154–11159

Takaishi S, Okumura T, Tu S et al (2009) Identification of gastric cancer stem cells using the cell surface marker CD44. Stem Cells 27:1006–1020

Tomuleasa C, Soritau O, Rus-Ciuca D et al (2010) Isolation and characterization of hepatic cancer cells with stem-like properties from hepatocellular carcinoma. J Gastrointestin Liver Dis 19:61–67

Turner C, Kohandel M (2010) Investigating the link between epithelial-mesenchymal transition and the cancer stem cell phenotype: A mathematical approach. J Theor Biol 265:329–335

Vega F, Davuluri Y, Cho-Vega et al (2010) Side population of a murine mantle cell lymphoma model contains tumor-initiating cells responsible for lymphoma maintenance and dissemination. J Cell Mol Med 14(6B):1532–1545

Wang J, Guo LP, Chen LZ et al (2007) Identification of cancer stem cell-like side population cells in human nasopharyngeal carcinoma cell line. Cancer Res 67:3716–3724

Wang T, Hu HS, Feng YX et al (2010) Characterisation of a novel cell line (CSQT-2) with high metastatic activity derived from portal vein tumour thrombus of hepatocellular carcinoma. Br J Cancer 102:1618–1626

Wang YH, Li F, Luo B et al (2009) A side population of cells from a human pancreatic carcinoma cell line harbors cancer stem cell characteristics. Neoplasma 56:371–378

Wesbuer S, Lanvers-Kaminsky C et al (2010) Association of telomerase activity with radio- and chemosensitivity of neuroblastomas. Radiat Oncol 5:66

Wesbuer S, Lanvers-Kaminsky C, Duran-Seuberth I et al (2010) Association of telomerase activity with radio- and chemosensitivity of neuroblastomas. Radiat Onco 15:66.

Xu JX, Morii E, Liu Y et al (2007) High tolerance to apoptotic stimuli induced by serum depletion and ceramide in side-population cells: high expression of CD55 as a novel character for side-population. Exp Cell Res 313:1877–1885

Xu Y, Stamenkovic I, Yu Q (2010) CD44 attenuates activation of the hippo signaling pathway and is a prime therapeutic target for glioblastoma. Cancer Res 70:2455–2464

Yamashita T, Ji J, Budhu A et al (2009) EpCAM-positive hepatocellular carcinoma cells are tumor-initiating cells with stem/progenitor cell features. Gastroenterology 136:1012–1024

Yang XR, Xu Y, Yu B et al (2010) High expression levels of putative hepatic stem/progenitor cell biomarkers related to tumour angiogenesis and poor prognosis of hepatocellular carcinoma. Gut 59:953–962

Yao J, Cai HH, Wei JS et al (2010) Side population in the pancreatic cancer cell lines SW1990 and CFPAC-1 is enriched with cancer stem-like cells. Oncol Rep 23:1375–1382

Yao J, Zhang T, Ren J et al (2009) Effect of CD133/prominin-1 antisense oligodeoxynucleotide on in vitro growth characteristics of Huh-7 human hepatocarcinoma cells and U251 human glioma cells. Oncol Rep 22:781–787

Yasuda H, Tanaka K, Saigusa S et al (2009) Elevated CD133, but not VEGF or EGFR, as a predictive marker of distant recurrence after preoperative chemoradiotherapy in rectal cancer. Oncol Rep 22:709–717

Yeung TM, Gandhi SC, Wilding JL et al (2010) Cancer stem cells from colorectal cancer-derived cell lines. Proc Natl Acad Sci USA 107:3722–3727

Zen Y, Fujii T, Yoshikawa S et al (2007) Histological and culture studies with respect to ABCG2 expression support the existence of a cancer cell hierarchy in human hepatocellular carcinoma. J Pathol 170:1750–1762

Zhang S, Balch C, Chan MW et al (2008) Identification and characterization of ovarian cancer-initiating cells from primary human tumors. Cancer Res 68:4311–4320

Zhang X, Jiang CL, Wang BS et al (2009) Primarily identification of the cell surface mark of ovarial cancer stem cells in a human ovarian cell line based on sorting side population cells. J S E U (Med Sci Edi) 28:800–803

Zhou XD, Wang XY, Qu FJ (2009) Detection of cancer stem cells from the C6 glioma cell line. J Int Med Res 37:503–510

Zhu Z, Hao X, Yan M et al (2010) Cancer stem/progenitor cells are highly enriched in CD133(+) CD44(+) population in hepatocellular carcinoma. Int J Cancer 126:2067–2078

Zlotnik A, Yoshie O. (2000) Chemokines: A new classification system and their role in immunity. Immunity 12:121–127

Chapter 5
Cancer Stem Cells and the Microenvironment

Alfonso Colombatti, Carla Danussi, Eliana Pivetta, and Paola Spessotto

Tumor Microenvironment

Primary and secondary tumor sites consist of a complex variety of cellular and extracellular components, i.e., soluble factors and extracellular matrix (ECM) constituents. The cellular compartment includes not only tumor cells themselves, but also blood or lymphatic endothelial cells (ECs), pericytes, smooth muscle cells, (myo)fibroblasts, adipocytes, immune and inflammatory cells (Albini and Sporn 2007). All these cells release promoting as well as inhibiting factors and cytokines. Thus, the initiation and progression of tumors depend not only on alterations in tumor cells but also on changes in their microenvironment (Joyce and Pollard 2009). In addition, fibroblasts associated with cancer tissue or cancer-associated fibroblasts (CAF) are structurally and functionally different from fibroblasts adjacent to normal epithelium (Dean and Nelson 2008). Similarly, the tumor infiltrating macrophages can either protect against (M1) or facilitate (M2) tumor development. Furthermore, both CAFs and TAMs promote tumor growth and alter drug response in vivo (Mantovani et al. 2006; Iwamoto et al. 2007).

Extracellular Matrix

Various components of the ECM directly and indirectly influence cellular behavior (Hynes 2009). Thus, the ECM is not simply an extracellular scaffold but represents a fundamental component of the microenvironment and influences cellular phenotype (Bissell et al. 2005); it also acts as a reservoir of biologically active molecules,

A. Colombatti (✉) • C. Danussi • E. Pivetta • P. Spessotto
Division of Experimental Oncology 2, National Cancer Institute IRCCS-CRO,
Via Franco Gallini 2, 33081 Aviano, Italy
e-mail: acolombatti@cro.it

such as growth factors and cytokines (Sternlicht and Werb 2001). Domains within ECM proteins are ligands for canonical growth factor receptors. The integrins, the ECM receptors, upon interaction with the respective ligand lead to signal transduction (Hynes 2002; Legate et al. 2009) and cross talks between integrins and various growth factor receptors are well documented (Alam et al. 2007). The coexistence in the same ECM proteins of sites for cell adhesion and binding sites for growth factors concentrates the growth factors close to the cell surface receptors. Their localized signaling contributes to the establishment of stable gradients within the microenvironment that are jointly composed of soluble, diffusible factors and ECM constituents both necessary for tumor cell behavior.

Tumor-Associated Cells

Numerous studies demonstrate that inflammation can support antitumor functions while others highlight the protumoral activity. This paradox reflects specific tumor microenvironments. The tumor-promoting role of TAMs was suggested by the high frequency of infiltrating TAMs and poor prognosis for many different human tumors (Bingle et al. 2002). Accordingly, genes of infiltrating macrophages were identified as part of molecular signatures associated with a poor prognosis and in response to different microenvironmental signals (Paik et al. 2004). The cross-talk between tumor cells and macrophages is instrumental for the activation switches during the course of progression. In established tumors, macrophages exhibit mainly the alternatively activated M2 phenotype with a peculiar chemokines expression pattern (e.g., CCL17, CCL22) and are engaged in immunosuppression and promotion of angiogenesis and metastasis (Sica et al. 2006). An established M2 profile correlates with poor prognosis and can predict progression (Dakhova et al. 2009) (Fig. 5.1a).

A significant fraction of the stromal cells in some tumors consists of CAFs (Bissell and Radisky 2001) and promote tumor cell growth compared with fibroblasts obtained from nonneoplastic locations. Bone marrow-derived mesenchymal stem cells (MSCs), the probable source of CAFs (Orimo et al. 2005; Mishra et al. 2008), exhibit sustained expression of CXCL12/SDF-1 and the ability to promote tumor cell growth both in vitro and in co-transplantation models. CAFs support aerobic glycolysis and cooperate with tumor cells by taking up the produced lactate and, after conversion to pyruvate, secrete it into the microenvironment where it can be used for oxidative phosphorylation (Samudio et al. 2008; Kroemer and Pouyssegur 2008). Given the extensive cross-talks between cancer cells and these components of the microenvironment, CAFs could harbor cancer-promoting mutations. Indeed the p53 response to radiation is attenuated in 70% of CAFs, whereas it is normal in the fibroblasts suggesting that alterations in the p53 pathway do occur (Hawsawi et al. 2008). Consequently, gene expression profiles of tumor stroma resulted in a novel improved prognostic predictor, the breast tumors stroma-derived prognosticator

5 Cancer Stem Cells and the Microenvironment

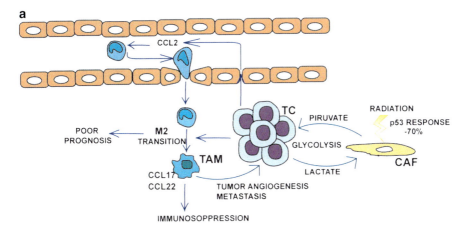

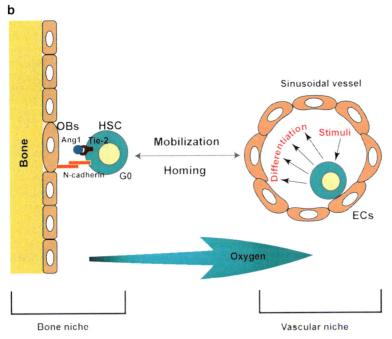

Fig. 5.1 Schematic view of the (**a**) contribution of tumor associated fibroblasts (CSF) and macrophages (TAM) to a tumor cell (TC) prone microenvironment and (**b**) the principal characteristics of the bone and vascular niches

(SDPR). Genes showing strong prognostic tendencies included those associated with differential immune responses and angiogenic and hypoxic responses underscoring the importance of stromal elements in tumor progression and clinical outcome (Finak et al. 2008).

Niche Concept

The first demonstration of a niche was obtained when cells newly introduced to the fly ovary remained germ line stem cells as long as they adhered to cap cells that function as a true stem cell niche (Xie and Spradling 2000). Germ line stem cells require a signal mediated by decapentaplegic (dpp), a member of the transforming growth factor (TGF)-β superfamily, in order to adhere to the cap cells and thus to maintain the stem cell condition and to control the frequency of cell division. Thus, the definition of a tissue-specific niche indicates a restricted place that supports self-renewing division of stem cells and prevents them from differentiating. It is composed of three basic elements: localized signaling cells and ECM-controlling stem cell behavior, specified signaling, and proper stem cell(s) (Dick 2008).

Embryonal Niche

It is known that embryonic stem cells sustain a microenvironment that facilitates a balance of self-renewal and differentiation. In addition, several studies have documented the ability of embryonic microenvironments to reprogram cancer cells to a less aggressive phenotype exemplified by diminished clonogenicity and tumorigenicity (Kasemeier-Kulesa et al. 2008; Utikal et al. 2009). Aggressive cancer cells respond to regulatory cues such as members of the Notch, Wingless, and TGF-β superfamilies (Hendrix et al. 2003; O'Connell and Weeraratna 2009) that control cell fate determination within the microenvironment of human embryonic stem cells (hESCs). Some tumor cells express the embryonic morphogen Nodal, which is essential to the maintenance of hESC pluripotency, however they lack Lefty, a negative regulator of Nodal. Down-regulation of Nodal expression via exposure to the hESC microenvironment (containing Lefty) results in reprogramming with decreased colony formation in soft agar concomitant with a marked abrogation of tumor formation in orthotopic mouse models (Topczewska et al. 2006). This embryological signaling pathway is aberrantly reexpressed in metastatic melanoma and breast carcinoma cells and could offer new therapeutic strategies to inhibit tumor progression by reprogramming aggressive tumor cells with unique embryonic regulator(s).

Osteoblastic Niche

During the process of hematopoiesis in bone marrow (BM), human stem cells (HSC) and osteoblasts bind each other via adhesion molecules such as N-cadherin. In addition, angiopoietin-1 produced by osteoblasts interacts with Tie-2, a type of receptor tyrosine kinase expressed in HSC: these interactions activate β1-integrin and N-cadherin and contribute to the maintenance of HSC in the endosteal microenvironment in a quiescent status (Arai et al. 2004). This microenvironment represents the osteoblastic niche. O_2 content is a functional component of the osteoblastic niche and maintains HSC in a hypoxic environment in BM (Parmar et al. 2007). The interaction between the bone morphogenetic protein and the parathyroid hormone with their receptor expressed in osteoblasts regulates the size (i.e., the number of osteoblasts) of the niche and hence the numbers of HSC (Zhang et al. 2003; Calvi et al. 2003) (Fig. 5.1b).

Vascular Niche

Along the ECs of the sinusoidal vessels in BM or spleen there is the vascular niche (Kiel et al. 2005). Its structure consists of a network of thin-walled fenestrated vessels that allow cells in the venous circulation to extravasate into hematopoietic tissues, support HSC development, proliferation, and mobilization to the peripheral blood circulation (Takakura et al. 1998). Sinusoidal ECs form a specialized microenvironment for the maintenance of HSCs homeostasis by delivering nutrients and through an instructive mechanism (Kopp et al. 2005; Coultas et al. 2005). One of the major differences between these osteoblastic and vascular niche is the O_2 level. O_2 availability is higher in the vascular than in the osteoblastic niche and in such a microenvironment the cell cycle of the stem cell resumes (Parmar et al. 2007). Thus, cells in a G0 state in the osteoblastic niche under regional hypoxia at a certain time move to the vascular niche and under appropriate stimuli undergo differentiation to provide the peripheral blood with the necessary supply of mature cells (Heissig et al. 2002).

Cancer Stem Cells

Cancer has been described as a "developmental disease," in which normal developmental pathways have been co-opted by oncogenic processes. Accordingly, the development of a tumor is considered analogous to the development of an aberrant organ. During normal organogenesis, a careful orchestration of stem cells results in a functional organ with heterogeneous cellular phenotypes. In tumorigenesis, the processes of self-renewal and differentiation are deregulated leading to the production of enhanced proliferation, aberrantly differentiated tumor cells composed of a heterogeneous population of cells different in morphology, marker expression, and proliferation ability. The CSC model proposes that only a small fraction of cells within a tumor possesses cancer-initiating potential and that only CSCs are able to initiate and sustain tumor growth. The normal stem cells support the cellular hierarchy of the tissue over the lifespan of an individual. CSCs self-renew while maintaining their ability to generate a progeny of both tumorigenic and nontumorigenic cancer cells through asymmetric division. The CSC model implies that the vast majority of the tumor cells lack self-renewal potential and, hence, do not possess the capacity to significantly perpetuate tumor growth which relies exclusively on rare cells

(Wang and Dick 2005; Clarke et al. 2006). An alternative view affirms that this heterogeneity is mainly explained by stochastic genetic events and microenvironmental influence leading to clonal selection (see below).

The CSC model has arisen primarily from xenotransplantation studies in which only very rare human tumor cells, in the order of 10^{-4} to 10^{-7} in samples of human AML, could transplant leukemia in sublethally irradiated immunodeficient (NOD-SCID) mice (Lapidot et al. 1994; Bonnet and Dick 1997; Wang and Dick 2005). Subsequently, several groups demonstrated that similar cells were present in solid cancers. Breast, colon, and brain tumors display a functional cellular heterogeneity with a potential hierarchy of differentiation (Al-Hajj et al. 2003; Taylor et al. 2005). The CSC model might provide a new approach to therapy (Clarke et al. 2006), but unfortunately, the largely quiescent CSCs are more refractory than other tumor cell populations to irradiation and chemotherapy (Wulf et al. 2001; Bao et al. 2006; Liu et al. 2006; Hambardzumyan et al. 2008). However, if all self-renewal depends on the CSC, they are the critical therapeutic targets, whereas elimination of the bulk of the tumor cells might have negligible effect on long-term patient survival.

CSCs and Epithelial–Mesenchymal Transition

Transition between epithelial and mesenchymal (EMT) states contributes to tumor progression and intratumoral heterogeneity. The EMT is triggered by a diverse set of stimuli including growth factor signaling, tumor–stromal cell interactions, and hypoxia. EMT results in cancer cells that have gained CSC-like qualities endowed with a propensity to invade surrounding tissue and are resistant to certain therapeutic interventions. There are characteristics of the niche that function to maintain tumor dormancy and render the niche relatively ineffective in order to support CSC proliferation. Then signaling pathways involved in the regulation of CSC function and niche–stem cell interactions can trigger EMT programs establishing and maintaining CSC-like characteristics. Notch signaling is involved in the regulation of EMT occurring during both embryogenesis and tumorigenesis. It involves multiple receptors, ligands, and downstream mediators. The outcome of its activation is cell-type specific and can be either oncogenic or tumor suppressive (Pui and Evans 2006). Due to the parallel expression of both stem cell markers and EMT factors in selected tumor cells at the invasive front, genes that regulate EMT, such as *TWIST*, *SNAI1*, and *ZEB1* can be misregulated (Brabletz et al. 2001; Mani et al. 2008). As an example, ZEB1 links EMT activation, stemness maintenance, and migrating CSCs by suppressing stemness inhibiting miR-200 that reciprocally controls ZEB1 in a feedback loop (Wellner et al. 2009; Bracken et al. 2008). Another miRNA, miR-203, controls the properties of skin stem cells through inhibition of the stem cell factor p63, thereby inducing terminal differentiation of skin stem cells into suprabasal cells. Accordingly, reduced expression of stemness inhibiting miRNAs maintains a stem cell phenotype. Less EMT allows less dissemination, and less expression of stemness maintaining factors results in less tumor- and metastasis-initiating capacity (Yi et al. 2008).

Challenges to the CSC Model

There are inconsistencies in putative CSC populations suggesting that the current clonal expansion model of a tumor driven solely through rare CSCs could be more complex (Hill 2006; Kern and Shibata 2007). How human tumor cells can home efficiently to an appropriate niche in the mouse is still unclear. Xenotransplantation is problematic because the growth of tumor cells requires an intricate network of interactions with diverse cells. By using highly immunocompromised NOD/SCID mice lacking the interleukin-2 gamma receptor (NOD/SCID$^{Il2rg-/-}$), melanoma tumors from a single human melanoma cell can be generated (Quintana et al. 2008). In addition, as few as ten unsorted mouse lymphoma cells reproduce the disease in congenic recipient mice (Kelly et al. 2007). This suggests that infrequent tumor cell engraftment may be a result of selective microenvironment pressures and could underestimate the population of tumorigenic cells in some cancers (Kelly et al. 2007). In addition, the potential for extrinsic factors such as tumor hypoxia, stromal derived cytokines, and tumor vasculature can alter the presence of CSCs (Li et al. 2009; Heddleston et al. 2010) to influence tumor "stemness" in several samples. Based on these observations a "stochastic" (Wang and Dick 2005) or "clonal evolution model" (Campbell and Polyak 2007), where many tumor cells are capable of self-renewal and can propagate tumors phenotypically similar to the parental tumor was proposed. Tumor heterogeneity depends on intraclonal genetic and epigenetic variation, differentiation as well as microenvironmental influences. Rather than lacking self-renewal activity, the nontransplantable human cell population might instead lack a critical feature for obtaining stromal support in the foreign microenvironment, such as a cytokine receptor responsive to mouse factors or a chemokine receptor that attracts the cells to an appropriate niche. Instead of being uniquely responsible for tumor growth, the transplantable cell population may have acquired (perhaps by epigenetic changes) more competitive properties that endow them with the ability to survive in the xenogenic microenvironment.

CSCs, Epigenetic Changes, and Tumor Microenvironment

Numerous evidences suggest that disruption of epigenetic processes can lead to altered gene function and malignant cellular transformation. Epigenetic abnormalities, which occur in normal stem or progenitor cells, are the earliest events in cancer initiation and involve DNA methylation, histone modifications, nucleosome positioning, and noncoding RNAs, specifically microRNA expression along with genetic alterations (Feinberg et al. 2006; Sharma et al. 2010). The accumulation of epigenetic abnormalities arises from very early alterations in the central control machinery and predisposes tumor cells to gain further epimutations as it occurs following defects in DNA repair machinery. Since epigenetic mechanisms are central to maintenance of stem cell identity, their disruption may give rise to high-risk aberrant progenitors that can undergo transformation following gatekeeper mutations (Meissner et al. 2008; Surani et al. 2007). Aberrant silencing of the so-called epigenetic gatekeeper genes such as p16, APC, SFRPs, under inflammatory conditions, confers stem/precursor cells infinite renewal capacity. These preinvasive stem cells are selected for and then form a pool of abnormal precursor cells that can undergo further genetic mutations, higher expression of pluripotency markers, enhanced "stemness" along with high proliferative capacity leading to tumorigenesis (Baylin and Ohm 2006). Polycomb proteins control the silencing of developmental regulators in embryonal cells and provide another important link between stem cell biology and cancer initiation. They are commonly upregulated in various forms of cancer (Valk-Lingbeek et al. 2004) and genes that are marked by polycomb repressive mark H3K27me3 in embryonal cells are often methylated in cancer and result in the permanent silencing of key regulatory genes that may contribute to cell proliferation and tumorigenesis (Gal-Yam et al. 2008). Such findings support the hypothesis of epigenetics playing a central role in early CSCs (Widschwendter et al. 2007).

The Tumor Niche

CSC and normal stem cells have much in common with regard to the maintenance within their niches. It is likely that there is a functional microenvironment to support CSC niche (Iwasaki and Suda 2009).

Lymphvascular Niche

Tumor-associated lymphangiogenesis is closely associated with tissue inflammation and actively promotes sentinel lymph node metastasis in several human cancers. In fact, primary tumors can alter draining lymph nodes by inducing lymphangiogenesis before they metastasize (Hirakawa 2009). The analysis of the lymphatic endothelium was favored by the recent identification of lymphatic vessel-specific markers and growth factors. This system likely promotes transport, migration, retention, and growth of metastatic tumor cells within lymph nodes suggesting that primary tumors can actively modify future metastatic sites for preferential relocation (Hirakawa 2009; Tammela and Alitalo 2010). Lymph node microenvironment is CXCL12/SDF-1-rich (Drayton et al. 2006) and this contributes to the formation of a lymphvascular niche that attracts and maintains a subset of CSCs that potentially initiate a new tumor at distant sites. However, whether tumor cell migration via lymphatics promotes further spreading, cell trapping, or just indicates that tumor cells transit there to go somewhere else is still a matter of investigation (Giampieri et al. 2009). The lymphatic endothelium of lymph nodes is composed of sinusoids with ECs lacking abundant ECM constituents in close contact with parenchymal cells. The structural similarity between the vascular niche in BM and spleen and the lymphvascular niche in the lymph nodes suggests that metastatic CSCs are retained and survive well in the lymphvascular niche. CAFs release hyaluronan and lymphangiogenic factors that stimulate further lymphangiogenesis (Koyama et al. 2008). Other constituents of the ECM regulate lymphangiogenesis under both normal as well as tumor development conditions (Danussi et al. 2008) and metastases formation (Danussi et al. submitted). For instance, lymphatic vessel density in benign tumors like lymphangiomas was significantly increased in $Emilin1^{-/-}$ mice lacking the ECM glycoprotein EMILIN1 compared with their wild type littermates. In addition, more and larger lymphatic vessels were detected in $Emilin1^{-/-}$ lymph nodes in skin-induced tumors indicating that lymphangiogenesis was more pronounced when EMILIN1 is absent. Consequently, RT-PCR of lymph node extracts for the K14 epidermal cells specific marker indicated that $Emilin1^{-/-}$ mice presented a ninefold increased percentage of positive lymph nodes compared to wild type mice (Danussi et al. submitted) suggesting a homeostatic role of this ECM glycoprotein in the skin as its absence promoted basal keratinocytes (and niche stem cells?) proliferation and in the formation of a prometastatic environment (i.e., niche) within the lymph nodes. Under appropriate conditions, specific proteolytic enzymes released by tumor cells and/or cells of the microenvironment degrade EMILIN1 and its loss results in a condition similar to that of the ablated molecule in KO mice leading to uncontrolled cell proliferation. Lymph node lymphangiogenesis could thus represent a crucial step able to specify different clinical categories: an early stage in which surgical resection of regional lymph nodes and primary site aims to cure; an advanced stage in which treatment can simply be aimed at prolonging life (Fig. 5.2).

Premetastatic Niche

Following experimental intravenous injection of malignant cells, a minority will successfully engraft in certain sites. This finding suggests that there are preexisting niches that do not need preparation by the primary tumor. If this is the case, are these related to physiological stem cell niches and do differences in the genetic makeup of the host influence the number, capacity, location, or efficiency of these niches? One could hypothesize that the behavior of CSCs and normal stem cells is regulated by the niche to different degrees (Li and Neaves 2006) also taking into account that CSCs possess intrinsic mutations. There are numerous examples on the diversity between tumor types in their requirement of premetastatic conditioning for dissemination to occur and a few will be briefly reported here. Cancer cells could produce their own favorable microenvironment, the future CSC niche, from a distance by secreting factors that influence their protein and cellular composition as seen for the lymph node lymphvascular niche. Bone metastasis of prostate cancer has been shown to be supported by urokinase-type plasminogen activator or PSA secreted by prostate cancer cells through alteration of growth factors in the bone microenvironment, thus increasing osteoblasts proliferation that serve as the CSC

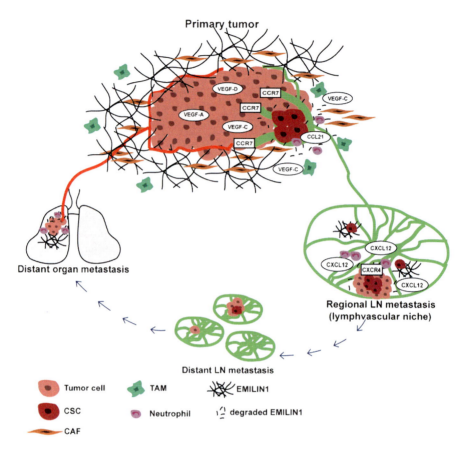

Fig. 5.2 The lymphvascular niche in the context of the natural history of a tumor from the primary site to distant metastases

bone niche (Logothetis and Lin 2005). Osteonectin or MMP2 are involved in similar mechanisms for lung metastasis of breast cancer (Minn et al. 2005). The oncogene MET is upregulated in hypoxic CSC and binding to its ligand HGF enhances plasminogen activator inhibitor type 1 and cyclooxygenase 2 transcription. This leads to enhanced blood coagulation and fibrin deposition, induction of vasculogenesis, supports the homing of CSCs and their proliferation, and thus serves as a CSC niche (Boccaccio et al. 2005). The formation of the premetastatic niche that is associated with several tumor types is favored by integrin $\alpha 4\beta 1$ and VEGFR-1 positive BM-derived cells (BMDC). In fact, BMDC co-transplanted with lung cancer or melanoma cells concentrate in the lung, creating a microenvironment that is highly receptive for cancer metastasis (Kaplan et al. 2005). Under more natural conditions, primary cancer cells secrete cytokines that positively regulate the expression of fibronectin (a ligand of $\alpha 4\beta 1$) at the sites of future premetastatic niches, which then induces the homing of VEGFR1-expressing BMDC, thus favoring CSCs seeding and growth at distant sites.

O_2 tension is tightly regulated and low oxygen tension is associated with maintenance of an undifferentiated cell state. Hypoxia regulates CSC self-renewal and tumor growth and converts and/or reprograms nonstem cells towards a CSC phenotype. Hypoxia promotes the self-renewal capability of the stem cells (Heddleston et al. 2010) and a more stem-like phenotype augmenting the tumorigenic potential of the nonstem population by the upregulation of important stem cell factors, such as OCT4, NANOG, and c-MYC. CSCs have greater plasticity and thus can dramatically change their phenotypes depending on microenvironmental cues (McCord et al. 2009). A representative example is observed in AML and its niche in BM. The molecular mechanisms resemble those of the interaction between normal HSC and the vascular niche. CD44-expressing CSCs adhere to the niche and bind to hyaluronic acid expressed by cells on the surface of sinusoidal endothelium or endosteum in BM maintaining the stem cell status. Consequently, CD44 antibody-treated NOD/SCID mice transplanted with AML cells exhibit a significantly lower rate of disease onset (Jin et al. 2006) suggesting that for AML CD44 is essential for the homing and engraftment of CSCs to the vascular (=premetastatic) niche. Another CSC marker, CD133 a cholesterol-binding glycoprotein associated with a membrane microdomain that determines the daughter cell's fate is worth mentioning. CD133-positive brain tumor cells are found near brain capillaries in a premetastatic vascular niche (Calabrese et al. 2007) and human CD133-positive medulloblastoma cells develop brain tumors only when co-transplanted with ECs suggesting that brain CSCs rely on ECs to form a vascular niche that maintains the capacity of the CSCs for self-renewal, differentiation, and proliferation. In conclusion, the specific localization of these premetastatic favorable niches within an organ is related primarily either to the secretion of specific factors by tumor cells or by the O_2 tension.

The Niche(s) and Anticancer Therapies

CSCs are insensitive to chemotherapy and developing modalities to destroy quiescent CSCs is a very promising therapeutic approach for future treatments that aim to completely cure cancer. This concept can be tested by altering CSC characteristics, such as inducing differentiation (Todaro et al. 2007) or resuming the cell cycle or obtaining a complete inhibition of CSC division. However, there is increasing interest in the possibility of manipulating the niche environment and exploiting the putative CSC niche for drug targeting (Davis and Desai 2008; Taylor and Risbridger 2008). In fact, targeting only CSCs may be insufficient to improve patient outcomes because the non-CSCs may acquire CSC characteristics due to effects of the microenvironment. Since CSCs can result in expansion of the normal niche as they proliferate, this may lead to an altered niche as the cells become independent of normal regulatory signals and produce extrinsic factors that deregulate niche-forming cells. Along these lines, the reversible nature of the epigenetic changes that occur has led to the possibility of epigenetic therapy as a treatment option (Yoo and Jones 2006). The aim of epigenetic therapy is to reverse the causal epigenetic aberrations that occur in CSCs, leading to the restoration of a "normal epigenome." DNA methylation inhibitors 5-azacytidine (5-aza-CR) or 5-aza-2′-deoxycytidine (5-aza-CdR) were among the first epigenetic drugs proposed for use as cancer therapeutics. The stem cell, whether normal or neoplastic, and its niche influence each other and understanding their regulatory system including O_2 levels could lead to novel therapeutic approaches that directly target CSCs or niches. As an example, the clinical application of antiangiogenic therapies remains to be optimized and methods of resistance are being identified. Bevacizumab, the neutralizing VEGF antibody, has been approved for the treatment of several solid cancers and recent work suggests that it targets CSC-induced angiogenesis (Bao et al. 2006) and disrupt the functional perivascular niche in which they reside (Calabrese et al. 2007). Freshly isolated CD133-positive CSC-enriched cells but not CD133-negative cells form highly vascular tumors in immunocompromised mice brains. Treatment of these CD133-positive cells with bevacizumab markedly inhibits their ability to initiate tumors in vivo and depletes both blood vessels and more importantly self-renewing CD133-positive cells from tumor xenografts. These studies suggest that glioblastoma CSCs release potent angiogenic activity and are maintained by signals from an aberrant vascular niche.

Changes in tumor stromal markers are significant predictors of prostate cancer recurrence, independent of Gleason grade and PSA levels (Ayala et al. 2003; Yanagisawa et al. 2008). While CSCs in breast and prostate cancer do not express estrogen and androgen receptors CAFs are positive. Since CSCs remain responsive to hormones through stromal-epithelial cell signaling, stromal constituents like CAFs are obvious therapeutic targets (Trimboli et al. 2009). Recent data suggest that radiotherapy could positively affect the tumor niche by likely acting also on the constituents of the microenvironment such as CAFs and/or TAMs. For instance, while the most common explanation for preferential localization of breast cancer recurrences at the surgical scar site is the presence of "residual" tumor cells, the extent of surgery has also been related to growth factor produced by the microenvironment during the wound healing process and may enhance tumor burden (Coussens and Werb 2002; Tsuchida et al. 2003; Tagliabue et al. 2006). This observation implies that several growth factors and cytokines secreted in the wound fluid (WF) participate in the stimulation of mammary tumor cells. It was formally demonstrated that WF harvested from breast cancer operated patients stimulate cell motility, invasion, and growth under three-dimensional contexts (Belletti et al. 2008). Improving local control positively affects overall survival and the status of the microenvironment at the surgery site may be a crucial prognosticator (Baum et al. 2005). TARGeted Intraoperative radioTherapy (TARGIT) almost completely abrogates the stimulatory effects of surgical WF on cancer cells in vitro, suggesting that it may affect the tumoricidal effect of radiotherapy by altering the various factors (e.g., IL-6, RANTES, HGF, or the STAT3 and p70[S6] kinase) released likely by TAMs and/or CAFs in the wound microenvironment, making it less favorable for cancer cell growth and invasion. These factors control tumor cell growth and motility and are potential targets of new anticancer therapies (Azenshtein et al. 2002; Ben-Baruch 2003). Whether these data can be interpreted as affecting the locally dormant or the distantly present breast CSCs is still to be formally proven but represents a plausible hypothesis. Nevertheless, TARGIT can be a way to reconstitute a less appropriate tumor microenvironment for CSCs and to facilitate development of innovative therapeutic approaches to control tumor growth by interfering with the interaction between diverse cellular components of solid tumors.

References

Albini A, Sporn MB (2007) The tumour microenvironment as a target for chemoprevention. Nat Rev Cancer 7:139–147

Alam N, Goel HL, Zarif MJ et al (2007) The integrin-growth factor receptor duet. J Cell Physiol 213:649–653

Al-Hajj M, Wicha MS, Benito-Hernandez A et al (2003) Prospective identification of tumorigenic breast cancer cells. Proc Natl Acad Sci USA 100:3983–3988

Arai F, Hirao A, Ohmura M et al (2004) Tie2/angiopoietin-1 signaling regulates hematopoietic stem cell quiescence in the bone marrow niche. Cell 118:149–161

Ayala G, Tuxhorn JA, Wheeler TM et al (2003) Reactive stroma as a predictor of biochemical-free recurrence in prostate cancer. Clin. Cancer Res 9:4792–4801

Azenshtein E, Luboshits G, Shina S et al (2002) The CC chemokine RANTES in breast carcinoma progression: regulation of expression and potential mechanisms of promalignant activity. Cancer Res 62:1093–1102

Bao S, Wu Q, McLendon RE et al (2006) Glioma stem cells promote radioresistance by preferential activation of the DNA damage response. Nature 444:756–760

Baum M, Demicheli R, Hrushesky W et al (2005) Does surgery unfavourably perturb the "natural history" of early breast cancer by accelerating the appearance of distant metastases? Eur J Cancer 41:508–515

Baylin SB, Ohm JE (2006) Epigenetic gene silencing in cancer—a mechanism for early oncogenic pathway addiction? Nat Rev Cancer 6:107–116

Belletti B, Vaidya JS, D'Andrea S et al (2008) Targeted intraoperative radiotherapy impairs the stimulation of breast cancer cell proliferation and invasion caused by surgical wounding. Clin Cancer Res. 14:1325–1332

Ben-Baruch A (2003) Inflammatory cells, cytokines and chemokines in breast cancer progression: reciprocal tumor-microenvironment interaction. Breast Cancer Res 5:31–36

Bingle L, Brown NJ, Lewis CE (2002) The role of tumour-associated macrophages in tumour progression: implications for new anticancer therapies. J Pathol 196:254–265

Bissell MJ, Kenny PA, Radisky DC (2005) Microenvironmental regulators of tissue structure and function also regulate tumor induction and progression: the role of extracellular matrix and its degrading enzymes. Cold Spring Harb Symp Quant Biol 70:343–356

Bissell MJ, Radisky D. (2001) Putting tumors in context. Nat Rev Cancer 1:46–54

Boccaccio C, Sabatino G, Medico E et al (2005) The MET oncogene drives a genetic programme linking cancer to haemostasis. Nature 434: 396–400.

Bonnet D, Dick J (1997) Human acute myeloid leukemia is organized as a hierarchy that originates from a primitive hematopoietic cell. Nat Med 3:730–737

Brabletz T, Jung A, Reu S et al (2001) Variable beta-catenin expression in colorectal cancer indicates a tumor progression driven by the tumor environment. Proc. Natl. Acad. Sci. USA 98: 10356–10361

Bracken CP, Gregory PA, Kolesnikoff N et al (2008) A double-negative feedback loop between ZEB1-SIP1 and the microRNA-200 family regulates epithelial-mesenchymal transition. Cancer Res. 68:7846–7854

Calabrese C, Poppleton H, Kocak M et al (2007) A perivascular niche for brain tumor stem cells. Cancer Cell 11:69–82

Calvi LM, Adams GB, Weibrecht KW et al (2003) Osteoblastic cells regulate the haematopoietic stem cell niche. Nature 425:841–846

Campbell LL, Polyak K (2007) Breast tumor heterogeneity: cancer stem cells or clonal evolution? Cell Cycle 6:2332–2338

Clarke MF, Dick JE, Dirks PB et al (2006) Cancer stem cells-perspectives on current status and future directions: AACR workshop on cancer stem cells. Cancer Res 66:9339–9344

Coultas L, Chawengsaksophak K, Rossant J (2005) Endothelial cells and VEGF in vascular development. Nature 438:937–945

Coussens LM, Werb Z (2002) Inflammation and cancer. Nature 420:860–867

Dakhova O, Ozen M, Creighton CJ et al (2009) Global gene expression analysis of reactive stroma in prostate cancer. Clin Cancer Res 15:3979–3989

Danussi C, Petrucco A, Wassermann B et al. EMILIN-negative microenvironment promotes tumor cell proliferation as well dissemination to lymph nodes. Submitted

Danussi C, Spessotto P, Petrucco A et al (2008) Emilin1 deficiency causes structural and functional defects of lymphatic vasculature. Mol Cell Biol 28:4026–4039

Davis ID, Desai J (2008) Clinical use of therapies targeting tumor vasculature and stroma. Curr. Cancer Drug Targets. 8:498–508

Dean JP, Nelson PS (2008) Profiling influences of senescent and aged fibroblasts on prostate carcinogenesis. Br J Cancer 98:245–249

Dick JE (2008) Stem cell concepts renew cancer research. Blood 112:4793–4807

Drayton DL, Liao S, Mounzer RH et al (2006) Lymphoid organ development: from ontogeny to neogenesis. Nat Immunol 7:344–353

Feinberg AP, Ohlsson R, Henikoff S (2006) The epigenetic progenitor origin of human cancer. Nat Rev Genet 7:21–33

Finak G, Bertos N, Pepin F et al (2008) Stromal gene expression predicts clinical outcome in breast cancer. Nat Med 14:518–527

Gal-Yam EN, Egger G, Iniguez L et al (2008) Frequent switching of Polycomb repressive marks and DNA hypermethylation in the PC3 prostate cancer cell line. Proc Natl Acad Sci USA 105:12979–12984

Giampieri S, Manning C, Hooper S et al (2009) Localized and reversible TGFbeta signalling switches breast cancer cells from cohesive to single cell motility. Nat Cell Biol 11:1287–1296

Hambardzumyan D, Becher OJ, Rosenblum MK et al (2008) PI3K pathway regulates survival of cancer stem cells residing in the perivascular niche following radiation in medulloblastoma in vivo. Genes Dev 22:436–448

Hawsawi NM, Ghebeh H, Hendrayani SF et al (2008) Breast carcinoma-associated fibroblasts and their counterparts display neoplastic-specific changes. Cancer Res 68:2717–2725

Heddleston JM, Li Z, Latria JD et al (2010) Hypoxia inducible factors in cancer stem cells. Br J Cancer 102:789–795

Heissig B, Hattori K, Dias S et al (2002) Recruitment of stem and progenitor cells from the bone marrow niche requires MMP-9 mediated release of Kit-ligand. Cell 109:625–637

Hendrix MJ, Seftor EA, Hess AR et al (2003) Vasculogenic mimicry and tumour-cell plasticity: Lessons from melanoma. Nat Rev Cancer 3:411–421

Hill RP (2006) Identifying cancer stem cells in solid tumors: case not proven. Cancer Res 66:1891–1895

Hirakawa S (2009) From tumor lymphangiogenesis to lymphvascular niche. Cancer Sci 100:983–989

Hynes RO (2002) Integrins: bidirectional, allosteric signaling machines. Cell 110:673–687

Hynes RO (2009) The extracellular matrix: not just pretty fibrils. Science 326:1216–1219

Iwamoto S, Mihara K, Dowining JR et al (2007) Mesenchymal cells regulate the response of acute lymphoblastic leukemia to asparaginase. J Clin Invest 117:1049–1057

Iwasaki H, Suda T (2009) Cancer stem cells and their niche. Proc Natl Acad Sci USA 100:1166–1172

Jin L, Hope KJ, Zhai Q et al (2006) Targeting of CD44 eradicates human acute myeloid leukemic stem cells. Nature Med 12:1167–1174

Joyce JA, Pollard JW (2009) Microenvironmental regulation of metastasis. Nat Rev Cancer 9:239–252

Kaplan RN, Riba RD, Zacharoulis S et al (2005) VEGFR1-positive haematopoietic bone marrow progenitors initiate the pre-metastatic niche. Nature 438:820–807

Kasemeier-Kulesa JC, Teddy JM, Postovit LM et al (2008) Reprogramming multipotent tumor cells with the embryonic neural crest microenvironment. Dev Dyn 237:2657–2666

Kelly PN, Dakic A, Adams JM et al (2007) Tumor growth need not be driven by rare cancer stem cells. Science 317:337

Kern SE, Shibata D (2007) The fuzzy math of solid tumor stem cells: a perspective. Cancer Res 67:8985–8988

Kiel MJ, Yilmaz OH, Iwashita T et al (2005) SLAM family receptors distinguish hematopoietic stem and progenitor cells and reveal endothelial niches for stem cells. Cell 121:1109–1121

Kopp HG, Avecilla ST, Hooper AT et al (2005) The bone marrow vascular niche: home of HSC differentiation and mobilization. Physiology (Bethesda) 20:349–356

Koyama H, Kobayashi N, Harada M et al (2008) Significance of tumor-associated stroma in promotion of intratumoral lymphangiogenesis: pivotal role of a hyaluronan-rich tumor microenvironment. Am J Pathol 172:179–193

Kroemer G, Pouyssegur J (2008) Tumor cell metabolism: cancer's Achilles' heel. Cancer Cell 13:472–482

Lapidot T, Sirard C, Vormoor J et al (1994) A cell initiating human acute myeloid leukaemia after transplantation into SCID mice. Nature 367:645–648

Legate KR, Wickstrom SA, Fassler R (2009) Genetic and cell biological analysis of integrin outside-in signaling. Genes Dev 23:397–418

Li Z, Bao S, Wu Q et al. (2009) Hypoxia-inducible factors regulate tumorigenic capacity of glioma stem cells. Cancer Cell 15:501–513

Li L, Neaves WB (2006) Normal stem cells and cancer stem cells: the niche matters. Cancer Res 66:4553–4557

Liu G, Yuan X, Zeng Z et al (2006) Analysis of gene expression and chemoresistance of CD133+ cancer stem cells in glioblastoma. Mol Cancer 5:67–78

Logothetis CJ, Lin SH (2005) Osteoblasts in prostate cancer metastasis to bone. Nature Rev 5:21–28

Mani SA, Guo W, Liao MJ et al (2008) The epithelial-mesenchymal transition generates cells with properties of stem cells. Cell 133:704–715

Mantovani A, Schioppa T, Porta C et al (2006) Role of tumor-associated macrophages in tumor progression and invasion. Cancer Metastasis Rev 25:315–322

McCord AM, Jamal M, Shankavarum UT et al. (2009) Physiologic oxygen concentration enhances the stem-like properties of CD133+ human glioblastoma cells in vitro. Mol Cancer Res 7:489–497

Meissner A, Mikkelsen TS, Gu H et al (2008) Genome-scale DNA methylation maps of pluripotent and differentiated cells. Nature 454:766–770

Minn AJ, Gupta GP, Siegel PM et al (2005) Genes that mediate breast cancer metastasis to lung. Nature 436:518–524

Mishra PJ, Mishra PJ, Humeniuk R et al (2008) Carcinoma-associated fibroblast-like differentiation of human mesenchymal stem cells. Cancer Res 68:4331–4339

O'Connell MP, Weeraratna AT (2009) Hear the Wnt Ror: how melanoma cells adjust to changes in Wnt. Pigment Cell Melanoma Res 22:724–739

Orimo A, Gupta PB, Sgroi DC et al (2005) Stromal fibroblasts present in invasive human breast carcinomas promote tumor growth and angiogenesis through elevated SDF-1/CXCL12 secretion. Cell 121:335–348

Paik S, Shak G, Tang G et al (2004) A multigene assay to predict recurrence of tamoxifen-treated, node-negative breast cancer. N Engl J Med 351:2817–2826

Parmar K, Mauch P, Vergilio JA et al (2007) Distribution of hematopoietic stem cells in the bone marrow according to regional hypoxia. Proc Natl Acad Sci USA 104:5431–5436

Pui CH, Evans WE (2006) Treatment of acute lymphoblastic leukemia. N Engl J Med 354:166–178

Quintana E, Shackleton M, Sabel MS et al (2008) Efficient tumour formation by single human melanoma cells. Nature 456:593–598

Samudio I, Fiegl M, McQueen T et al (2008) The Warburg effect in leukemia-stroma cocultures is mediated by mitochondrial uncoupling associated with uncoupling protein-2 activation. Cancer Res 68:5198–5205

Sharma S, Kelly TK, Jones PA (2010) Epigenetics in cancer. Carcinogenesis 31:27–36

Sica A, Schioppa T, Mantovani A et al (2006) Tumour-associated macrophages are a distinct M2 polarised population promoting tumour progression: potential targets of anti-cancer therapy. Eur J Cancer 42:717–727

Sternlicht MD, Werb Z (2001) How matrix metalloproteinases regulate cell behavior. Annu Rev Cell Dev Biol 17:463–516

Surani MA, Hayashi K, Hajkova P (2007) Genetic and epigenetic regulators of pluripotency. Cell 128:747–762

Tagliabue E, Agresti R, Casalini P et al (2006) Linking survival of HER2-positive breast carcinoma patients with surgical invasiveness. Eur J Cancer 42:1057–1061

Takakura N, Huang XL, Naruse T et al (1998) Critical role of the TIE2 endothelial cell receptor in the development of definitive hematopoiesis. Immunity 9:677–686

Tammela T, Alitalo K (2010) Lymphangiogenesis: Molecular mechanisms and future promise. Cell 140:460–476

Taylor MD, Poppleton H, Fuller C et al (2005) Radial glia cells are candidate stem cells of ependymoma. Cancer Cell 8:323–835

Taylor RA, Risbridger GP (2008) Prostatic tumor stroma: a key player in cancer progression. Curr. Cancer Drug Targets. 8:490–497

Todaro M, Alea MP, Di Stefano AB et al (2007) Colon cancer stem cells dictate tumor growth and resist cell death by production of interleukin-4. Cell Stem Cell 1:389–402

Topczewska JM, Postovit LM, Margaryan NV et al (2006) Embryonic and tumorigenic pathways converge via Nodal signaling: Role in melanoma aggressiveness. Nat Med 12:925–932

Trimboli AJ, Cantemir-Stone CZ, Li F et al (2009) Pten in stromal fibroblasts suppresses mammary epithelial tumours. Nature 461:1084–1091

Tsuchida Y, Sawada S, Yoshioka I et al (2003) Increased surgical stress promotes tumor metastasis. Surgery 133:547–555

Utikal J, Maherali N, Kulalert W et al (2009) Sox2 is dispensable for the reprogramming of melanocytes and melanoma cells into induced pluripotent stem cells. J Cell Sci 122:3502–3510

Valk-Lingbeek ME, Bruggeman SWM, Van Lohuizen M et al (2004) Stem cells and cancer; the polycomb connection. Cell 118:409–418

Vogelstein B, Kinzler KW (2004) Cancer genes and the pathways they control. Nat Med 10:789–799

Wellner U, Schubert J, Burk UC et al (2009) The EMT-activator ZEB1 promotes tumorigenicity by repressing stemness-inhibiting microRNAs. Nat Cell Biol 11:1487–1495

Wang JC, Dick JE (2005) Cancer stem cells: lessons from leukemia. Trends Cell Biol 15:494–501

Widschwendter M, Fiegl H, Egle D et al (2007) Epigenetic stem cell signature in cancer. Nat Genet 39:157–158

Wulf GG, Wang RY, Kuehnle I et al (2001) A leukemic stem cell with intrinsic drug efflux capacity in acute myeloid leukemia. Blood 98:1166–1173

Xie T, Spradling AC (2000) A niche maintaining germ line stem cells in the Drosophila ovary. Science 290:328–330

Yanagisawa N, Li R, Rowley D et al (2008) Stromogenic prostatic carcinoma pattern (carcinomas with reactive stromal grade 3) in needle biopsies predicts biochemical recurrence-free survival in patients after radical prostatectomy. Hum Pathol 39:282–291

Yi R, Poy MN, Stoffel M et al (2008) A skin microRNA promotes differentiation by repressing 'stemness'. Nature 452:225–229

Yoo CB, Jones PA (2006) Epigenetic therapy of cancer: past, present and future. Nat Rev Drug Discov 5:37–50

Zhang J, Niu C, Ye L et al (2003) Identification of the haematopoietic stem cell niche and control of the niche size. Nature 425:836–841

Chapter 6
Leukemia Stem Cells

Steven W. Lane and David A. Williams

Definition of LSC

It has been known for many years that different cell populations within tumors of the hematopoietic system vary in their functional properties, including the ability to form colonies in vitro or cause tumors in transplanted recipient mice (Bruce and Van Der Gaag 1963; Griffin and Lowenberg 1986). More recently, the development and use of fluorescence-activated cell sorting to prospectively identify hematopoietic stem (HSC) and progenitor cell populations by surface immunophenotype (Spangrude et al. 1988; Morrison and Weissman 1994), has enabled similar experiments in the context of leukemia. This technology, used in parallel with murine transplantation experiments, has led to the prospective isolation and characterization of cells that possess the ability to initiate acute myeloid leukemia (AML) in vivo. These leukemia-initiating cells, known also as leukemia stem cells (LSC) are able to reconstitute a hierarchy of malignant cells that is somewhat analogous to the hierarchy found in normal hematopoiesis (Bonnet and Dick 1997). As with normal HSC, LSC are stringently defined by functional attributes including the ability to initiate, sustain and serially propagate leukemia in vivo and are able to differentiate into more mature, committed progeny that lack this ability. Furthermore, LSC may be identified using surface markers and the ability to undergo serial rounds of replating

S.W. Lane (✉)
Division of Immunology, Queensland Institue of Medical Research,
Brisbane, Australia
e-mail: steven.lane@gimr.edu.au

D.A. Williams
Division of Hematology/Oncology, Children's Hospital Boston, Department of Pediatrics,
Harvard Medical School, Boston, MA, USA

Department of Pediatrics Oncology, Dana-Farber Cancer Institute,
Harvard Stem Cell Institute, Boston, MA, USA

in cytokine-enriched methylcellulose media, demonstrating limitless self-renewal in vitro (Bonnet and Dick 1997; Jordan et al. 2000; Huntly et al. 2004).

A purification strategy for LSC from human AML samples was initially described by Lapidot (1994) and subsequently refined by Bonnet in John Dick's laboratory in Toronto (Bonnet and Dick 1997). They identified a subpopulation of human AML cells, expressing CD34 but negative for CD38 surface expression that were able to serially transplant leukemia in a mouse xenograft model. The more committed blast cells, (representing the bulk tumor population and expressing CD38) lacked this potential. Using this methodology, the frequency of LSC varied greatly between different AML samples, ranging from 1 in 10^4 to 1 in 10^7 cells (Bonnet and Dick 1997). Importantly, the LSC identified in this xenograft model were not limited to their ability to cause leukemia, but also gave rise to progeny that lost leukemia-initiating activity, leading to the conclusion that AML is arranged in a hierarchy with the leukemia-initiating LSC at the apex and the more "differentiated" blasts representing the bulk, tumor population. This hierarchical model differs from the original model based on the hypothesis that rare cells found randomly within tumors stochastically possessed or acquired the ability to form colonies and transplant disease (Bruce and Van Der Gaag 1963; Griffin and Lowenberg 1986).

Support for this hierarchical model of leukemia has come from subsequent murine transplantation experiments. For example, the fusion oncogene *MLLT3-MLL* (also known as *MLL-AF9*) was able to transform committed progenitors cells and this gave rise to a transplantable AML in vivo (Somervaille and Cleary 2006; Krivtsov et al. 2006). The leukemia-initiating activity in these leukemias was predominantly found within the cKit^{high} population, whereas the differentiated, bulk tumor population expressed lower cKit levels (Krivtsov et al. 2006). In other retrovirus models, AML LSC may also be marked by aberrant lineage marking (e.g., the B-lymphoid antigen B220) that is not present in the bulk tumor population (Deshpande et al. 2006). Finally, in a retroviral model of chronic myelogenous leukemia (CML), the LSC were found in an immunophenotypic compartment that normally contains HSC and progenitors, lineage^{low}cKit$^+$Sca1$^+$ cells (Hu et al. 2009).

LSC Cell of Origin

The term "leukemia stem cell" has been criticized as potentially misleading, leading to an assumption a hematopoietic *stem cell* has undergone transformation to become its leukemic counterpart. While this was not the claim of the work from Dick's group, certain early models of LSC biology appeared to support this theory (Bonnet and Dick 1997). However, it has become apparent that this is not always the case prompting vigorous debate (Clarke et al. 2006). Based on more recent work, it appears that LSC do not need to be derived from their corresponding tissue stem cell (i.e., HSC) and may share most phenotypic characteristics with more committed downstream progenitors. However, LSC often share functional characteristics and components of the gene expression program (i.e., expression signature) seen in HSC that appears to control self-renewal (Krivtsov et al. 2006).

Murine models provide strong direct evidence that the cell of origin of LSC may be a progenitor, corresponding to a more phenotypically mature cell than the primitive HSC. For example, using retrovirus vectors containing fusion oncogenes such as *MLL-AF9*, committed progenitors may be transformed leading to LSC that express immunophenotypic markers of more mature progenitor cells, when compared to HSC. This is in contrast to other oncogenes characterized by constitutively active tyrosine kinase domains (such as *BCR-ABL1*, the result of t(9;22) (q34.1;q11.23) and found in patients with CML, AML, and acute lymphoblastic leukemia) that are only able to transform HSC (Huntly et al. 2004). This latter group of oncogenic alleles provide a proliferative advantage but are unable to engender the property of self-renewal in committed progenitors (Huntly et al. 2004). Rather, self-renewal appears to be regulated in LSC by transcription factors and the epigenetic changes that control these. In keeping with this observation, the LSC in murine AML generated by retroviral transformation of committed progenitors with *MLL-AF9*, *MLLT1-MLL* or *MYST3-NCOA2* (also known as *MLL-ENL* and *MOZ-TIF2*, respectively) did not express the stem cell antigen Sca1 (Krivtsov et al. 2006; Scholl et al. 2007) and had an immunophenotype similar to normal granulocyte-macrophage progenitors (GMP) (Huntly et al. 2004; Krivtsov et al. 2006; Cozzio et al. 2003). In some cases, LSC may express a limited array of lineage markers such as CD11b (Mac1) in *MLL*-translocation-induced AML (Somervaille and Cleary 2006; Cozzio et al. 2003) or in a transgenic model of AML induced by mutated CCAAT/enhancer-binding protein alpha (*C/EBPα*) (Kirstetter et al. 2008). Additionally, other lineage markers, such as Gr1 (a marker of mature myeloid cells) have been described on LSC from a transgenic model of murine acute promyelocytic leukemia. Acute promyelocytic leukemia is considered the most phenotypically mature form of AML and is usually associated with the t(15;17) translocation leading to *PML–RARA* fusion (Guibal et al. 2009; Wojiski et al. 2009). The LSC found in certain transgenic models offer further biological observations relevant to human disease. For example, in contrast to the retroviral model, the putative LSC in a *MLL-AF9* transgenic model of AML was enriched within the compartment phenotypically, corresponding with HSC and multipotent progenitors (Chen et al. 2008). To more accurately determine LSC identity in these transgenic models and knock-in approaches, lineage, and developmentally specified expression of the oncogene will be informative.

In correlative xenograft studies, most groups have documented leukemia-initiating activity within the CD34$^+$CD38$^-$ fraction of AML bone marrow, an immunophenotypic profile that is similar to normal HSC (Bonnet and Dick 1997; Ishikawa et al. 2007). It is important to note that although phenotypic and morphologic studies may link LSC to HSC, human LSC do not express CD90 (Thy1) (Blair et al. 1997). This immunophenotype (CD34$^+$CD38$^-$CD90$^-$) is more consistent with the multipotent progenitor (MPP) compartment that is more differentiated and lacks the limitless self-renewal capability of long-term HSC. Despite this, leukemogenic oncogenes can have effects on long-term HSC that may contribute to leukemogenesis. Pathogenic fusion oncogenes, such as *RUNX1-RUNX1T1* (also known as *AML1-ETO*) have been

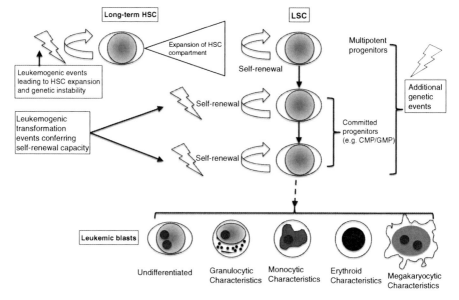

Fig. 6.1 Hierarchy of leukemia stem cells (LSC). Transforming events (i.e., oncogenic mutations) may occur in either long-term hematopoietic stem cells (HSC) or in more committed progenitors (such as granulocyte-macrophage progenitors, GMP). In long-term HSC, these mutations may give rise to a preleukemic state with expansion of HSC numbers and predisposing to genetic instability. Subsequent genetic events may then confer the full leukemic phenotype. Conversely, mutations may occur within downstream progenitors that confer the property of limitless self-renewal to those cells (e.g., expression of the *MLL-AF9* fusion oncogene) directly giving rise to these leukemias. A hierarchical structure is retained within the leukemia with the putative LSC at the apex of this and the bulk population (leukemic blasts) lacking in their ability to give rise to leukemia in vivo (figure reproduced from Lane et al. 2009)

found in preleukemic samples in the CD90$^+$ HSC-enriched compartment (Miyamoto et al. 2000), documenting the presence of a primitive preleukemic clone that can presumably predispose to subsequent additional mutations engendering the full LSC phenotype in downstream hematopoietic precursors. Evidence supporting this hypothesis was also generated using a murine transgenic model of AML (induced by expressing a mutated form of *C/EBPα* from the endogenous promoter). In this model, there was expansion of normal HSC compartment prior to the development of leukemia arising from a downstream progenitor (Bereshchenko et al. 2009). A similar model, describing this "preleukemic phase" characterized by HSC expansion and acquisition of mutations has also been provided from recent observations in acute lymphoblastic leukemia (Fig. 6.1) (Hong et al. 2008; Mullighan et al. 2008).

It is important to prospectively identify and isolate cell populations enriched for leukemia or cancer-initiating activity if the ultimate goal of successfully incorporating new therapeutic modalities that specifically target the LSC population is to be realized.

Properties of LSC

There are intrinsic properties of HSC that enable their long-term survival. Two such properties are the maintenance of a quiescent state and resistance to the effects of cytotoxic agents. LSC, like their normal counterparts, appear to utilize some of these properties to facilitate their long-term maintenance. For example, LSC express the p-glycoprotein multidrug resistance efflux pump, ABCB1 (also known as MDR1) that can remove potentially toxic agents, including chemotherapy drugs, from the cell (Mahadevan and List 2004). By reducing the stress from cytotoxic agents, LSC may become a reservoir for the selection of additional mutants that are resistant to targeted or conventional therapy (Heidel et al. 2006).

LSC are characterized by limitless self-renewal and recent experimental evidence implicates key developmentally conserved self-renewal pathways such as Bmi-1 (Lessard and Sauvageau 2003), Wnt/β-catenin (Hu et al. 2009; Zhao et al. 2007; Wang et al. 2010) and Hedgehog (Dierks et al. 2008; Zhao et al. 2009) in this phenotype. Additionally, an increase in the expression of *Hox* genes, in particular *HoxA9*, has been demonstrated to be essential for the pathogenesis of *MLL-AF9*-induced AML (Krivtsov et al. 2006; Ferrando et al. 2003). The dependence on specific self-renewal pathways may be context and oncogene dependent as evidenced by two recent papers. An intact hedgehog signaling pathway was found to be essential for the maintenance of LSC in CML (Dierks et al. 2008; Zhao et al. 2009) but not required for LSC survival in *MLL-AF9*-induced AML (Hofmann et al. 2009). The maintenance of canonical Wnt signaling may also have differential requirements for the survival of LSC and adult HSC (Wang et al. 2010). Another pathway by which LSC may evade apoptosis is by the upregulation of NF-κB (a pro-survival factor) (Guzman et al. 2001, 2005) or by evasion of programmed cell death mediated by Fas/CD95 interactions (Costello et al. 2000).

In contrast to the shared mechanisms of self-renewal and cytoprotection found in HSC, the normal maintenance of long telomeres in HSC may be lost or attenuated in LSC. Telomerase is required for the maintenance of chromosomal telomere length and telomere shortening leads to cellular senescence. Telomerase activity is high in HSC and this contributes to the long-term maintenance of self-renewal in a tightly regulated manner (Morrison et al. 1996). In contrast, telomerase activity (in particular the hTERT catalytic subunit) appears to be reduced in some studies of CML (Drummond et al. 2005; Campbell et al. 2006) leading to shortened telomeres. In support of this observation, shortened telomere length has been described in some myeloproliferative neoplasms (MPN) and this length inversely correlates with some measures of disease burden (Bernard et al. 2009). Finally, mutations in the TERT catalytic subunit of telomerase have been described in rare families that demonstrate a predisposition to AML (Kirwan et al. 2009). Based on these observations it has been hypothesized that accelerated telomere shortening may predispose to the progression of MPN to more advanced disease such as AML or therapy-induced myelodysplastic syndrome, possibly through the effects of increased chromosomal recombination caused by telomere shortening (Chakraborty et al. 2009).

As discussed previously, LSC utilize many shared cell-intrinsic mechanisms that facilitate the progression of malignant disease and simultaneously protect from the effects of chemotherapy. However, in addition to these, it has recently been found that LSC use novel mechanisms to evade the host innate immune system from clearing circulating LSC. In recent work from the laboratory of Irving Weissman, LSC were shown to express CD47, a surface protein that interacts with the macrophage receptor signal regulatory protein alpha (SIRPα) to inhibit phagocytosis. This molecule was selectively expressed on normal HSC upon mobilization and exit from the bone marrow niche (Jaiswal et al. 2009). LSC were shown to up-regulate surface expression of CD47, thereby mimicking normal mobilized HSC and providing a "don't eat me" signal to host macrophages and evading the host's innate immune response in vivo. The presence of high levels of CD47 on patient's leukemic cells was demonstrated to predict an inferior outcome after conventional therapy, suggesting that this mechanism of LSC clearance may have biological significance (Jaiswal et al. 2009; Majeti et al. 2009).

The Relevance of the Hematopoietic Microenvironment to LSC

There is substantial evidence that LSC reside within and utilize the normal bone marrow hematopoietic microenvironment (HM), taking refuge in the sanctuary of this niche during chemotherapy and consequently re-emerging to initiate disease relapse. To best understand the role of this niche in the setting of LSC, it is important to first detail the specific mechanisms of support between normal HSC and the HM. The HSC niche is an overarching term used to describe the multiple bone marrow biochemical and physical structures that are essential for the maintenance of the long-term HSC pool (Scadden 2007). There appear to be at least two anatomically defined HSC niches in the medullary cavity of the bone: one is comprised of endosteal (Adams et al. 2006; Zhang et al. 2003) and the other perivascular structures (Kiel et al. (2005) that appear to have overlapping roles.

The initial hypothesis of a HSC niche came from the observations of Schofield and was based on the findings that murine long-term repopulating stem cells were deferentially located near bone cortex containing the endosteum (Schofield 1978). The endosteal niche was further defined in localization studies that demonstrated most HSC reside in immediate proximity to trabecular or cortical bone (Nilsson et al. 2001). These observational studies were supported by functional assays revealing that osteoblasts provided essential support to HSC in vivo. In these studies, osteoblasts were ablated by the expression of herpes thymidine kinase from an osteoblast-specific promoter and the subsequent administration of ganciclovir. When mature osteoblasts were ablated using this novel approach, there was a marked reduction in the number of primitive hematopoietic cells, although transplantation studies were not performed to document the effects on long-term repopulating cells (Visnjic et al. 2001). Subsequently, two concurrent studies showed that manipulation of osteoblasts could increase HSC number as well, either through expression of a constitutively active parathyroid hormone (*PTH*) receptor or through Mx1-Cre-mediated excision of the conditionally expressed bone morphogenic protein 1a (*BMP1a*) receptor (Zhang et al. 2003; Calvi et al. 2003). However, not all models with abnormal osteoblast numbers demonstrate a HSC phenotype. For example, biglycan-deficient mice have reduced osteoblasts but have qualitatively and quantitatively normal HSC (Kiel et al. 2007). Conversely, treatment with strontium increases osteoblasts without effects on HSC numbers (Lymperi et al. 2008). Moreover, mice with chronic inflammatory arthritis have functionally defective osteoblasts, but normal hematopoietic function (Ma et al. 2009). The explanation for these findings may lie in functional heterogeneity of osteoblast/niche cells. In addition to osteoblasts, bone marrow matrix proteins such as osteopontin regulate HSC numbers within the niche (Stier et al. 2005; Nilsson et al. 2005) and osteoclasts regulate HSC engraftment and mobilization (Kollet et al. 2006). The interaction between fibronectin and stromal vascular cell adhesion molecule 1 (VCAM-1) in bone marrow matrix and very late antigen-4 (VLA-4) is also critical in HSC homing and engraftment into the niche (Williams et al. 1991; Papayannopoulou et al. 1995; Papayannopoulou and Nakamoto 1993).

The other major niche component is defined by proximity to sinusoidal vascular endothelium, also known as the perivascular niche. The initial studies utilized in vivo immunofluorescence and the identification of HSC by "SLAM" (signaling lymphocyte activation molecule) markers showing HSC residing in proximity to endovascular structures (Kiel et al. 2005). This vascular niche appears dependent on the interactions between chemokine receptor 4 (CXCR4) on HSC and chemokine ligand 12 (CXCL12, also known as stromal-derived factor 1 alpha, SDF1α), highly expressed on mesenchymal stromal cells (Sugiyama et al. 2006; Ara et al. 2003; Sacchetti et al. 2007) and the binding of integrins (such as VLA-4) to VCAM-1 (Avecilla et al. 2004). The Rac family of Rho GTPases are critical downstream effectors of these interactions and thereby integrate combined critical pathways in HSC retention and engraftment (Cancelas et al. 2005). Indeed, one paradoxical observation is that simultaneous deletion of Rac1 and Rac2 lead to massive mobilization of HSC/P in spite of the fact that these cells appear to be totally deficient in migratory behavior. In addition to the previously mentioned pathways, the vascular niche is also regulated by effects of the sympathetic nervous system, leading to circadian oscillations in HSC mobilization (Mendez-Ferrer et al. 2008; Lucas et al. 2008). There remains some ongoing controversy regarding the validity of the endosteal vs. perivascular niche models; however, recent evidence has demonstrated an intimate association between bone marrow vascular and endosteal structures (Lo Celso et al. 2009; Xie et al. 2009). This suggests that there may be significant overlap between the previously envisioned dichotomous models and remains a subject of ongoing interest in the field.

LSC home to and engraft the bone marrow niche and therefore the importance of HSC–niche interactions is noteworthy in leukemia (Lane et al. 2011). Within this niche, LSC appear to be protected from the effects of chemotherapy in part mediated through niche-induced LSC quiescence (as many chemotherapeutic agents target actively cycling cells) (Ishikawa et al. 2007). LSC–niche interactions are essential for the proper "engraftment" or at least retention of LSC and interruption of this inhibits AML in xenograft models (Jin et al. 2006). In a xenograft transplantation model of human AML, the LSC that resided adjacent to endosteal cells were more quiescent and also resistant to the effects of conventional chemotherapy (cytarabine) (Ishikawa et al. 2007). An additional explanation for the cytoprotection may be gleaned from an observation that bone marrow stromal cells can secrete enzymes such as asparagine synthetase. In this latter example, the asparagine synthetase production may directly induce resistance in acute lymphoblastic leukemia (ALL) cells to a commonly used chemotherapeutic agent, L-asparaginase (Iwamoto et al. 2007).

It is tempting to speculate that manipulation of the microenvironment may be effective in the reduction or elimination of LSC as an adjunct to normal chemotherapy. In further support of this, LSC receive vital cues from the bone marrow HM that dictate their behavior and eventual disease phenotype. In a human xenograft model of *MLL-AF9* leukemia, the immunophenotype of the blast cells could be altered between lymphoid, biphenotypic or myeloid by expression of human cytokines *KITLG*, *CSF-2* and *IL3* (stem cell factor, granulocyte-macrophage colony-stimulating factor and interleukin 3 respectively) in the recipient microenvironment (Wei et al. 2008). Many of the specific HSC–niche pathways previously discussed are important in LSC–niche interactions as well. For example, *MLL-AF9* transformed LSC exhibited altered migration to CXCL-12, in part mediated through increased activity of the Rho GTPases Cdc42 and Rac (Somervaille and Cleary 2006). As with HSC, the relationship between LSC and the niche need not be unidirectional and there is some evidence to suggest that normal HSC can be altered by signals within a pathological niche to cause hematopoietic dyscrasias (Walkley et al. 2007a, b). In addition to this, LSC may circumvent normal constraints and create their own distinct niche at the expense of normal HSC leading to disproportionate impairment of HSC engraftment and hematopoietic function (Colmone et al. 2008).

Implications for Diagnosis, Prognosis, and Therapy

The existence of a defined population within leukemia (i.e., LSC) that is responsible for the initiation, propagation and maintenance of leukemia has substantial implications for the diagnosis and management of patients with leukemia. Obviously, tumor therapy must effectively eliminate the LSC or even large reductions in tumor burden may still be associated with relapsed disease. In addition the ability to prospectively identify and study LSC will yield new therapeutic targets and may have important implications for "personalized medicine" approaches. For example, the immunophenotype of LSC may facilitate recognition of this population at the diagnosis of AML in patients, either through LSC-specific surface antigens such as CD123 (Jin et al. 2009) or CD96 (Hosen et al. 2007) that are not found on normal HSC, or through identification of rare cell populations with aberrant surface marker expression (Deshpande et al. 2006). Although considerable variability may be expected between patients, the identification of such antigens in a diagnostic samples derived from a patient with AML may provide a unique, patient specific LSC signature. This signature may be used to facilitate the use of highly sensitive tests (such as multiparameter flow cytometry) to enable longitudinal surveillance of treatment success or the detection of low level AML burden (preceding relapse) much more efficiently than conventional morphological or cytogenetic methods. Although molecular genetic methods (real-time quantitative PCR of specific fusion genes) may be even more sensitive for detecting minimal residual disease (MRD) (Lane et al. 2008), monitoring of LSC-associated antigens would provide a direct link between MRD detection and a crucial functional attribute of the leukemia.

The number of LSC within a particular patient sample at diagnosis may also provide prognostic information. For example, LSC frequency, defined by immunophenotype as $CD34^+ CD38^-$ percentage at diagnosis, was shown to correlate with increased levels of persistent residual disease after chemotherapy and was associated with inferior survival in patients with AML (van Rhenen et al. 2005). Similarly, functional assays of LSC frequency may provide similar prognostic information. In one study, patients whose AML samples readily engrafted NOD/SCID immunocompromised mice in xenograft transplantation assays (the conventional functional assay of LSC frequency), were found to have a poorer prognosis (Monaco et al. 2004). These preliminary studies will require confirmation by the prospective evaluation of LSC markers or functional assays with proper consideration or balancing for other known adverse prognostic factors such as age, cytogenetics, treatment received, and molecular markers (Schlenk et al. 2008). For example, samples with higher LSC number and function were less likely to have favorable risk cytogenetic profiles (Cheung et al. 2007).

Therapeutic targeting of LSC remains the ambition of many researchers who hope for new approaches in AML, a disease where the long-term survival of patients has improved more slowly during the preceding 40 years than other cancers (such as pediatric ALL). Consistent with this goal, a variety of compounds have entered preclinical and early phase clinical trials, but most of these have been limited by moderate efficacy and/or dose-limiting toxicity. Monoclonal antibodies targeting the specific epitopes of adhesion molecules expressed on LSC, rather than HSC appear logical to target LSC in vivo and preclinical models have provided encouraging results to support the further development of these agents. For example, treatment with a monoclonal antibody to CD44 (the cell surface receptor for hyaluronic acid, osteopontin, and other bone marrow niche components) was shown to prevent engraftment of LSC in vivo in murine models of both AML and CML (Jin et al. 2006; Krause et al. 2006). The lack of engraftment was shown to be as a result of defective LSC homing, as directly implanted LSC retained the ability to instigate leukemia. This observation that anti-CD44 therapy does not affect LSC within the bone marrow niche somewhat tempers enthusiasm for clinical translation and limits the consideration of this type of therapy to the transplantation setting. Perhaps of more direct clinical applicability, the expression of CD47 by LSC appears to be an important mechanism to evade the host's innate immune response. In these studies as noted above, blockade of CD47 with a specific monoclonal antibody led to increased phagocytosis and reduced engraftment of LSC with concomitant reduction in leukemic burden (Majeti et al. 2009). Treatment of BCR-ABL transformed murine stem cells and CD34⁺ cells from CML patients and AML cells with an inhibitor of Rac GTPases has been shown to inhibit these cells in vitro and in vivo (Somervaille and Cleary 2006; Wei et al. 2008; Thomas et al. 2007; Muller et al. 2008). Whether these affects are due to the inhibition of Rac-dependent cell adhesion and migration is not yet clear. Finally, specific targeting of the LSC-specific interleukin-3 receptor alpha (IL-3Rα) chain (CD123) with a monoclonal antibody has been demonstrated to impair homing to the bone marrow and may activate host innate immune responses. Treatment with this antibody in preclinical murine models led to longer overall survival in recipient mice (Jin et al. 2009). The results of ongoing clinical trials testing LSC-specific agents such as these will be highly anticipated.

Arsenic trioxide has been reported to degrade the protein encoded by the *Promyelocytic Leukemia* (*PML*) gene, leading to specific effects on LSC. This has been effective in eradication of LSC in an experimental model of CML, where arsenic caused a reduction of endogenous PML protein (Ito et al. 2008), and also in a murine model of APL, where arsenic increased degradation of the PML–RARA oncoprotein (Nasr et al. 2008). The therapeutic relevance of this approach is immediately obvious, as arsenic is already used in the therapy of acute promyelocytic leukemia with considerable efficacy and generally acceptable toxicity (Soignet et al. 1998; Shen et al. 1997). The role of pro-survival pathways in LSC may also provide an opportunity to specifically target these cells. For example, drugs such as parthenolide (and its derivatives) or proteasome inhibitors are postulated to act by inhibiting the NF-κB anti-apoptotic pathway as well as other pathways (such as through reactive oxygen species) (Guzman et al. 2005, 2007).

Direct targeting of the interactions between LSC and the HM represents a promising new paradigm for LSC-targeted therapy. Two recent reports have demonstrated the proof of principle that disruption of the LSC–niche interaction may have therapeutic utility. Interruption of CXCR4-mediated LSC adhesion was shown to cause LSC mobilization and a profound sensitization to the effects of chemotherapy (Nervi et al. 2009; Zeng et al. 2009). A similar concept has been described in human studies examining the effects of priming leukemia cells with granulocyte-colony stimulating factor (G-CSF) prior to the commencement of chemotherapy. In a pivotal trial, G-CSF treatment administered prior to chemotherapy was shown to improve disease-free and overall survival in patients with AML (Lowenberg et al. 2003). The exact mechanism of this effect remains unclear. Priming agents may act through a synergistic combination of cytotoxicity with chemotherapy (e.g., by the activation of cytokine-dependent growth pathways), prevention of stromal cell–LSC interactions (analogous to the mobilization of HSC by G-CSF) or by the specific targeting of LSC by some other means (such as interference with a quiescent, long-term LSC population) (Ito et al. 2008). Proteasome inhibitors, such as bortezomib have also been shown to inhibit AML blast cell migration in response to stromal cell-derived CXCL-12 (Liesveld et al. 2005).

A significant barrier to the development of novel compounds has been the underlying nature of LSC that precludes their long-term ex vivo culture without a substantial reduction in their biologically relevant leukemia-initiating activity and concomitant changes in surface marker expression (Huntly et al. 2004; Krivtsov et al. 2006). This is interesting in that the same limitation has been problematic in normal HSC studies. Surrogate assays have been proposed, such as in vitro colony formation in cytokine-enriched methylcellulose media; however, these assays likely do not accurately reflect the most primitive LSC compartment and certainly exclude the presence of LSC–HM interactions. An alternative to this is heterotypic co-culture assays that have been extensively validated in HSC biology (Dexter 1982; Ploemacher et al. 1989; Moore et al. 1997). Briefly, these assays comprise the growth of hematopoietic (or leukemic) stem cells on a supportive stromal cell layer (either cell lines or primary bone marrow-derived stromal cells). The frequency of primitive cells that survive and proliferate within these conditions (visualized as cobblestone area-forming units or enumerated in methylcellulose colony forming assays) has been shown to correlate with the frequency of long-term HSC in vivo (Ploemacher et al. 1989). A clear benefit of using this approach is that the LSC–HM interactions are evaluable in this model. Preliminary work supports the utility of this assay in measuring LSC (Ito et al. 2008), although further validation is necessary. Recently, other high-throughput approaches to the screening of cancer stem cells (CSC) have been described. A breast cancer model was used in which the induction of an epithelial–mesenchymal transition was shown to greatly enhance CSC numbers. A novel compound, salinomycin was identified as a specific inhibitor of CSC (Gupta et al. 2009). It is hoped that similar approaches may prove fruitful for LSC; however, the development of LSC-based heterotypic cell culture assays with careful in vivo validation or RNA interference based in vivo models appears necessary for such progress.

Controversies

There exist a number of controversies regarding the frequency and generation of LSC that require further discussion. The initial studies that described LSC identified LSC as rare cells that uniquely possessed the ability to instigate and perpetuate the leukemia in vivo (Bonnet and Dick 1997). However, further evidence has suggested that LSC were not necessarily rare and that the measured frequency may depend upon the assay utilized (Kelly et al. 2007). Furthermore, there may be functional heterogeneity within hematopoietic tumors that may also depend on a graded (rather than absolute) ability to contribute to tumor maintenance and respond to external cues (Adams et al. 2008). This clonal evolution theory therefore implies that many of the malignant cells can contribute to the growth and maintenance of tumors; however, different tumor subclones may possess varying proliferative potential and this differential growth can lead to the outgrowth of the most potent tumor subclone. In this chapter, we have already discussed in detail the convincing evidence supporting the LSC theory. However, of significance, there are some apparent exceptions regarding LSC frequency and the evolution of LSC clones over time.

The clonal evolution theory is based around the premise that mutations occur randomly within individual tumor cells. These mutations occasionally provide a sequential growth advantage to a subclone of the tumor that then eventually outgrows and dominates the overall population. There are data to support this theory in human models of leukemia. For example, committed downstream progenitors (such as GMP) may acquire leukemia-initiating properties through mutations in alternative splicing in GSK-3β (Abrahamsson et al. 2009; Jamieson et al. 2004). These mutations lead to the activation of Wnt signaling and transformation from chronic phase to blast crisis in CML. Notably, using this example, the two theories (LSC vs. clonal evolution) are not mutually exclusive and the putative LSC may change in potency or identity with clonal evolution throughout the course of disease (Clarke et al. 2006).

Another contention between the two theories relates to the frequency of cells within an individual leukemia that are capable of leukemia initiation. The LSC theory has traditionally argued that LSC are rare (albeit of widely varying frequency) and the counter-argument has asserted that tumor-initiating activity may be found within most leukemia cells. To support the latter contention, there are a number of compelling models that have been demonstrated to have a very high percentage of cells (10–20%) with cancer-initiating activity. Such models include a Eμ-Nras transgenic model of T-cell lymphoma, Eμ-Myc-induced lymphoma in transgenic mice, AML caused by knockout of PU.1 in mice (Kelly et al. 2007) or even in some examples of *MLL-AF9*-induced AML (Somervaille and Cleary 2006). One explanation for the discrepancy between LSC frequency in transgenic mouse models and xenograft assays is that engraftment of AML cells into xenograft models may be impaired by residual host innate immunity in NOD/SCID mice where limited NK-cell function remains and apropos of the findings discussed in this chapter the species differences in supporting microenvironments. It has also been revealed that certain antibodies used to identify LSC (i.e., the HIT2 and AT13/5 clones of anti-CD38 but not their corresponding F(ab′)2 fragments) can encourage Fc-receptor-mediated clearance of LSC, masking potential leukemia-initiating activity within the CD34$^+$CD38$^+$ compartment (Taussig et al. 2008).

As mentioned above, the divergence between these two models may relate to the inherent limitations of xenograft transplantation as an assay of stem cell frequency. LSC are believed to be dependent on the bone marrow microenvironment for long-term self-renewal; however, in xenograft models the cytokines that signal LSC chemotaxis and homing or the pathways that regulate self-renewal may be incompatible between species (Adams et al. 2008). While it remains possible, even likely, that the frequency of LSC by current xenograft assays is an underestimate, it is also clear, however, that not all syngeneic models of leukemia are characterized by a high frequency of LSC (Krivtsov et al. 2006; Deshpande et al. 2006; Kirstetter et al. 2008;

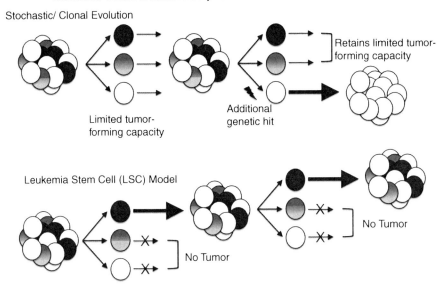

Fig. 6.2 Stochastic/Clonal evolution theory vs. hierarchical (LSC) model of leukemogenesis. Clonal evolution theory asserts that each cell within the leukemia has an equal, yet limited ability to recapitulate the leukemia. The additional genetic hits lead to a proliferative advantage and consequent evolution of a dominant clone that may alter the disease phenotype. The LSC model states that there is a defined population of cells that possess the ability to instigate, maintain and serially propagate the leukemia. LSC may also give rise to more differentiated progeny that lack this ability

Guibal et al. 2009; Wojiski et al. 2009; Chen et al. 2008; Yilmaz et al. 2006). Therefore, we would propose that both models provide complementary and important information that is dependent on the specific experimental model or context in which each model is applied (Fig. 6.2).

Further steps should be considered to optimize current xenograft assays to better estimate true LSC frequency. First, assays should endeavor to use the most permissive available strain for LSC engraftment and phenotypic analysis of the transplanted leukemia. Currently this would be the neonatal NOD/SCID/IL2Rγ$^{-/-}$ (carrying a complete null mutation for the interleukin-2 common gamma chain) model (Ishikawa et al. 2007). The humanization of cytokine/chemokine interactions or the immune system may further facilitate engraftment within these models. Second, pretreatment with intravenous gamma globulin or anti-CD122 can be used to minimize the antiengraftment effects of the antibodies used to enrich for LSC and any residual innate immune response (Taussig et al. 2008). Direct intrafemoral injection (Jin et al. 2006) may reduce the inefficiency of LSC homing and minimize splenic or pulmonary sequestration of cells. Finally, co-transferred supporting cells (such as bone marrow stromal cells) or transplantable microenvironments such as matrigel (Clarke et al. 2006; Quintana et al. 2008) may provide a species or tumor-specific microenvironment that enhances the efficiency of engraftment of tumor-initiating cells.

The Future of LSC Research

The ongoing opportunity and most stringent test of the relevance of LSC research may primarily be in the development and application of effective LSC-specific therapies that improve the outcome of patients with leukemia and related disorders. To achieve such lofty goals, the identification of novel therapeutic targets by prospective screening platforms that interrogate LSC biology followed by rigorous in vivo validation will be required.

Disclosure of Conflicts of Interest S.W.L and D.A.W. have no relevant conflicts of interest to declare.

Acknowledgments We gratefully acknowledge the insightful comments from Drs. Claudia Scholl, Stefan Fröhling and Michael Milsom. S.W.L. has received funding support from the National Health and Medical Research Council Australia, Australia/U.S. Fulbright Commission, Haematology Society of Australia and New Zealand and Royal Brisbane and Women's Hospital Foundation. D.A.W. received funding support from the US National Institute of Health (NIH; Bethesda, MD).

References

Bruce WR, Van Der Gaag H. A Quantitative Assay for the Number of Murine Lymphoma Cells Capable of Proliferation in Vivo. Nature 1963;199:79–80.

Griffin JD, Lowenberg B. Clonogenic cells in acute myeloblastic leukemia. Blood 1986;68: 1185–95.

Spangrude GJ, Heimfeld S, Weissman IL. Purification and characterization of mouse hematopoietic stem cells. Science 1988;241:58–62.

Morrison SJ, Weissman IL. The long-term repopulating subset of hematopoietic stem cells is deterministic and isolatable by phenotype. Immunity 1994;1:661–73.

Bonnet D, Dick JE. Human acute myeloid leukemia is organized as a hierarchy that originates from a primitive hematopoietic cell. Nat Med 1997;3:730–7.

Jordan CT, Upchurch D, Szilvassy SJ, Guzman ML, Howard DS, Pettigrew AL, et al. The interleukin-3 receptor alpha chain is a unique marker for human acute myelogenous leukemia stem cells. Leukemia 2000;14:1777–84.

Huntly BJ, Shigematsu H, Deguchi K, Lee BH, Mizuno S, Duclos N, et al. MOZ-TIF2, but not BCR-ABL, confers properties of leukemic stem cells to committed murine hematopoietic progenitors. Cancer Cell 2004;6:587–96.

Lapidot T, Sirard C, Vormoor J, Murdoch B, Hoang T, Caceres-Cortes J, et al. A cell initiating human acute myeloid leukaemia after transplantation into SCID mice. Nature 1994;367: 645–8.

Somervaille TC, Cleary ML. Identification and characterization of leukemia stem cells in murine MLL-AF9 acute myeloid leukemia. Cancer Cell 2006;10:257–68.

Krivtsov AV, Twomey D, Feng Z, Stubbs MC, Wang Y, Faber J, et al. Transformation from committed progenitor to leukaemia stem cell initiated by MLL-AF9. Nature 2006;442:818–22.

Deshpande AJ, Cusan M, Rawat VP, Reuter H, Krause A, Pott C, et al. Acute myeloid leukemia is propagated by a leukemic stem cell with lymphoid characteristics in a mouse model of CALM/AF10-positive leukemia. Cancer Cell 2006;10:363–74.

Dexter, TM. Stromal cell associated haemopoiesis. J Cell Physiol 1982;1:87–94.

Hu Y, Chen Y, Douglas L, Li S. beta-Catenin is essential for survival of leukemic stem cells insensitive to kinase inhibition in mice with BCR-ABL-induced chronic myeloid leukemia. Leukemia 2009;23:109–16.

Clarke MF, Dick JE, Dirks PB, Eaves CJ, Jamieson CH, Jones DL, et al. Cancer stem cells--perspectives on current status and future directions: AACR Workshop on cancer stem cells. Cancer Res 2006;66:9339–44.

Scholl C, Bansal D, Dohner K, Eiwen K, Huntly BJ, Lee BH, et al. The homeobox gene CDX2 is aberrantly expressed in most cases of acute myeloid leukemia and promotes leukemogenesis. J Clin Invest 2007;117:1037–48.

Cozzio A, Passegue E, Ayton PM, Karsunky H, Cleary ML, Weissman IL. Similar MLL-associated leukemias arising from self-renewing stem cells and short-lived myeloid progenitors. Genes Dev 2003;17:3029–35.

Kirstetter P, Schuster MB, Bereshchenko O, Moore S, Dvinge H, Kurz E, et al. Modeling of C/EBPalpha mutant acute myeloid leukemia reveals a common expression signature of committed myeloid leukemia-initiating cells. Cancer Cell 2008;13:299–310.

Guibal FC, Alberich-Jorda M, Hirai H, Ebralidze A, Levantini E, Di Ruscio A, et al. Identification of a myeloid committed progenitor as the cancer initiating cell in acute promyelocytic leukemia. Blood 2009.

Wojiski S, Guibal FC, Kindler T, Lee BH, Jesneck JL, Fabian A, et al. PML-RARalpha initiates leukemia by conferring properties of self-renewal to committed promyelocytic progenitors. Leukemia 2009;23:1462–71.

Chen W, Kumar AR, Hudson WA, Li Q, Wu B, Staggs RA, et al. Malignant transformation initiated by Mll-AF9: gene dosage and critical target cells. Cancer Cell 2008;13:432–40.

Ishikawa F, Yoshida S, Saito Y, Hijikata A, Kitamura H, Tanaka S, et al. Chemotherapy-resistant human AML stem cells home to and engraft within the bone-marrow endosteal region. Nat Biotechnol 2007;25:1315–21.

Blair A, Hogge DE, Ailles LE, Lansdorp PM, Sutherland HJ. Lack of expression of Thy-1 (CD90) on acute myeloid leukemia cells with long-term proliferative ability in vitro and in vivo. Blood 1997;89:3104–12.

Miyamoto T, Weissman IL, Akashi K. AML1/ETO-expressing nonleukemic stem cells in acute myelogenous leukemia with 8;21 chromosomal translocation. Proc Natl Acad Sci USA 2000;97:7521–6.

Bereshchenko O, Mancini E, Moore S, Bilbao D, Mansson R, Luc S, et al. Hematopoietic Stem Cell Expansion Precedes the Generation of Committed Myeloid Leukemia-Initiating Cells in C/EBPalpha Mutant AML. Cancer Cell 2009;16:390–400.

Hong D, Gupta R, Ancliff P, Atzberger A, Brown J, Soneji S, et al. Initiating and cancer-propagating cells in TEL-AML1-associated childhood leukemia. Science 2008;319:336–9.

Mullighan CG, Phillips LA, Su X, Ma J, Miller CB, Shurtleff SA, et al. Genomic analysis of the clonal origins of relapsed acute lymphoblastic leukemia. Science 2008;322:1377–80.

Mahadevan D, List AF. Targeting the multidrug resistance-1 transporter in AML: molecular regulation and therapeutic strategies. Blood 2004;104:1940–51.

Heidel F, Solem FK, Breitenbuecher F, Lipka DB, Kasper S, Thiede MH, et al. Clinical resistance to the kinase inhibitor PKC412 in acute myeloid leukemia by mutation of Asn-676 in the FLT3 tyrosine kinase domain. Blood 2006;107:293–300.

Lessard J, Sauvageau G. Bmi-1 determines the proliferative capacity of normal and leukaemic stem cells. Nature 2003;423:255–60.

Lane SW, Wang YJ, Lo Celso C, Ragu C, Bullinger L, Sykes SM, et al. Differential niche and Wnt requirements during acute myeloid leukemia progression. Blood 2011; Jul 15 (Epub).

Zhao C, Blum J, Chen A, Kwon HY, Jung SH, Cook JM, et al. Loss of beta-catenin impairs the renewal of normal and CML stem cells in vivo. Cancer Cell 2007;12:528–41.

Wang Y, Krivtsov AV, Sinha AU, North TE, Goessling W, Feng Z, et al. The Wnt/beta-catenin pathway is required for the development of leukemia stem cells in AML. Science 2010;327:1650–3.

Dierks C, Beigi R, Guo GR, Zirlik K, Stegert MR, Manley P, et al. Expansion of Bcr-Abl-positive leukemic stem cells is dependent on Hedgehog pathway activation. Cancer Cell 2008;14:238–49.

Zhao C, Chen A, Jamieson CH, Fereshteh M, Abrahamsson A, Blum J, et al. Hedgehog signalling is essential for maintenance of cancer stem cells in myeloid leukaemia. Nature 2009;458:776–9.

Ferrando AA, Armstrong SA, Neuberg DS, Sallan SE, Silverman LB, Korsmeyer SJ, et al. Gene expression signatures in MLL-rearranged T-lineage and B-precursor acute leukemias: dominance of HOX dysregulation. Blood 2003;102:262–8.

Hofmann I, Stover EH, Cullen DE, Mao J, Morgan KJ, Lee BH, et al. Hedgehog signaling is dispensable for adult murine hematopoietic stem cell function and hematopoiesis. Cell Stem Cell 2009;4:559–67.

Guzman ML, Rossi RM, Karnischky L, Li X, Peterson DR, Howard DS, et al. The sesquiterpene lactone parthenolide induces apoptosis of human acute myelogenous leukemia stem and progenitor cells. Blood 2005;105:4163–9.

Guzman ML, Neering SJ, Upchurch D, Grimes B, Howard DS, Rizzieri DA, et al. Nuclear factor-kappaB is constitutively activated in primitive human acute myelogenous leukemia cells. Blood 2001;98:2301–7.

Costello RT, Mallet F, Gaugler B, Sainty D, Arnoulet C, Gastaut JA, et al. Human acute myeloid leukemia CD34+/CD38- progenitor cells have decreased sensitivity to chemotherapy and Fas-induced apoptosis, reduced immunogenicity, and impaired dendritic cell transformation capacities. Cancer Res 2000;60:4403–11.

Morrison SJ, Prowse KR, Ho P, Weissman IL. Telomerase activity in hematopoietic cells is associated with self-renewal potential. Immunity 1996;5:207–16.

Drummond MW, Hoare SF, Monaghan A, Graham SM, Alcorn MJ, Keith WN, et al. Dysregulated expression of the major telomerase components in leukaemic stem cells. Leukemia 2005;19:381–9.

Campbell LJ, Fidler C, Eagleton H, Peniket A, Kusec R, Gal S, et al. hTERT, the catalytic component of telomerase, is downregulated in the haematopoietic stem cells of patients with chronic myeloid leukaemia. Leukemia 2006;20:671–9.

Bernard L, Belisle C, Mollica L, Provost S, Roy DC, Gilliland DG, et al. Telomere length is severely and similarly reduced in JAK2V617F-positive and -negative myeloproliferative neoplasms. Leukemia 2009;23:287–91.

Kirwan M, Vulliamy T, Marrone A, Walne AJ, Beswick R, Hillmen P, et al. Defining the pathogenic role of telomerase mutations in myelodysplastic syndrome and acute myeloid leukemia. Hum Mutat 2009;30:1567–73.

Chakraborty S, Sun CL, Francisco L, Sabado M, Li L, Chang KL, et al. Accelerated telomere shortening precedes development of therapy-related myelodysplasia or acute myelogenous leukemia after autologous transplantation for lymphoma. J Clin Oncol 2009;27:791–8.

Jaiswal S, Jamieson CH, Pang WW, Park CY, Chao MP, Majeti R, et al. CD47 is upregulated on circulating hematopoietic stem cells and leukemia cells to avoid phagocytosis. Cell 2009;138:271–85.

Majeti R, Chao MP, Alizadeh AA, Pang WW, Jaiswal S, Gibbs KD, Jr., et al. CD47 is an adverse prognostic factor and therapeutic antibody target on human acute myeloid leukemia stem cells. Cell 2009;138:286–99.

Scadden DT. The stem cell niche in health and leukemic disease. Best Pract Res Clin Haematol 2007;20:19–27.

Adams GB, Chabner KT, Alley IR, Olson DP, Szczepiorkowski ZM, Poznansky MC, et al. Stem cell engraftment at the endosteal niche is specified by the calcium-sensing receptor. Nature 2006;439:599–603.

Zhang J, Niu C, Ye L, Huang H, He X, Tong WG, et al. Identification of the haematopoietic stem cell niche and control of the niche size. Nature 2003;425:836–41.

Kiel MJ, Yilmaz OH, Iwashita T, Yilmaz OH, Terhorst C, Morrison SJ. SLAM family receptors distinguish hematopoietic stem and progenitor cells and reveal endothelial niches for stem cells. Cell 2005;121:1109–21.

Schofield R. The relationship between the spleen colony-forming cell and the haemopoietic stem cell. Blood Cells 1978;4:7–25.

Nilsson SK, Johnston HM, Coverdale JA. Spatial localization of transplanted hemopoietic stem cells: inferences for the localization of stem cell niches. Blood 2001;97:2293–9.

Visnjic D, Kalajzic I, Gronowicz G, Aguila HL, Clark SH, Lichtler AC, et al. Conditional ablation of the osteoblast lineage in Col2.3deltatk transgenic mice. J Bone Miner Res 2001;16:2222–31.

Calvi LM, Adams GB, Weibrecht KW, Weber JM, Olson DP, Knight MC, et al. Osteoblastic cells regulate the haematopoietic stem cell niche. Nature 2003;425:841–6.

Kiel MJ, Radice GL, Morrison SJ. Lack of evidence that hematopoietic stem cells depend on N-cadherin-mediated adhesion to osteoblasts for their maintenance. Cell Stem Cell 2007; 1:204–17.

Lymperi S, Horwood N, Marley S, Gordon MY, Cope AP, Dazzi F. Strontium can increase some osteoblasts without increasing hematopoietic stem cells. Blood 2008;111:1173–81.

Ma YD, Park C, Zhao H, Oduro KA, Jr., Tu X, Long F, et al. Defects in osteoblast function but no changes in long term repopulating potential of hematopoietic stem cells in a mouse chronic inflammatory arthritis model. Blood 2009.

Stier S, Ko Y, Forkert R, Lutz C, Neuhaus T, Grunewald E, et al. Osteopontin is a hematopoietic stem cell niche component that negatively regulates stem cell pool size. J Exp Med 2005; 201:1781–91.

Nilsson SK, Johnston HM, Whitty GA, Williams B, Webb RJ, Denhardt DT, et al. Osteopontin, a key component of the hematopoietic stem cell niche and regulator of primitive hematopoietic progenitor cells. Blood 2005;106:1232–9.

Kollet O, Dar A, Shivtiel S, Kalinkovich A, Lapid K, Sztainberg Y, et al. Osteoclasts degrade endosteal components and promote mobilization of hematopoietic progenitor cells. Nat Med 2006;12:657–64.

Williams DA, Rios M, Stephens C, Patel VP. Fibronectin and VLA-4 in haematopoietic stem cell-microenvironment interactions. Nature 1991;352:438–41.

Papayannopoulou T, Craddock C, Nakamoto B, Priestley GV, Wolf NS. The VLA4/VCAM-1 adhesion pathway defines contrasting mechanisms of lodgement of transplanted murine hemopoietic progenitors between bone marrow and spleen. Proc Natl Acad Sci USA 1995; 92:9647–51.

Papayannopoulou T, Nakamoto B. Peripheralization of hemopoietic progenitors in primates treated with anti-VLA4 integrin. Proc Natl Acad Sci U S A 1993;90:9374–8.

Sugiyama T, Kohara H, Noda M, Nagasawa T. Maintenance of the hematopoietic stem cell pool by CXCL12-CXCR4 chemokine signaling in bone marrow stromal cell niches. Immunity 2006;25:977–88.

Ara T, Tokoyoda K, Sugiyama T, Egawa T, Kawabata K, Nagasawa T. Long-term hematopoietic stem cells require stromal cell-derived factor-1 for colonizing bone marrow during ontogeny. Immunity 2003;19:257–67.

Sacchetti B, Funari A, Michienzi S, Di Cesare S, Piersanti S, Saggio I, et al. Self-renewing osteoprogenitors in bone marrow sinusoids can organize a hematopoietic microenvironment. Cell 2007;131:324–36.

Avecilla ST, Hattori K, Heissig B, Tejada R, Liao F, Shido K, et al. Chemokine-mediated interaction of hematopoietic progenitors with the bone marrow vascular niche is required for thrombopoiesis. Nat Med 2004;10:64–71.

Cancelas JA, Lee AW, Prabhakar R, Stringer KF, Zheng Y, Williams DA. Rac GTPases differentially integrate signals regulating hematopoietic stem cell localization. Nat Med 2005;11:886–91.

Mendez-Ferrer S, Lucas D, Battista M, Frenette PS. Haematopoietic stem cell release is regulated by circadian oscillations. Nature 2008;452:442–7.

Lucas D, Battista M, Shi PA, Isola L, Frenette PS. Mobilized hematopoietic stem cell yield depends on species-specific circadian timing. Cell Stem Cell 2008;3:364–6.

Lo Celso C, Fleming HE, Wu JW, Zhao CX, Miake-Lye S, Fujisaki J, et al. Live-animal tracking of individual haematopoietic stem/progenitor cells in their niche. Nature 2009;457:92–6.

Xie Y, Yin T, Wiegraebe W, He XC, Miller D, Stark D, et al. Detection of functional haematopoietic stem cell niche using real-time imaging. Nature 2009;547:97–101.

Jin L, Hope KJ, Zhai Q, Smadja-Joffe F, Dick JE. Targeting of CD44 eradicates human acute myeloid leukemic stem cells. Nat Med 2006;12:1167–74.

Iwamoto S, Mihara K, Downing JR, Pui CH, Campana D. Mesenchymal cells regulate the response of acute lymphoblastic leukemia cells to asparaginase. J Clin Invest 2007;117:1049–57.

Wei J, Wunderlich M, Fox C, Alvarez S, Cigudosa JC, Wilhelm JS, et al. Microenvironment determines lineage fate in a human model of MLL-AF9 leukemia. Cancer Cell 2008; 13:483–95.

Walkley CR, Olsen GH, Dworkin S, Fabb SA, Swann J, McArthur GA, et al. A microenvironment-induced myeloproliferative syndrome caused by retinoic acid receptor gamma deficiency. Cell 2007;129:1097–110.

Walkley CR, Shea JM, Sims NA, Purton LE, Orkin SH. Rb regulates interactions between hematopoietic stem cells and their bone marrow microenvironment. Cell 2007;129:1081–95.

Colmone A, Amorim M, Pontier AL, Wang S, Jablonski E, Sipkins DA. Leukemic cells create bone marrow niches that disrupt the behavior of normal hematopoietic progenitor cells. Science 2008;322:1861–5.

Jin L, Lee EM, Ramshaw HS, Busfield SJ, Peoppl AG, Wilkinson L, et al. Monoclonal antibody-mediated targeting of CD123, IL-3 receptor alpha chain, eliminates human acute myeloid leukemic stem cells. Cell Stem Cell 2009;5:31–42.

Hosen N, Park CY, Tatsumi N, Oji Y, Sugiyama H, Gramatzki M, et al. CD96 is a leukemic stem cell-specific marker in human acute myeloid leukemia. Proc Natl Acad Sci USA 2007; 104:11008–13.

Lane S, Saal R, Mollee P, Jones M, Grigg A, Taylor K, et al. A> or =1 log rise in RQ-PCR transcript levels defines molecular relapse in core binding factor acute myeloid leukemia and predicts subsequent morphologic relapse. Leuk Lymphoma 2008;49:517–23.

van Rhenen A, Feller N, Kelder A, Westra AH, Rombouts E, Zweegman S, et al. High stem cell frequency in acute myeloid leukemia at diagnosis predicts high minimal residual disease and poor survival. Clin Cancer Res 2005;11:6520–7.

Monaco G, Konopleva M, Munsell M, Leysath C, Wang RY, Jackson CE, et al. Engraftment of acute myeloid leukemia in NOD/SCID mice is independent of CXCR4 and predicts poor patient survival. Stem Cells 2004;22:188–201.

Schlenk RF, Dohner K, Krauter J, Frohling S, Corbacioglu A, Bullinger L, et al. Mutations and treatment outcome in cytogenetically normal acute myeloid leukemia. N Engl J Med 2008; 358:1909–18.

Cheung AM, Wan TS, Leung JC, Chan LY, Huang H, Kwong YL, et al. Aldehyde dehydrogenase activity in leukemic blasts defines a subgroup of acute myeloid leukemia with adverse prognosis and superior NOD/SCID engrafting potential. Leukemia 2007;21:1423–30.

Krause DS, Lazarides K, von Andrian UH, Van Etten RA. Requirement for CD44 in homing and engraftment of BCR-ABL-expressing leukemic stem cells. Nat Med 2006;12:1175–80.

Thomas EK, Cancelas JA, Chae HD, Cox AD, Keller PJ, Perrotti D, et al. Rac guanosine triphosphatases represent integrating molecular therapeutic targets for BCR-ABL-induced myeloproliferative disease. Cancer Cell 2007;12:467–78.

Muller LU, Schore RJ, Zheng Y, Thomas EK, Kim MO, Cancelas JA, et al. Rac guanosine triphosphatases represent a potential target in AML. Leukemia 2008;22:1803–6.

Ito K, Bernardi R, Morotti A, Matsuoka S, Saglio G, Ikeda Y, et al. PML targeting eradicates quiescent leukaemia-initiating cells. Nature 2008;453:1072–8.

Nasr R, Guillemin MC, Ferhi O, Soilihi H, Peres L, Berthier C, et al. Eradication of acute promyelocytic leukemia-initiating cells through PML-RARA degradation. Nat Med 2008;14:1333–42.

Soignet SL, Maslak P, Wang ZG, Jhanwar S, Calleja E, Dardashti LJ, et al. Complete remission after treatment of acute promyelocytic leukemia with arsenic trioxide. N Engl J Med 1998;339:1341–8.

Shen ZX, Chen GQ, Ni JH, Li XS, Xiong SM, Qiu QY, et al. Use of arsenic trioxide (As2O3) in the treatment of acute promyelocytic leukemia (APL): II. Clinical efficacy and pharmacokinetics in relapsed patients. Blood 1997;89:3354–60.

Guzman ML, Rossi RM, Neelakantan S, Li X, Corbett CA, Hassane DC, et al. An orally bioavailable parthenolide analog selectively eradicates acute myelogenous leukemia stem and progenitor cells. Blood 2007;110:4427–35.

Nervi B, Ramirez P, Rettig MP, Uy GL, Holt MS, Ritchey JK, et al. Chemosensitization of acute myeloid leukemia (AML) following mobilization by the CXCR4 antagonist AMD3100. Blood 2009;113:6206–14.

Zeng Z, Shi YX, Samudio IJ, Wang RY, Ling X, Frolova O, et al. Targeting the leukemia microenvironment by CXCR4 inhibition overcomes resistance to kinase inhibitors and chemotherapy in AML. Blood 2009;113:6215–24.

Lowenberg B, van Putten W, Theobald M, Gmur J, Verdonck L, Sonneveld P, et al. Effect of priming with granulocyte colony-stimulating factor on the outcome of chemotherapy for acute myeloid leukemia. N Engl J Med 2003;349:743–52.

Liesveld JL, Rosell KE, Lu C, Bechelli J, Phillips G, Lancet JE, et al. Acute myelogenous leukemia--microenvironment interactions: role of endothelial cells and proteasome inhibition. Hematology 2005;10:483–94.

Ploemacher RE, van der Sluijs JP, Voerman JS, Brons NH. An in vitro limiting-dilution assay of long-term repopulating hematopoietic stem cells in the mouse. Blood 1989;74:2755–63.

Moore KA, Ema H, Lemischka IR. In vitro maintenance of highly purified, transplantable hematopoietic stem cells. Blood 1997;89:4337–47.

Gupta PB, Onder TT, Jiang G, Tao K, Kuperwasser C, Weinberg RA, et al. Identification of selective inhibitors of cancer stem cells by high-throughput screening. Cell 2009;138:645–59.

Kelly PN, Dakic A, Adams JM, Nutt SL, Strasser A. Tumor growth need not be driven by rare cancer stem cells. Science 2007;317:337.

Adams JM, Kelly PN, Dakic A, Carotta S, Nutt SL, Strasser A. Role of "cancer stem cells" and cell survival in tumor development and maintenance. Cold Spring Harb Symp Quant Biol 2008;73:451–9.

Abrahamsson AE, Geron I, Gotlib J, Dao KH, Barroga CF, Newton IG, et al. Glycogen synthase kinase 3beta missplicing contributes to leukemia stem cell generation. Proc Natl Acad Sci USA 2009;106:3925–9.

Jamieson CH, Ailles LE, Dylla SJ, Muijtjens M, Jones C, Zehnder JL, et al. Granulocyte-macrophage progenitors as candidate leukemic stem cells in blast-crisis CML. N Engl J Med 2004;351:657–67.

Taussig DC, Miraki-Moud F, Anjos-Afonso F, Pearce DJ, Allen K, Ridler C, et al. Anti-CD38 antibody-mediated clearance of human repopulating cells masks the heterogeneity of leukemia-initiating cells. Blood 2008;112:568–75.

Yilmaz OH, Valdez R, Theisen BK, Guo W, Ferguson DO, Wu H, et al. Pten dependence distinguishes haematopoietic stem cells from leukaemia-initiating cells. Nature 2006;441:475–82.

Quintana E, Shackleton M, Sabel MS, Fullen DR, Johnson TM, Morrison SJ. Efficient tumour formation by single human melanoma cells. Nature 2008;456:593–8.

Lane SW, Gilliland DG. Leukemia stem cells. Semin Cancer Biol 2009.

Chapter 7
Cancer Stem Cells and the Central Nervous System

Serdar Korur, Maria Maddalena Lino, and Adrian Merlo

Cancer and Cancer Stem Cells

Cancer is the result of a malignant transformation originating in a single cell. Tumors develop through the accumulation of mutations leading to uncontrolled cell proliferation and an elevated apoptotic threshold (Lino and Merlo 2009). Two developmental theories regarding tumorigenesis have been proposed, firstly, all tumor cells have the same tumorigenic potential, and secondly, only a rare subset of cells within the tumor have significant proliferative capacity while the others represent more differentiated cells (Bonnet and Dick 1997; Reya et al. 2001). This second hypothesis states that only a subset of the tumor cells has the capacity to divide indefinitely while the majority of cells have limited tumorigenic potential, thereby establishing the concept of CSCs. The CSC hypothesis suggests that tumors, including GBM, can be established, expanded, and perpetuated by a sub-population of cells bearing stem cell properties, aberrant growth, and tumor-initiating capabilities (Ailles and Weissman 2007). CSCs have been isolated in most tumor types (hematological and solid malignancies). They share characteristics with normal stem cells, specifically the ability of extensive cell renewal, and the possibility to give rise to different tissue-specific cell types according to their tissue of origin.

Already at the end of the nineteenth century, the idea that cancers are derived from displaced placental tissue or activated germinal cells in adult tissue has been discussed (Colnhein 1889; Oberling 1944). Nowadays, the prominent idea is that most tumors arise from maturation arrest of a cellular lineage derived from tissue specific stem cells (Sell and Pierce 1994). The hypothesis of CSCs was first established in hematological malignancies with the detection of leukemia-initiating cells

S. Korur • M.M. Lino • A. Merlo (✉)
Laboratory of Molecular Neuro-Oncology, University Hospital Basel,
Buchserstrasse 26, Bern CH-3006, Switzerland
e-mail: adrian.merlo@gmx.ch

that were able to reproduce leukemia in immunodeficient mice (Bonnet and Dick 1997; Hope et al. 2004). CSCs have the ability to self-renew, giving rise to other CSCs, or generating more differentiated progeny. The origin of these CSCs is still a matter of debate, however, the concept of CSCs has also been extended to solid tumors, including malignant brain neoplasms. All these studies paralleled the discovery of the generation of new cells persisting into adulthood within discrete areas of the brain (Doetsch et al. 1999; Morshead et al. 1994). These cells may therefore be the cellular source for transformation giving rise to tumor stem cells. In 2002, the first data proving the existence of brain CSCs in GBM was published (Hemmati et al. 2003; Ignatova et al. 2002; Singh et al. 2004).

It has been shown that CSCs are resistant to conventional chemotherapy that may be more active on the "more differentiated cell" that constitutes the bulk of the tumor. The rare CSCs persist in tumors and are responsible for the relapse or progression if not specifically eliminated. Stem cells are embedded in a special micro-environment called "the stem cell niche" which is tightly regulated and contains adult stem cells in a quiescent state which are re-activated by specific signals. Cell-to-cell or cell-to-ECM (extracellular matrix) interactions, paracrine signals, and oxygen levels are the most important factors in the regulation of the stem cell response. This regulation of the stem cell niche is of crucial importance, and its malfunctioning contributes to tumorigenesis. CSCs are believed to either be derived from a mutated stem cell or from de-differentiation of more mature progenitor cells (Voog and Jones, 2010).

Glioblastoma

Gliomas are the most common primary tumors of the central nervous system (CNS) in adults (Davis and McCarthy 2001). Glioblastoma (GBM, WHO grade IV) accounts for approximately 50% of all glial tumor types (Newton 1994, 2004) and manifests with an incidence of about 5/100,000 belonging to the group of orphan diseases. These aggressive, highly invasive, and neurologically destructive tumors are among the deadliest of human cancers, with a median survival ranging from 9 to 12 months (Newton 1994, 2004).

Despite treatment efforts including new technological advances in neurosurgery, radiation therapy, and clinical trials with novel therapeutic agents, median survival has not significantly changed over the past three decades. More sophisticated drugs interfering with the specific molecular targets are being tested clinically in addition to conventional cytotoxic chemotherapeutics (Merlo et al. 1999, 2003). In high-grade gliomas, several genes, and pathways are altered due to a severe mutator phenotype that leads to the accumulation of mutations in critical regulatory genes. The most frequent mutations involve the following pathways regulating: cell cycle INK4a (50%)/CDK4 (14%)/RB1 (12%), apoptosis ARF (50%)/TP53 (40%)/HDM2/HDM4, growth PI3KCA (10%)/PTEN (30%)/PKB, and for EGFR (37%) that

7 Cancer Stem Cells and the Central Nervous System

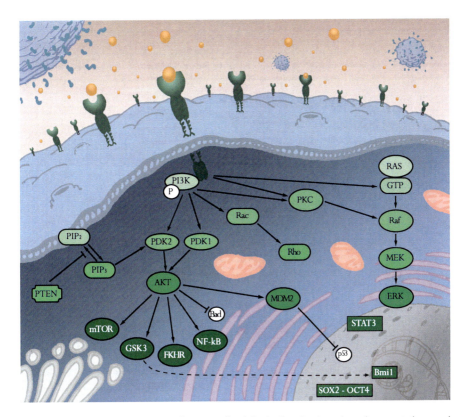

Fig. 7.1 Aberrant signaling in malignant cells: inherited and selected random mutations and epigenetic dysregulation disturb normal cell signaling. This image schematically shows frequently affected key pathways in a transformed cell, e.g., PI3K/Akt/mTOR and the MAPK. Maintenance of stem cell features leads to upregulation of critical developmental regulatory factors such as SOX2, Nestin, and many others

impinges on several pathways including MAPK and migration via Ras/Rac/Rho (Knobbe et al. 2002, 2005; Parsons et al. 2008) (Fig. 7.1). Besides classic mutations, epigenetic silencing of tumor suppressor genes frequently leads to dysregulation of signaling pathways promoting tumorigenesis. To identify the genetic alterations in GBMs, 20,661 protein coding genes were sequenced in a recent study to determine the presence of amplifications and deletions and to define gene expression profiles. This comprehensive analysis confirmed the known mutations and a variety of genes that were not known to be altered in GBMs were discovered, however, at low frequency (Parsons et al. 2008). Interestingly, mutations in the active site of isocitrate dehydrogenase 1 (IDH1) were detected in 12% of GBM patients, mostly young patients with secondary GBMs.

Brain Cancer Stem Cells in GBM

Estimated CSCs' frequency varies depending on the tissue of origin, technique of isolation, and recipient mice adopted. These observations suggest that the stemness of CSCs is not strictly an inherent cell property, but also the result of the interaction with the environmental milieu. A series of publications proposed the CD133-antigen as the stem cell marker in hematopoietic stem cells, endothelial progenitor cells, glioblastomas, neuronal and glial stem cells, and some other cell types. CD133 is a transmembrane glycoprotein also known as prominin-1 (PROM1). In 2004, Singh et al. showed that as few as 100 CD133-positive cells isolated from a GBM and transplanted in NOD-SCID mice brain produced a tumor that was a phenocopy of the original tumors. On the other hand, engraftment of 10^5 CD133-negative cells did not cause a tumor (Singh et al. 2004).

Subsequent reports contradicted the hypothesis that CD133-positive cells are the only cellular source capable to induce tumor formation. Although the CD133 marker is widely used as specific stem cell marker, it has been shown that both the CD133-positive and CD133-negative cells share similar stemness and tumorigenic properties. Clement et al. showed that neither the expression of stemness genes nor the capability for long-term self-renewal between CD133-positive and CD133-negative cells were significantly different (Clement et al. 2009). The CD133 marker therefore lacks specificity and is not sufficient to tag the entire self-renewing tumor cell reservoir.

Joo et al. showed that both CD133-positive and CD133-negative cells purified from GBM patients give rise to GBM tumors in NOD-SCID mouse brains. The CD133-negative cells showed even more pronounced proliferative and angiogenic features compared with the CD133-positive cells (Joo et al. 2008). More recently, CD133-negative cells were also found to have stemness characteristics distinct from the CD133-positive cells. Beier et al. proved that the CD133-positive CSC maintain only a subset of primary GBM. CD133-negative tumor cells also possess stem cell-like characteristics but with distinct molecular profiles and growth characteristics (Beier et al. 2007). Interestingly, Wang et al. showed that CD133-negative cells are tumorigenic, and that CD133-positive cells can be obtained from the tumors formed by the CD133-negative cells. CD133-positive cells start to appear during angiogenesis and display shorter survival. This suggests that they are not required for tumor initiation, but are involved during brain tumor progression (Wang et al. 2008a). Griguer et al. showed that expression of CD133 is upregulated in hypoxic conditions and mitochondrial dysfunction suggests that CD133 is a marker of bioenergetic stress in GBM. Therefore, the concept that CD133 is a CSC marker needs to be revised (Griguer et al. 2008).

Other researchers try to distinguish the CSC pool according to the spatial presentation of tumor cells. For example, Piccirillo et al. describe the existence of distinct pools of CSC in glioblastoma, one from the GBM periphery (p-GBM) and one from the tumor core (c-GBM) (Piccirillo et al. 2009). Both subpopulations are multipotent but differ in terms of clonogenicity and growth kinetics, which is higher for the CSC contained in the GBM core. Moreover, orthotopic transplantation from c-GBM cells induced tumor formation while p-GBM cells did not. p-GBM cells do share common genetic aberrations with c-GBM, such as trisomy 7, monosomy 10, t(1;9)(q31;p13), t(7;15)(q32;q21-22), but also display specific alterations. c- and p-GBM may be derived from common ancestor cells which then accumulate further genetic aberrations, defining cellular characteristics (Piccirillo et al. 2009).

Pathways Regulating Stem and Cancer Stem Cells

Many proteins that are implicated in normal stem cells such as Bmi-1, Notch, Shh, and Wnt are also implicated to play a role in tumorigenesis. In this section, we analyze critical proteins associated with glioma CSCs.

The Polycomb Group of Repressors Bmi1 and EZH2

Bmi1 is a member of the Polycomb group of transcriptional repressors involved in nervous system development (Leung et al. 2004). Polycomb group proteins maintain adult and embryonic stem cells by repressing specific sets of genes important for differentiation (Molofsky et al. 2003; Orlando 2003; Park et al. 2003; Valk-Lingbeek et al. 2004). Bmi1 is implicated in several cancers such as non-small-cell lung cancer, colorectal carcinoma, nasopharyngeal carcinoma, medulloblastoma, lymphoma, multiple myeloma, and neuroblastoma (Haupt et al. 1993; Leung et al. 2004; Vonlanthen et al. 2001; Kim et al. 2004; Nowak et al. 2006; Song et al. 2006). It is believed to regulate cell proliferation and senescence through the Ink4a/arf locus (Jacobs et al. 1999). In differentiated cells, Bmi1 levels decrease, while Ink4a/Arf protein levels increase (Molofsky et al. 2006). As the Ink4a/Arf locus is frequently deleted in brain tumors (Labuhn et al. 2001), the role of Bmi1 overexpression in GBM cells appears to be distinct from repression of the Ink4a/Arf locus. We showed that downregulation of Bmi1 did not change Ink4a/Arf protein levels in tumor cells that retained the Ink4a/Arf locus (Korur et al. 2009). This suggests that, in GBM cells, Bmi1 targets a different pathway. We further showed that Bmi1 down-regulation induced GBM cell differentiation, limiting the developmental capacity of glioblastoma cells. We found this effect to be mediated by GSK3beta protein (Korur et al. 2009). In addition, microRNA-128 has been shown to inhibit proliferation and self-renewal in glioma, in part by downregulating Bmi1 (Godlewski et al. 2008).

Another member of the polycomb group proteins EZH2 (enhancer of zeste homologue 2) is involved in the initiation of epigenetic gene-silencing mechanisms and implicated in glioma CSC maintenance (Suva et al. 2009). It was shown that treatment of glioma CSCs with 3-deazaneplanocin – an inhibitor which depletes cells of EZH2 activity – dramatically reduced their in vitro-clonogenic potential and in vivo-tumor-forming ability. The authors further identified c-myc as an important target for EZH2 complex in maintaining tumorigenicity of glioma CSCs (Suva et al. 2009).

ABCG2 Multidrug-Resistance Gene

ABCB1, ABCC1, and ABCG2 are the three main multidrug-resistance genes overexpressed in multiple cancers including GBM. In addition to the efflux of drugs, these pumps also possess the ability to exclude fluorescent dyes, such as the Hoechst 33342. Stem cells are frequently identified as the "side population" by flow cytometry based on ABCG2-mediated efflux of Hoechst dye (Goodell et al. 1996). In this side population, Akt, but not its downstream target mTOR, regulates ABCG2 activity, and loss of PTEN increases the "side population." Temozolomide, frequently used as chemotherapeutic agent for GBM, is not an ABCG2 substrate, but also increases the "side population" in glioma cells, indicating an adaptive reaction of GBM cells to the therapeutic challenge. This phenomenon was more pronounced in GBM cells lacking functional PTEN (Bleau et al. 2009a, b). ABCG2 or ABCC2 modulation influenced the Tie 2 receptor expression (Bleau et al. 2009b; Martin et al. 2009). GBM show an abnormally high expression of the Tie2 receptor. Tie2 activation results in increased expression of ATP-binding cassette (ABC) transporters and downmodulation of ABCG2 or ABCC2 abolishing the ability of Tie2 activation to induce a chemoresistant phenotype (Martin et al. 2009).

The Notch Proteins

Notch encodes a transmembrane receptor that upon cleavage releases its intracellular domain (NICD) which controls transcription by RBPJk/CSL (Bray 2006). The Notch signaling pathway is required for both brain tumor and non-neoplastic neural stem cells. GBM contain stem-like cells with higher Notch activity. Fan et al. described that CSC in brain tumors are selectively vulnerable to inhibition of the Notch pathway. Notch blockade more selectively induced apoptosis in the nestin-positive population and reduced the CD133-positive cell fraction (Androutsellis-Theotokis et al. 2006; Fan et al. 2006; Hitoshi et al. 2002; Purow et al. 2005; Shen et al. 2004). Blocking the Notch pathway with a γ-secretase inhibitor has been shown to induce cell differentiation in colon adenomas (van Es et al. 2005) and to deplete CSC in GBM (Fan et al. 2006; van Es et al. 2005). Similarly, blocking antibodies against the Notch ligand Delta-like 4 inhibit tumor growth by acting on angiogenesis. Wang et al. suggest that Notch signaling influences radioresistance of glioma stem cells (Wang et al. 2009b). Inhibiting the Notch pathway with gamma-secretase inhibitors (GSI) renders the glioma stem cells more sensitive to radiation and impairs clonogenic survival of glioma stem cells but not non-stem cell-like glioma cells, by reducing pAkt and Mcl-1 levels. Similarly, expression of the constitutively active intracellular domain of Notch1 or Notch2 protects glioma stem cells against radiation (Wang et al. 2009b). Notch blockade by GSI reduced neurosphere growth and clonogenicity in vitro, while expression of an active form of Notch2 increased tumor growth (van Es et al. 2005). The CD133-marker, nestin, Bmi1, and Olig2 are also reduced following Notch blockade. Moreover, GSI-treated cells implanted in mice did not lead to tumor formation (Fan et al. 2006, 2009). Notch pathway inhibition depleted stem-like cancer cells through reduced proliferation and increased apoptosis associated with decreased phosphorylation of Akt and STAT3 (Fan et al. 2009). Notch, Wnt, and SHH interact together on other signaling pathways as bone morphogenetic proteins (BMP) produced by CSC. BMP4 has been shown to induce differentiation of CD133-positive cells into astrocyte-like cells and reduced their tumor-forming ability in a preclinical model (Piccirillo et al. 2006).

SHH

SHH has been shown to regulate cerebellar neurogenesis and is implicated in the generation of medulloblastoma (Goodrich et al. 1997; Palma et al. 2005). Bar et al. described that GBM-derived neurospheres treated with cyclopamine lose the ability to form neurospheres and tumors when orthotopically implanted (Bar et al. 2007). On the contrary, radiation therapy increased neurospere formation. Both SHH-dependent and -independent brain tumor growth required phosphoinositide 3-kinase-mTOR signaling. In human GBMs, the levels of SHH and PTCH1 expression are significantly higher in PTEN-expressing tumors than in PTEN-deficient tumors. Moreover, SHH-GLI signaling in PTEN co-expressing human GBM is associated with an especially poor prognosis (Xu et al. 2008).

c-MYC

c-Myc has been suggested to have a role in regulating proliferation and survival of glioma stem cells (Wang et al. 2008b). c-Myc is highly expressed in glioma stem cells and knockdown of c-Myc lead to reduce proliferation and increased apoptosis. Furthermore, glioma stem cells with decreased c-Myc levels fail to in vitro form neurospheres or tumors in orthotopically transplanted mice (Wang et al. 2008b).

STAT3

Signal transducer and activator of transcription 3 (STAT3) is an important regulator of various cellular processes such as cell growth, differentiation, and apoptosis, and is frequently targeted during tumorigenesis (Bromberg 2002). STAT3 was recently shown to be an important regulator of glioma stem cell proliferation and maintenance (Sherry et al. 2009). Biochemical or biological inhibition of STAT3 protein inhibited neurosphere-forming ability, decreased stem cell-related proteins, and induced markers of differentiation. These data suggested that STAT3 regulates self-renewal of glioma stem cells and might be an attractive therapeutic target (Sherry et al. 2009). In a recent study it has been shown that IFN-beta suppresses proliferation, self-renewal, and tumorigenesis of CSC via STAT3 signaling by inducing terminal differentiation of mature oligodendroglia-like cells (Yuki et al. 2009).

It has been demonstrated that STAT3 is a downstream mediator of the prosurvival factor IL6 which is expressed in CSC. Perturbation of IL6 signaling in CSCs leads to reduced growth and neurosphere formation, and increased apoptosis by interfering with STAT3 signaling. High expression of IL6 ligand and receptor are associated with poor glioma patient survival, suggesting contribution to gliomagenesis (Wang et al. 2009a).

Nestin

Nestin is an intermediate filament protein and is expressed by neural precursor cells located in the subventricular zone (Lendahl et al. 1990). Upon differentiation of precursor cells into the neural lineage, nestin becomes downregulated and is replaced either by neuron-specific neurofilaments or by the glial fibrillary acidic protein (GFAP) according to the respective lineage-specific fate. Nestin is re-expressed in the adult during pathological situations such as the formation of the glial scar after CNS injury and during regeneration of injured muscle tissue. Signaling pathways operative in GBM such as Notch, Bmi1, and GSK3beta regulate CSCs by modulating nestin expression (Shih and Holland 2006; Korur et al. 2009).

Musashi

Musashi is an RNA-binding protein critical for asymmetric division in neural stem cells (Okano et al. 2005). It has been suggested to act as a translational repressor and to regulate Notch signaling (Bachman et al. 2004; Hemmati et al. 2003; Nakamura et al. 1994; Thon et al. 2008). Musashi is expressed in brain tumor stem cells (Hemmati et al. 2003), GBM, and medulloblastoma. Its downregulation negatively affects tumor cell proliferation (Hemmati et al. 2003; Kong et al. 2008; Strojnik et al. 2007; Yokota et al. 2004).

GSK3Beta

Glycogen synthase kinase 3 (GSK3) is a serine/threonine kinase that regulates numerous signaling pathways involved in cell cycle control, proliferation, differentiation, and apoptosis (Cheung et al. 2000; Cohen and Goedert 2004). We have shown that Bmi1 regulates glioma cell identity and maintenance of a stem cell-like phenotype through GSK3beta. Inhibition of GSK3beta mimicked downregulation of Bmi1 and induced differentiation of glioma CSCs (Korur et al. 2009). Thus, GSK3beta is an important regulator in GBM and is required for the maintenance of glioma CSCs. In-depth analysis of GSK3beta function in GBM is likely to open new therapeutic perspectives for GBM.

SOX

Sox4 is a HMG box containing DNA-binding protein which acts as a transcriptional activator involved in the development of the CNS (Cheung et al. 2000). Overexpression of SOX4 has been found to be associated with several cancers, including glioma. The mechanism of action of Sox4 has not been yet clarified (Aaboe et al. 2006; Lee et al. 2002; Liao et al. 2008; Pramoonjago et al. 2006). However, a recent report identified Sox4 as a target of TGF-β which is required for tumorigenecity of CSC together with Sox2 (Ikushima et al. 2009).

Sox2 is one of the transcription factors together with Oct4 and Klf4 that can directly reprogram somatic cells to a pluripotent stem cell state (Okita et al. 2007; Takahashi et al. 2007). Sox2 protein is widely expressed in the early neural plate and early neural tube of several species (Wegner 1999). In the developing CNS, Sox2 expression becomes restricted to the neuroepithelial cells of the ventricular layer which continue to divide presenting an immature phenotype throughout life. Cells that leave the ventricular layer stop expressing Sox2 (Graham et al. 2003; Wegner 1999), and Sox2 deficiency impaired neurogenesis in the adult mouse brain (Ferri et al. 2004). Interestingly, Sox2 has also been implicated in gliomagenesis (Gangemi et al. 2009; Ikushima et al. 2009) since downregulation of Sox2 reduced tumorigenicity in glioma CSC. Ikushima et al. specifically showed that Sox2 is required for tumorigenicity of glioma CSC and is regulated by TGF-β which directly induced its transcriptional activator Sox4 (Ikushima et al. 2009). Therefore, Sox2 has been proposed as a new GBM therapeutic target (Gangemi et al. 2009; Ikushima et al. 2009; Korur et al. 2009).

Hide et al. recently showed that downregulation of Sox11 correlated with a significant decrease in survival while its overexpression prevented tumorigenesis. Sox11 prevents gliomagenesis by blocking the expression of oncogenic plagl1 (Hide et al. 2009).

TGF-Beta

Transforming growth factor β (TGF-β) is a member of a cytokine family that regulates organism development (Wu and Hill 2009). TGF-β evolved to regulate expanding systems of neural and epithelial tissues (Massague 2008). TGF-β is emerging as an important regulator of glioblastoma CSC. Although TGF-β shows anti-proliferative effects in certain types of carcinoma cells and is a well-known tumor suppressor. It promotes proliferation of some non-epithelial tumors such as glioma through the induction of PDGF-B (Bruna et al. 2007). Several recent reports suggested an important role of TGF-β in glioma CSC maintenance through different mechanisms. Penuelas et al. suggested that TGF-β increases CSC self-renewal via induction of leukemia inhibitory factor (LIF) (Ikushima et al. 2009; Penuelas et al. 2009). Ikushima et al. showed that tumorigenicity of glioma CSC are maintained by TGF-β via Sox4–Sox2 (Ikushima et al. 2009; Penuelas et al. 2009). Moreover, glioma cells are less aggressive in transplantation assays upon blocking of TGF-β (Ikushima et al. 2009; Penuelas et al. 2009).

New Markers

An important bottle neck for specific targeting of CSCs is the lack of reliable cell surface markers since CD133 has proven inefficient as 40% of freshly isolated GBM cell populations do not contain CD133-positive cells (Son et al. 2009). Myung Jin Son proposed stage-specific embryonic antigen 1 (SSEA-1/LeX) as a glioma CSC enrichment marker which was present in majority of GBM cells fulfilling the functional criteria for CSCs (Son et al. 2009). Interestingly, in a Ptch(+/−)-medulloblastoma mouse model, CSCs were identified to express the SSEA-1 antigen, but not CD133 (Read et al. 2009; Ward et al. 2009). Given the genetic and epigenetic heterogeneity of GBM cells, there might exist several markers to identify CSCs. Nonetheless, future work on additional glioma stem cells markers will allow to better identify those cells and investigate molecular mechanisms governing their stemness behavior and therapeutic resistance. Interference with the stemness-regulatory network will help to eradicate those "primordial" malignant cells.

Focusing on CSC Therapy

CSCs have evolved strategies to evade intrinsic and extrinsic cell death mechanisms. After initial response to chemotherapy, relapse is frequently observed. The CSC resistance to drugs involves mechanisms like the expression of multidrug-resistance proteins, deficiency in DNA repair, and strategies to evade apoptosis (Kvinlaug and Huntly 2007). CSCs stay within niches which might respond to signals either by maintaining a state of quiescence or by stimulating proliferation. One important factor regulating these niches is hypoxia which leads to HIF1α (hypoxia-inducing factor alpha) upregulation enhancing self-renewal of the CD133-positive CSC and inhibiting differentiation. Moreover, knockdown of HIF1α abrogates the expansion of hypoxia-mediated CD133-positive CSC. Similarly, blocking the Akt or ERK1/2 pathway also reduced the hypoxia-driven CD133 expansion, suggesting that these signaling cascades may modulate the hypoxic response (Soeda et al. 2009). HIF 2α influences proliferation through inhibition of c-Myc and mTOR while stimulating p53 (Li et al. 2009). It was recently reported that physiological oxygen levels differentially induced hypoxia inducible factor-2α (HIF2α) levels in CSCs. Hypoxia promotes the self-renewal capability of the stem and non-stem populations by upregulating important stem cell factors, such as OCT4, NANOG, and c-MYC. While HIF1α influenced proliferation and survival of all cancer cells, HIF2α was found to be mainly essential in CSCs (Li et al. 2009). Moreover, increased HIF2α levels augment the tumorigenic potential of the non-stem population (Heddleston et al. 2009). Interestingly, Pistollato et al. describe a new network between Hypoxia-p53-BMP-SMAD in pediatric high-grade gliomas. Hypoxia inhibits p53 activation and BMP signaling by blocking astroglial differentiation of glioma precursors. An acute increase in oxygen tension led to Smad activation and silencing of HIF1α (Pistollato et al. 2009).

CSC also express high levels of anti-apoptotic genes such as BCL-2, BCL-XL, and IAP family members, and are particularly resistant to drugs and toxins (Jin et al. 2008; Liu et al. 2006). This phenomenon is mainly due to the high expression of ABC drug transporters which protect cells from cytotoxic agents (Dean et al. 2005). Tumor recurrence may be mostly due to the presence of these CSC with high expression of ABC transporters. New therapeutic compounds should aim to alter ABC transporters to reach a better clinical outcome. Increased telomerase activity has been reported in up to 90% of malignant tumors (Shay and Keith 2008). All these specific CSC characteristics should be taken in consideration to develop targeted therapies. It represents a very difficult task since CSC constitute an heterogeneous population according to genetic, epigenetic, and environmental factors within each individual patient. In addition, there is individual variation of the spectrum of somatic mutations and the degree of genetic instability. CSC are also relatively resistant to oxidative or DNA damage (Diehn et al. 2009). Moreover, CSC reside in niches, which may be difficult to be reached by drugs due to impaired perfusion as a consequence of increased interstitial pressure (Jain et al. 2007). Although it is essential to eliminate CSC, the tumor bulk is constituted by non-CSC cells which should also be removed since they cause the major mass effect. In addition, it cannot be excluded that CSC are generated through an inverse process of de-differentiation (Gupta et al. 2009). Recently we proposed GSK3 inhibitory drugs including LiCl as possible first- and/or second-line treatments complementing standard cancer therapy. We described that combining the GSK3 inhibitor LiCl and with an alkylating agent leads to sensitization due to the induction of differentiation by interference with GSK3 activity. Epidemiological studies in psychiatric patients have shown a lower cancer prevalence in LiCl-treated patients when compared to the general population, suggesting a protective effect of the drug (Cohen et al. 1998). Future clinical trials will have to show whether long-term LiCl therapy in stabilized GBM patients may delay tumor recurrence from the residual CSC pool by driving CSCs into differentiation and apoptosis.

Conclusion

Conventional therapies may reduce the tumor mass mainly by killing cells with limited proliferative potential. This leads to a transient clinical response followed by tumor recurrence or progression of GBM. Effective therapy aims to kill CSC which would render the tumor unable to regrow. CSC are more resistant to chemotherapy than mature cell types from the same tissue, probably due to the expression of multidrug resistance genes and high levels of anti-apoptotic proteins. An important challenge now is to identify and characterize the properties of these CSC. Once characterized, the therapeutic goal will be induction of apoptosis or differentiation. Antiangiogenetic, antiproliferative, and anti-invasive strategies represent promising adjuvant strategies. In the future, combination therapies using tumor-targeted drugs and more advanced cytotoxic agents that target CSC with simultaneous or sequential hits onto their specific niches may become a promising strategy. Regarding the brain, we have also to take into consideration the many obstacles of drug distribution within the target area. Advances in molecular disease imaging are needed to get direct answers on therapeutic effects and the degree of drug penetration within the tumor to avoid collateral damage to healthy stem cells.

References

Aaboe M, Birkenkamp-Demtroder K, Wiuf C, Sorensen FB, Thykjaer T, Sauter G, Jensen KM, Dyrskjot L, Orntoft T (2006) SOX4 expression in bladder carcinoma: clinical aspects and in vitro functional characterization. Cancer research 66: 3434–3442

ahttp://perssearch.unibas.ch/perssearch/search Gangemi RM, Griffero F, Marubbi D, Perera M, Capra MC, Malatesta P, Ravetti GL, Zona GL, Daga A, Corte G (2009) SOX2 silencing in glioblastoma tumor-initiating cells causes stop of proliferation and loss of tumorigenicity. Stem cells (Dayton, Ohio) 27: 40–48

Ailles LE, Weissman IL (2007) Cancer stem cells in solid tumors. Curr Opin Biotechnol 18: 460–466

Androutsellis-Theotokis A, Leker RR, Soldner F, Hoeppner DJ, Ravin R, Poser SW, Rueger MA, Bae SK, Kittappa R, McKay RD (2006) Notch signalling regulates stem cell numbers in vitro and in vivo. Nature 442: 823–826

Bachman KE, Argani P, Samuels Y, Silliman N, Ptak J, Szabo S, Konishi H, Karakas B, Blair BG, Lin C, Peters BA, Velculescu VE, Park BH (2004) The PIK3CA gene is mutated with high frequency in human breast cancers. Cancer Biol Ther 3: 772–775

Bar EE, Chaudhry A, Lin A, Fan X, Schreck K, Matsui W, Piccirillo S, Vescovi AL, DiMeco F, Olivi A, Eberhart CG (2007) Cyclopamine-mediated hedgehog pathway inhibition depletes stem-like cancer cells in glioblastoma. Stem cells (Dayton, Ohio) 25: 2524–2533

Beier D, Hau P, Proescholdt M, Lohmeier A, Wischhusen J, Oefner PJ, Aigner L, Brawanski A, Bogdahn U, Beier CP (2007) CD133(+) and CD133(−) glioblastoma-derived cancer stem cells show differential growth characteristics and molecular profiles. Cancer research 67: 4010–4015

Bleau AM, Hambardzumyan D, Ozawa T, Fomchenko EI, Huse JT, Brennan CW, Holland EC (2009) PTEN/PI3K/Akt pathway regulates the side population phenotype and ABCG2 activity in glioma tumor stem-like cells. Cell stem cell 4: 226–235

Bleau AM, Huse JT, Holland EC (2009) The ABCG2 resistance network of glioblastoma. Cell Cycle 8: 2936–2944

Bonnet D, Dick JE (1997) Human acute myeloid leukemia is organized as a hierarchy that originates from a primitive hematopoietic cell. Nat Med 3: 730–737

Bray SJ (2006) Notch signalling: a simple pathway becomes complex. Nat Rev Mol Cell Biol 7: 678–689

Bromberg J (2002) Stat proteins and oncogenesis. J Clin Invest 109: 1139–1142

Bruna A, Darken RS, Rojo F, Ocana A, Penuelas S, Arias A, Paris R, Tortosa A, Mora J, Baselga J, Seoane J (2007) High TGFbeta-Smad activity confers poor prognosis in glioma patients and promotes cell proliferation depending on the methylation of the PDGF-B gene. Cancer cell 11: 147–160

Cheung M, Abu-Elmagd M, Clevers H, Scotting PJ (2000) Roles of Sox4 in central nervous system development. Brain research 79: 180–191

Clement V, Dutoit V, Marino D, Dietrich PY, Radovanovic I (2009) Limits of CD133 as a marker of glioma self-renewing cells. Int J Cancer 125: 244–248

Cohen P, Goedert M (2004) GSK3 inhibitors: development and therapeutic potential. Nature reviews 3: 479–487

Cohen Y, Chetrit A, Sirota P, Modan B (1998) Cancer morbidity in psychiatric patients: influence of lithium carbonate treatment. Med Oncol 15: 32–36

Cohnhein J (1889) Lectures in general pathology. London: The New Sydenham Society

Davis FG, McCarthy BJ (2001) Current epidemiological trends and surveillance issues in brain tumors. Expert Rev Anticancer Ther 1: 395–401

Dean M, Fojo T, Bates S (2005) Tumour stem cells and drug resistance. Nat Rev Cancer 5: 275–284

Diehn M, Cho RW, Lobo NA, Kalisky T, Dorie MJ, Kulp AN, Qian D, Lam JS, Ailles LE, Wong M, Joshua B, Kaplan MJ, Wapnir I, Dirbas FM, Somlo G, Garberoglio C, Paz B, Shen J, Lau SK, Quake SR, Brown JM, Weissman IL, Clarke MF (2009) Association of reactive oxygen species levels and radioresistance in cancer stem cells. Nature 458: 780–783

Doetsch F, Caille I, Lim DA, Garcia-Verdugo JM, Alvarez-Buylla A (1999) Subventricular zone astrocytes are neural stem cells in the adult mammalian brain. Cell 97: 703–716

Fan X, Matsui W, Khaki L, Stearns D, Chun J, Li YM, Eberhart CG (2006) Notch pathway inhibition depletes stem-like cells and blocks engraftment in embryonal brain tumors. Cancer research 66: 7445–7452

Fan X, Khaki L, Zhu TS, Soules ME, Talsma CE, Gul N, Koh C, Zhang J, Li YM, Maciaczyk J, Nikkhah G, Dimeco F, Piccirillo S, Vescovi AL, Eberhart CG (2009) Notch Pathway Blockade Depletes CD133-Positive Glioblastoma Cells and Inhibits Growth of Tumor Neurospheres and Xenografts. Stem cells (Dayton, Ohio)

Ferri AL, Cavallaro M, Braida D, Di Cristofano A, Canta A, Vezzani A, Ottolenghi S, Pandolfi PP, Sala M, DeBiasi S, Nicolis SK (2004) Sox2 deficiency causes neurodegeneration and impaired neurogenesis in the adult mouse brain. Development (Cambridge, England) 131: 3805–3819

Godlewski J, Nowicki MO, Bronisz A, Williams S, Otsuki A, Nuovo G, Raychaudhury A, Newton HB, Chiocca EA, Lawler S (2008) Targeting of the Bmi-1 oncogene/stem cell renewal factor by microRNA-128 inhibits glioma proliferation and self-renewal. Cancer research 68: 9125–9130

Goodell MA, Brose K, Paradis G, Conner AS, Mulligan RC (1996) Isolation and functional properties of murine hematopoietic stem cells that are replicating in vivo. J Exp Med 183: 1797–1806

Goodrich LV, Milenkovic L, Higgins KM, Scott MP (1997) Altered neural cell fates and medulloblastoma in mouse patched mutants. Science 277: 1109–1113

Graham V, Khudyakov J, Ellis P, Pevny L (2003) SOX2 functions to maintain neural progenitor identity. Neuron 39: 749–765

Griguer CE, Oliva CR, Gobin E, Marcorelles P, Benos DJ, Lancaster JR, Jr., Gillespie GY (2008) CD133 is a marker of bioenergetic stress in human glioma. PLoS One 3: e3655

Gupta PB, Onder TT, Jiang G, Tao K, Kuperwasser C, Weinberg RA, Lander ES (2009) Identification of selective inhibitors of cancer stem cells by high-throughput screening. Cell 138: 645–659

Haupt Y, Bath ML, Harris AW, Adams JM (1993) bmi-1 transgene induces lymphomas and collaborates with myc in tumorigenesis. Oncogene 8: 3161–3164

Heddleston JM, Li Z, McLendon RE, Hjelmeland AB, Rich JN (2009) The hypoxic microenvironment maintains glioblastoma stem cells and promotes reprogramming towards a cancer stem cell phenotype. Cell Cycle 8: 3274–3284

Hemmati HD, Nakano I, Lazareff JA, Masterman-Smith M, Geschwind DH, Bronner-Fraser M, Kornblum HI (2003) Cancerous stem cells can arise from pediatric brain tumors. Proc Natl Acad Sci U S A 100: 15178–15183

Hide T, Takezaki T, Nakatani Y, Nakamura H, Kuratsu J, Kondo T (2009) Sox11 prevents tumorigenesis of glioma-initiating cells by inducing neuronal differentiation. Cancer research 69: 7953–7959

Hitoshi S, Alexson T, Tropepe V, Donoviel D, Elia AJ, Nye JS, Conlon RA, Mak TW, Bernstein A, van der Kooy D (2002) Notch pathway molecules are essential for the maintenance, but not the generation, of mammalian neural stem cells. Genes Dev 16: 846–858

Hope KJ, Jin L, Dick JE (2004) Acute myeloid leukemia originates from a hierarchy of leukemic stem cell classes that differ in self-renewal capacity. Nat Immunol 5: 738–743

Ignatova TN, Kukekov VG, Laywell ED, Suslov ON, Vrionis FD, Steindler DA (2002) Human cortical glial tumors contain neural stem-like cells expressing astroglial and neuronal markers in vitro. Glia 39: 193–206

Ikushima H, Todo T, Ino Y, Takahashi M, Miyazawa K, Miyazono K (2009) Autocrine TGF-beta signaling maintains tumorigenicity of glioma-initiating cells through Sry-related HMG-box factors. Cell stem cell 5: 504–514

Jacobs JJ, Kieboom K, Marino S, DePinho RA, van Lohuizen M (1999) The oncogene and Polycomb-group gene bmi-1 regulates cell proliferation and senescence through the ink4a locus. Nature 397: 164–168

Jain RK, di Tomaso E, Duda DG, Loeffler JS, Sorensen AG, Batchelor TT (2007) Angiogenesis in brain tumours. Nat Rev Neurosci 8: 610–622

Jin F, Zhao L, Zhao HY, Guo SG, Feng J, Jiang XB, Zhang SL, Wei YJ, Fu R, Zhao JS (2008) Comparison between cells and cancer stem-like cells isolated from glioblastoma and astrocytoma on expression of anti-apoptotic and multidrug resistance-associated protein genes. Neuroscience 154: 541–550

Joo KM, Kim SY, Jin X, Song SY, Kong DS, Lee JI, Jeon JW, Kim MH, Kang BG, Jung Y, Jin J, Hong SC, Park WY, Lee DS, Kim H, Nam DH (2008) Clinical and biological implications of CD133-positive and CD133-negative cells in glioblastomas. Lab Invest 88: 808–815

Kim JH, Yoon SY, Kim CN, Joo JH, Moon SK, Choe IS, Choe YK, Kim JW (2004) The Bmi-1 oncoprotein is overexpressed in human colorectal cancer and correlates with the reduced p16INK4a/p14ARF proteins. Cancer Lett 203: 217–224

Knobbe CB, Merlo A, Reifenberger G (2002) Pten signaling in gliomas. Neuro-oncol 4: 196–211

Knobbe CB, Trampe-Kieslich A, Reifenberger G (2005) Genetic alteration and expression of the phosphoinositol-3-kinase/Akt pathway genes PIK3CA and PIKE in human glioblastomas. Neuropathol Appl Neurobiol 31: 486–490

Kong DS, Kim MH, Park WY, Suh YL, Lee JI, Park K, Kim JH, Nam DH (2008) The progression of gliomas is associated with cancer stem cell phenotype. Oncol Rep 19: 639–643

Korur S, Huber RM, Sivasankaran B, Petrich M, Morin P, Jr., Hemmings BA, Merlo A, Lino MM (2009) GSK3beta regulates differentiation and growth arrest in glioblastoma. PLoS One 4: e7443

Kvinlaug BT, Huntly BJ (2007) Targeting cancer stem cells. Expert Opin Ther Targets 11: 915–927

Labuhn M, Jones G, Speel EJ, Maier D, Zweifel C, Gratzl O, Van Meir EG, Hegi ME, Merlo A (2001) Quantitative real-time PCR does not show selective targeting of p14(ARF) but concomitant inactivation of both p16(INK4A) and p14(ARF) in 105 human primary gliomas. Oncogene 20: 1103–1109

Lee CJ, Appleby VJ, Orme AT, Chan WI, Scotting PJ (2002) Differential expression of SOX4 and SOX11 in medulloblastoma. Journal of neuro-oncology 57: 201–214

Lendahl U, Zimmerman LB, McKay RD (1990) CNS stem cells express a new class of intermediate filament protein. Cell 60: 585–595

Leung C, Lingbeek M, Shakhova O, Liu J, Tanger E, Saremaslani P, Van Lohuizen M, Marino S (2004) Bmi1 is essential for cerebellar development and is overexpressed in human medulloblastomas. Nature 428: 337–341

Li Z, Bao S, Wu Q, Wang H, Eyler C, Sathornsumetee S, Shi Q, Cao Y, Lathia J, McLendon RE, Hjelmeland AB, Rich JN (2009) Hypoxia-inducible factors regulate tumorigenic capacity of glioma stem cells. Cancer cell 15: 501–513

Liao YL, Sun YM, Chau GY, Chau YP, Lai TC, Wang JL, Horng JT, Hsiao M, Tsou AP (2008) Identification of SOX4 target genes using phylogenetic footprinting-based prediction from expression microarrays suggests that overexpression of SOX4 potentiates metastasis in hepatocellular carcinoma. Oncogene 27: 5578–5589

Lino M, Merlo A (2009) Translating biology into clinic: the case of glioblastoma. Curr Opin Cell Biol 21: 311–316

Liu G, Yuan X, Zeng Z, Tunici P, Ng H, Abdulkadir IR, Lu L, Irvin D, Black KL, Yu JS (2006) Analysis of gene expression and chemoresistance of CD133+ cancer stem cells in glioblastoma. Mol Cancer 5: 67

Martin V, Xu J, Pabbisetty SK, Alonso MM, Liu D, Lee OH, Gumin J, Bhat KP, Colman H, Lang FF, Fueyo J, Gomez-Manzano C (2009) Tie2-mediated multidrug resistance in malignant gliomas is associated with upregulation of ABC transporters. Oncogene 28: 2358–2363

Massague J (2008) TGFbeta in Cancer. Cell 134: 215–230

Merlo A, Hausmann O, Wasner M, Steiner P, Otte A, Jermann E, Freitag P, Reubi JC, Muller-Brand J, Gratzl O, Macke HR (1999) Locoregional regulatory peptide receptor targeting with the diffusible somatostatin analogue 90Y-labeled DOTA0-D-Phe1-Tyr3-octreotide (DOTATOC): a pilot study in human gliomas. Clin Cancer Res 5: 1025–1033

Merlo A, Mueller-Brand J, Maecke HR (2003) Comparing monoclonal antibodies and small peptidic hormones for local targeting of malignant gliomas. Acta Neurochir Suppl 88: 83–91

Molofsky AV, Pardal R, Iwashita T, Park IK, Clarke MF, Morrison SJ (2003) Bmi-1 dependence distinguishes neural stem cell self-renewal from progenitor proliferation. Nature 425: 962–967

Molofsky AV, Slutsky SG, Joseph NM, He S, Pardal R, Krishnamurthy J, Sharpless NE, Morrison SJ (2006) Increasing p16(INK4a) expression decreases forebrain progenitors and neurogenesis during ageing. Nature 443: 448–452

Morshead CM, Reynolds BA, Craig CG, McBurney MW, Staines WA, Morassutti D, Weiss S, van der Kooy D (1994) Neural stem cells in the adult mammalian forebrain: a relatively quiescent subpopulation of subependymal cells. Neuron 13: 1071–1082

Nakamura M, Okano H, Blendy JA, Montell C (1994) Musashi, a neural RNA-binding protein required for Drosophila adult external sensory organ development. Neuron 13: 67–81

Newton HB (1994) Primary brain tumors: review of etiology, diagnosis and treatment. Am Fam Physician 49: 787–797

Newton HB (2004) Molecular neuro-oncology and development of targeted therapeutic strategies for brain tumors. Part 2: PI3K/Akt/PTEN, mTOR, SHH/PTCH and angiogenesis. Expert Rev Anticancer Ther 4: 105–128

Nowak K, Kerl K, Fehr D, Kramps C, Gessner C, Killmer K, Samans B, Berwanger B, Christiansen H, Lutz W (2006) BMI1 is a target gene of E2F-1 and is strongly expressed in primary neuroblastomas. Nucleic acids research 34: 1745–1754

Oberling (ed) (1944) The riddle of cancer. New Heaven : Yale Univ. Press

Okano H, Kawahara H, Toriya M, Nakao K, Shibata S, Imai T (2005) Function of RNA-binding protein Musashi-1 in stem cells. Exp Cell Res 306: 349–356

Okita K, Ichisaka T, Yamanaka S (2007) Generation of germline-competent induced pluripotent stem cells. Nature 448: 313–317

Orlando V (2003) Polycomb, epigenomes, and control of cell identity. Cell 112: 599–606

Palma V, Lim DA, Dahmane N, Sanchez P, Brionne TC, Herzberg CD, Gitton Y, Carleton A, Alvarez-Buylla A, Ruiz i Altaba A (2005) Sonic hedgehog controls stem cell behavior in the postnatal and adult brain. Development (Cambridge, England) 132: 335–344

Park IK, Qian D, Kiel M, Becker MW, Pihalja M, Weissman IL, Morrison SJ, Clarke MF (2003) Bmi-1 is required for maintenance of adult self-renewing haematopoietic stem cells. Nature 423: 302–305

Parsons DW, Jones S, Zhang X, Lin JC, Leary RJ, Angenendt P, Mankoo P, Carter H, Siu IM, Gallia GL, Olivi A, McLendon R, Rasheed BA, Keir S, Nikolskaya T, Nikolsky Y, Busam DA, Tekleab H, Diaz LA, Jr., Hartigan J, Smith DR, Strausberg RL, Marie SK, Shinjo SM, Yan H, Riggins GJ, Bigner DD, Karchin R, Papadopoulos N, Parmigiani G, Vogelstein B, Velculescu VE, Kinzler KW (2008) An Integrated Genomic Analysis of Human Glioblastoma Multiforme. Science 321: 1807–1812

Penuelas S, Anido J, Prieto-Sanchez RM, Folch G, Barba I, Cuartas I, Garcia-Dorado D, Poca MA, Sahuquillo J, Baselga J, Seoane J (2009) TGF-beta increases glioma-initiating cell self-renewal through the induction of LIF in human glioblastoma. Cancer cell 15: 315–327

Piccirillo SG, Reynolds BA, Zanetti N, Lamorte G, Binda E, Broggi G, Brem H, Olivi A, Dimeco F, Vescovi AL (2006) Bone morphogenetic proteins inhibit the tumorigenic potential of human brain tumour-initiating cells. Nature 444: 761–765

Piccirillo SG, Combi R, Cajola L, Patrizi A, Redaelli S, Bentivegna A, Baronchelli S, Maira G, Pollo B, Mangiola A, DiMeco F, Dalpra L, Vescovi AL (2009) Distinct pools of cancer stem-like cells coexist within human glioblastomas and display different tumorigenicity and independent genomic evolution. Oncogene 28: 1807–1811

Pistollato F, Chen HL, Rood BR, Zhang HZ, D'Avella D, Denaro L, Gardiman M, te Kronnie G, Schwartz PH, Favaro E, Indraccolo S, Basso G, Panchision DM (2009) Hypoxia and HIF1alpha repress the differentiative effects of BMPs in high-grade glioma. Stem cells (Dayton, Ohio) 27: 7–17

Pramoonjago P, Baras AS, Moskaluk CA (2006) Knockdown of Sox4 expression by RNAi induces apoptosis in ACC3 cells. Oncogene 25: 5626–5639

Purow BW, Haque RM, Noel MW, Su Q, Burdick MJ, Lee J, Sundaresan T, Pastorino S, Park JK, Mikolaenko I, Maric D, Eberhart CG, Fine HA (2005) Expression of Notch-1 and its ligands, Delta-like-1 and Jagged-1, is critical for glioma cell survival and proliferation. Cancer research 65: 2353–2363

Read TA, Fogarty MP, Markant SL, McLendon RE, Wei Z, Ellison DW, Febbo PG, Wechsler-Reya RJ (2009) Identification of CD15 as a marker for tumor-propagating cells in a mouse model of medulloblastoma. Cancer cell 15: 135–147

Reya T, Morrison SJ, Clarke MF, Weissman IL (2001) Stem cells, cancer, and cancer stem cells. Nature 414: 105–111

Sell S, Pierce GB (1994) Maturation arrest of stem cell differentiation is a common pathway for the cellular origin of teratocarcinomas and epithelial cancers. Lab Invest 70: 6–22

Shay JW, Keith WN (2008) Targeting telomerase for cancer therapeutics. Br J Cancer 98: 677–683

Shen Q, Goderie SK, Jin L, Karanth N, Sun Y, Abramova N, Vincent P, Pumiglia K, Temple S (2004) Endothelial cells stimulate self-renewal and expand neurogenesis of neural stem cells. Science 304: 1338–1340

Sherry MM, Reeves A, Wu JK, Cochran BH (2009) STAT3 is required for proliferation and maintenance of multipotency in glioblastoma stem cells. Stem cells (Dayton, Ohio) 27: 2383–2392

Shih AH, Holland EC (2006) Notch signaling enhances nestin expression in gliomas. Neoplasia (New York, NY 8: 1072–1082

Singh SK, Hawkins C, Clarke ID, Squire JA, Bayani J, Hide T, Henkelman RM, Cusimano MD, Dirks PB (2004) Identification of human brain tumour initiating cells. Nature 432: 396–401

Soeda A, Park M, Lee D, Mintz A, Androutsellis-Theotokis A, McKay RD, Engh J, Iwama T, Kunisada T, Kassam AB, Pollack IF, Park DM (2009) Hypoxia promotes expansion of the CD133-positive glioma stem cells through activation of HIF-1alpha. Oncogene 28: 3949–3959

Son MJ, Woolard K, Nam DH, Lee J, Fine HA (2009) SSEA-1 is an enrichment marker for tumor-initiating cells in human glioblastoma. Cell stem cell 4: 440–452

Song LB, Zeng MS, Liao WT, Zhang L, Mo HY, Liu WL, Shao JY, Wu QL, Li MZ, Xia YF, Fu LW, Huang WL, Dimri GP, Band V, Zeng YX (2006) Bmi-1 is a novel molecular marker of nasopharyngeal carcinoma progression and immortalizes primary human nasopharyngeal epithelial cells. Cancer research 66: 6225–6232

Strojnik T, Rosland GV, Sakariassen PO, Kavalar R, Lah T (2007) Neural stem cell markers, nestin and musashi proteins, in the progression of human glioma: correlation of nestin with prognosis of patient survival. Surg Neurol 68: 133–143; discussion 143–134

Suva ML, Riggi N, Janiszewska M, Radovanovic I, Provero P, Stehle JC, Baumer K, Le Bitoux MA, Marino D, Cironi L, Marquez VE, Clement V, Stamenkovic I (2009) EZH2 Is Essential for Glioblastoma Cancer Stem Cell Maintenance. Cancer research 69: 9211–9218

Takahashi K, Tanabe K, Ohnuki M, Narita M, Ichisaka T, Tomoda K, Yamanaka S (2007) Induction of pluripotent stem cells from adult human fibroblasts by defined factors. Cell 131: 861–872

Thon N, Damianoff K, Hegermann J, Grau S, Krebs B, Schnell O, Tonn JC, Goldbrunner R (2008) Presence of pluripotent CD133(+) cells correlates with malignancy of gliomas. Mol Cell Neurosci 43: 51–59

Valk-Lingbeek ME, Bruggeman SW, van Lohuizen M (2004) Stem cells and cancer; the polycomb connection. Cell 118: 409–418

van Es JH, van Gijn ME, Riccio O, van den Born M, Vooijs M, Begthel H, Cozijnsen M, Robine S, Winton DJ, Radtke F, Clevers H (2005) Notch/gamma-secretase inhibition turns proliferative cells in intestinal crypts and adenomas into goblet cells. Nature 435: 959–963

Vonlanthen S, Heighway J, Altermatt HJ, Gugger M, Kappeler A, Borner MM, van Lohuizen M, Betticher DC (2001) The bmi-1 oncoprotein is differentially expressed in non-small cell lung cancer and correlates with INK4A-ARF locus expression. Br J Cancer 84: 1372–1376

Voog J, Jones DL (2010) Stem cells and the niche: a dynamic duo. Cell stem cell 6: 103–115

Wang H, Lathia JD, Wu Q, Wang J, Li Z, Heddleston JM, Eyler CE, Elderbroom J, Gallagher J, Schuschu J, MacSwords J, Cao Y, McLendon RE, Wang XF, Hjelmeland AB, Rich JN (2009) Targeting interleukin 6 signaling suppresses glioma stem cell survival and tumor growth. Stem cells (Dayton, Ohio) 27: 2393–2404

Wang J, Sakariassen PO, Tsinkalovsky O, Immervoll H, Boe SO, Svendsen A, Prestegarden L, Rosland G, Thorsen F, Stuhr L, Molven A, Bjerkvig R, Enger PO (2008) CD133 negative glioma cells form tumors in nude rats and give rise to CD133 positive cells. Int J Cancer 122: 761–768

Wang J, Wang H, Li Z, Wu Q, Lathia JD, McLendon RE, Hjelmeland AB, Rich JN (2008) c-Myc is required for maintenance of glioma cancer stem cells. PLoS One 3: e3769

Wang J, Wakeman TP, Lathia JD, Hjelmeland AB, Wang XF, White RR, Rich JN, Sullenger BA (2009) Notch Promotes Radioresistance of Glioma Stem Cells. Stem cells (Dayton, Ohio) 28: 17–28

Ward RJ, Lee L, Graham K, Satkunendran T, Yoshikawa K, Ling E, Harper L, Austin R, Nieuwenhuis E, Clarke ID, Hui CC, Dirks PB (2009) Multipotent CD15+ cancer stem cells in patched-1-deficient mouse medulloblastoma. Cancer research 69: 4682–4690

Wegner M (1999) From head to toes: the multiple facets of Sox proteins. Nucleic acids research 27: 1409–1420

Wu MY, Hill CS (2009) Tgf-beta superfamily signaling in embryonic development and homeostasis. Dev Cell 16: 329–343

Xu Q, Yuan X, Liu G, Black KL, Yu JS (2008) Hedgehog signaling regulates brain tumor-initiating cell proliferation and portends shorter survival for patients with PTEN-coexpressing glioblastomas. Stem cells (Dayton, Ohio) 26: 3018–3026

Yokota N, Mainprize TG, Taylor MD, Kohata T, Loreto M, Ueda S, Dura W, Grajkowska W, Kuo JS, Rutka JT (2004) Identification of differentially expressed and developmentally regulated genes in medulloblastoma using suppression subtraction hybridization. Oncogene 23: 3444–3453

Yuki K, Natsume A, Yokoyama H, Kondo Y, Ohno M, Kato T, Chansakul P, Ito M, Kim SU, Wakabayashi T (2009) Induction of oligodendrogenesis in glioblastoma-initiating cells by IFN-mediated activation of STAT3 signaling. Cancer Lett 284: 71–79

Chapter 8
Cancer Stem Cells and Glioblastoma Multiforme: Pathophysiological and Clinical Aspects

Akio Soeda, Mark E. Shaffrey, and Deric M. Park

Introduction

Classification and Grading of Gliomas

Gliomas are classified by the World Health Organization (WHO) into four distinct grades based on histological features of cellularity, nuclear morphology, mitotic activity, and presence of necrosis and vascular proliferation (Louis et al. 2007) (Table 8.1). Although initially named after histological resemblance to normal glial cells such as astrocytes–astrocytoma and oligodendrocytes–oligodendroglioma, there is no compelling evidence that the corresponding type of glia represent the cell of origin. Grade I gliomas are often well-circumscribed and potentially curable by complete surgical resection. Patients with grade II tumors, also known as low-grade gliomas, may on occasion experience a protracted clinical course, but the infiltrating nature of the disease precludes a surgical cure. These tumors eventually transform into a higher grade over time. The median survival for patients with grade II tumors is 5 years (DeAngelis 2001); "low grade" is a histological description, not one intended to describe the clinical course. Grade III or anaplastic tumors exhibit mitotic figures and greater cellular density compared to grade II gliomas. Unfortunately, the most common type, grade IV or glioblastoma multiforme (GBM) is also the most aggressive. Even with multimodal treatment of surgery and chemoradiation (concurrent radiation and temozolomide), median survival of patients with GBM is approximately 1 year with occasional "long-term" survivors (Stupp et al. 2005). The observation that some patients live longer than the majority speaks to disease heterogeneity. It was suggested many years ago by Hans Joachim Scherer that GBM may develop by progressive dedifferentiation of lower-grade tumors (secondary GBM) or arise "de novo" without

---

A. Soeda • M.E. Shaffrey • D.M. Park (✉)
Department of Neurological Surgery, University of Virginia, PO Box 800212 Charlottesville, VA 22908, USA
e-mail: dmp3j@virginia.edu

Table 8.1 WHO grade of gliomas

Grade I	Pilocytic astrocytoma
	Subependymal giant cell astrocytoma
	Ependymoma
	Choroid plexus papilloma
Grade II	Astrocytoma (fibrillary, protoplasmic, gemistocytic)
	Oligodendroglioma
Grade III	Anaplastic astrocytoma
	Anaplastic oligodendroglioma
Grade IV	Glioblastoma multiforme
	Medulloblastoma
	Pineoblastoma

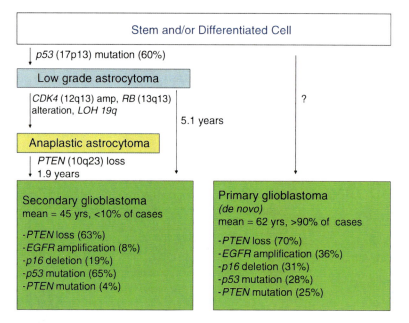

Fig. 8.1 Scherer suggested the presence of at least two distinct glioblastomas based on age, precursor lesion, and prognosis. This chart illustrates the timing and frequency of genetic changes. Reproduced with permission from the World Health Organization Press

a precursor lesion (primary GBM), an observation since supported by comparative molecular analyses (Fig. 8.1) (Peiffer and Kleihues 1999).

Clinical Features

Clinical symptoms and signs caused by the underlying brain tumor depend on the location of the tumor within the central nervous system (CNS) and can be aggravated by surrounding cerebral edema in more aggressive gliomas. Patients often present with seizures of focal onset or with non-localizing neurological symptoms, such as headache. Gliomas typically do not metastasize beyond the CNS, but they can spread via the cerebrospinal fluid and cause "drop metastases" along the spinal cord.

Treatment

Multimodality treatment of glioma consists of surgery and chemoradiation. Tissue sampling is necessary for histologic confirmation and assignment of grade. Although this can be achieved by a needle biopsy, extensive resection avoids the problem of possible under-sampling. There is also evidence suggesting better prognosis associated with aggressive tumor removal (Lacroix et al. 2001). Because surgical cure is not possible for infiltrating gliomas (grades II–IV), chemoradiation is often used. Fractionated external beam irradiation and/or chemotherapy prolong survival of patients with malignant glioma, although disease relapse is inevitable (Stupp et al. 2005; DeAngelis 2001). Treatment of recurrent glioma is tailored to the particular case, and may consist of surgery, focused irradiation, and medical therapy. There is no standard therapy for recurrent gliomas. The recent Food and Drug Administration (FDA) of the United States approval of bevacizumab, a neutralizing antibody directed against the vascular endothelial growth factor (VEGF), for recurrent GBM is potentially welcome news for those treating this challenging disease (Vredenburgh et al. 2007b).

Cancer Stem Cells

Neural Stem Cells

Tripotent neural stem cells (NSC) that are capable of differentiation into neurons, astrocytes, and oligodendrocytes have been isolated from various regions within the adult mammalian brain (Renfranz et al. 1991; Reynolds and Weiss 1992; Androutsellis-Theotokis et al. 2009). NSC can be propagated in vitro as an adherent monolayer with appropriate substratum or as unattached neurospheres in the absence of serum and presence of epidermal growth factor (EGF) and basic fibroblast growth factor (bFGF) (Reynolds et al. 1992; Doetsch et al. 2002; Johe et al. 1996; Ravin et al. 2008). In addition to multipotency, cells must exhibit an undifferentiated phenotype and a capacity for extensive self-renewal to satisfy the "neural stem cell" requirement. A variety of markers to identify the undifferentiated phenotype of NSC has been proposed. These markers include nestin, glial fibrillary acidic protein, CD133-prominin, CD15, notch, sox2, mushashi, and others (Lendahl et al. 1990; Doetsch et al. 1999; Uchida et al. 2000; Capela and Temple 2002; Androutsellis-Theotokis et al. 2006). However, the identity of the definitive marker for NSC remains elusive. Self-renewal is a necessary property for neural stem cell because the capacity of a cell to make a carbon copy of itself while producing a differentiated progeny, a process known as asymmetric division, is essential to prevent stem cell exhaustion. Cells that may resemble NSC in relation to expression of markers and multipotency, but with limited self-renewal capacity are referred to as "transit amplifying cells." Therefore, the assay needed to distinguish NSC from the transit amplifying cells is one of function, not expression of a particular marker.

CSC Background

Cancer stem cell biology is an area of intense interest of many investigators. Although attaining the technical feasibility to engage in the detailed study of stem cell biology is a relatively recent achievement, the concept that cancers share features of stem cells dates back many years. Rudolf Virchow, the noted German pathologist, suggested as early as the mid-nineteenth century that cancers originate from tissues with embryonic properties (Virchow 1858). Comparative histologic analyses convinced subsequent investigators to conclude that failed development of "embryonal rests" led to formation of cancers (Conheim 1875). Pathologic descriptions of cancers such as "blastoma" and "poorly differentiated" suggest the role of improper regional tissue specification. Therefore, it was suspected for quite some time that cancer may originate from lineage-uncommitted, developmentally primitive cells.

The development of technical abilities to support the growth of cells dissociated from tissue in a plastic dish and ability to recognize the identity of the cells have contributed to better understanding of both normal and cancer biology. In vivo studies of a melanoma cell line indicated heterogeneity as to the metastatic potential (Fidler and Kripke 1977). Although such observations do not necessarily suggest the presence of cancer cells with properties of "stemness," it does validate the idea that cancers may be composed of cells with heterogeneous functions. Using developmental markers associated with hematopoiesis, John Dick and colleagues identified a CD34+CD38− subpopulation of immature leukemia cells capable of recapitulating the disease in immunodeficient mice (Lapidot et al. 1994). This report prompted others to investigate different cancer types using developmental markers associated with stemness. Tumorigenic cancer cells with a stem cell phenotype were subsequently shown to be present in tumors of the brain, breast, lung, prostate, and colon (Ignatova et al. 2002; Singh et al. 2004; Al-Hajj et al. 2003; Collins et al. 2005; Kim et al. 2005; O'Brien et al. 2007; Park et al. 2007b). Some investigators have taken issue with the CSC concept because of lack of clear evidence that stem cells are the cell of cancer origin, and offer alternative nomenclature such as stem-like cancer cells, tumor-initiating cancer cells, and malignant progenitor cells. However, such argument is largely semantic as the cancer stem cell hypothesis neither implies CSC are derived from stem cells nor represent a rare population. The model merely suggests the presence of a cellular hierarchy based on differentiation status that correlates to tumor initiation, an idea not incompatible with a superimposed stochastic process of cellular diversity. Nevertheless, in spite of the interest in the field, there are no uniform criteria defining CSC.

Table 8.2 Proposed criteria for GCSC

Cancer-initiating ability upon orthotopic implantation (tumors should be a phenocopy of the tumor of origin)
Extensive self-renewal ability, demonstrated either ex vivo (by showing both sequential-clonogenic and population-kinetic analyses or in vivo (by serial, orthotopic transplantation)
Karyotypic or genetic alterations
Aberrant differentiation properties
Capacity to generate non-tumorigenic end cells
Multilineage differentiation capacity[a]

---
[a] Not a defining characteristic in all circumstances

Glioblastoma Stem Cells

GBM is an aggressive incurable cancer. Recognizing that extensive infiltration into surrounding normal white matter is a key barrier to surgical cure, attempts at removing the entire afflicted hemisphere were carried out (Dandy 1928). However, even such shockingly bold intervention failed, with tumor recurrence observed over time in the contralateral half of the brain. Because the clinically intractable behavior extends to therapies that can potentially expose the entire brain, GBM are thought of as chemoradiation-resistant due to the intrinsic heterogeneity of the cancer cells. A possible consideration of CSC hypothesis is that glioblastoma treatments may fail because they are directed at incorrect cellular targets (non-stem cell). The CSC concept suggests that because CSC are resistant to chemoradiation, current therapies will eventually lead to tumor recurrence, as has been seen in xenograft models. Experimental evidence indicates that GCSC are resistant to irradiation through enhanced capacity to regulate DNA damage responders (Bao et al. 2006a). In that specifically targeting the CSC may lead to more effective and durable clinical response, there is considerable interest in better understanding the identity and biology of GCSC (Park et al. 2007a; Rich and Eyler 2008; Park and Rich 2009).

Origin of GCSC

"Blastoma" is commonly used in the histopathologic classification of aggressive brain tumors such as glioblastoma, medulloblastoma, and pineoblastoma, suggesting a correlation between developmental immaturity of the cancer cells and poor outcome. Bailey and Cushing (1926) recognized early that a common pediatric brain tumor, medulloblastoma, might arise from undifferentiated embryonal cells. The expression of nestin, a marker of neural progenitors, has been demonstrated in a variety of brain tumors (Valtz et al. 1991; Tohyama et al. 1992). Subsequent studies showed that glioma cells with expression of stem cell markers can be propagated on plastic dishes and serially passaged in immunodeficient animals (Ignatova et al. 2002; Singh et al. 2003). Although the tumorigenic property was initially thought to be endowed only to CD133+ cells (Singh et al. 2004), that assertion has been called into question (Beier et al. 2007; Joo et al. 2008; Ogden et al. 2008; Wang et al. 2008). Table 8.2 outlines proposed criteria for defining GCSC, requirements that are more functional in nature than dependent on expression of specific markers (Vescovi et al. 2006).

The existence of cancer cells bearing stem cell markers has been demonstrated repeatedly (Ignatova et al. 2002; Singh et al. 2003, 2004; Galli et al. 2004; Lubensky et al. 2006). Yet it would be a fallacy to assume that cancer cells with stem cell markers originate from stem cells as deregulated genomic program associated with cancer can lead to ectopic expression of variety of proteins. In spite of the obvious challenges, the interest in determining the cell of origin is difficult to ignore because of potential impact on elucidating pathogenesis and improving therapy.

The stem cell origin model in which the cancer cells might exist in a hierarchical model is supported by both observation and experimental data. It has been suggested that only the native stem cells within the tissue of interest have been in existence for a sufficient period of time to accumulate necessary genetic damage for neoplastic transformation (Hanahan and Weinberg 2000; Dalerba et al. 2007). Apart from the time period required for development of tumors, stem cells appear to be more vulnerable to oncogene-induced transformation. Combined activation of *Ras* and *Akt*, two well-known oncogenes, can drive formation of tumors in neural progenitors, but not from differentiated astrocytes (Holland et al. 2000). Similar results are seen with loss of two tumor suppressor genes. In mice engineered to sequentially disrupt expression of *p53* and *NF1*, tumor formation was restricted to the subventricular zone, a region of the brain populated by NSC (Zhu et al. 2005). Also, activation of the platelet-derived growth factor receptor signaling can lead to appearance of hyperplastic lesions resembling gliomas in the subventricular zone (Jackson et al. 2006). Based on such observations, NSC have been proposed to be a suitable candidate for malignant transformation.

There is compelling experimental evidence to make a case for non-stem cells as the cell of origin for cancers. Although proponents of a stem cell origin point out that the longevity of stem cells make them vulnerable to necessary genetic defects, because stem cells are in most cases mitotically quiescent it is unlikely that sufficient genomic disruptions can accumulate during the limited number of mitotic events. As discussed above, coactivation of *Ras* and *Akt* did not lead to neoplastic transformation of differentiated astrocytes. However, the same investigators found that activation of *Ras* in the setting of disrupted *Ink4a-Arf*, a tumor suppressor gene commonly deleted in biallelic fashion in GBM, was of sufficient tumorigenic signal to transform both neural progenitors and differentiated astrocytes (Uhrbom et al. 2002). Similar results were obtained by a different group investigating the combined effect of activating the EGF receptor signaling with *INK4a-Arf* disruption (Bachoo et al. 2002). Experiments such these suggest that with an appropriate combination of signals, lineage-restricted differentiated cells can transform and attain tumorigenic capacity.

Review of experimental data indicates that the cell of origin for glioma may be both NSC and lineage-restricted cells. However, the studies are far from conclusive. It remains unclear how relevant these different mice models may be to human gliomagenesis. One potentially amusing interpretation of the experimental models is that they provide data to support both hierarchical and stochastic models

8 Cancer Stem Cells and Glioblastoma Multiforme: Pathophysiological...

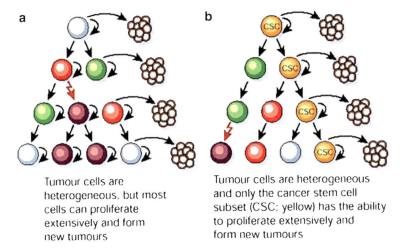

Fig. 8.2 The two models of cellular heterogeneity in cancer is illustrated. The stochastic model suggests that many different types of tumor cells have the potential to proliferate and form tumors while the hierarchical model states that only a small subpopulation of tumor cells possess proliferative and tumorigenic properties. Reproduced with permission from the Nature Publishing Group

(Fig. 8.2). The hierarchical model posits that cancer stem cells are at the hierarchy of differentiation from which most differentiated cancer cells are subsequently derived because only the CSC retain the capacity for extensive divisions (Reya et al. 2001). Such a view can explain why transplantation of CSC-enriched population leads to recapitulation of the parental tumor phenotype, while use of equal number of randomly chosen tumor cells is incapable of establishing a viable graft. Accordingly, failure of conventional cancer treatment is due to persistence of CSC. The stochastic model predicts that within the pool of cancer cells with diverse phenotype, any particular type can wield proliferative capacity. In this paradigm, cancer cells without expression of stem cell markers may divide and generate progenies with expression of stem cell markers. This model may be helpful in explaining the experiments indicating formation of tumors from lineage-restricted cells and the clinical observation of disease progression from relatively well-differentiated low-grade gliomas to poorly differentiated malignant glioma that contain greater proportion of identifiable CSC. Although it is likely that both hierarchical and stochastic processes are at work in gliomagenesis and progression, investigations directed to better define how the two processes interact should prove worthwhile (Rich and Eyler 2008; Lagasse 2008; Park and Rich 2009).

GCSC Xenograft Models

The defining feature of the murine hematopoietic stem cell is the ability of a single donor cell to rescue and establish long-term reconstitution of all blood cells in the recipient (Osawa et al. 1996). Such a simple assay does not exist for GCSC xenograft model because it has not yet been possible to recapitulate the parental tumor with injection of single cancer cell. Instead, one can demonstrate that a pool of glioma cells as few as 100, if tumorigenic, is enriched with glioma cancer stem cells (Singh et al. 2004). The tumorigenic efficiency appears to be variable for different solid tumors, as a recently reported study of single cell injections of melanoma cells into highly immunodeficient mice found that 25% of tumor cells were tumorigenic (Quintana et al. 2008). The investigators using animals that have features of both subacute combined immunodeficiency and interleukin-2 receptor gamma-null observed a lack of correlation between particular surface marker expressions with tumorigenicity, raising the possibility that a stochastic model may be more relevant for melanomas. Whether the inability to establish a glioma in animals with a single cell speaks to technical issues that can eventually be met or the underlying distinctive biology of GCSC remains unclear. Also, mere tumorigenicity is inadequate. Rather the CSC should recapitulate the heterogeneous cellular constituents of the tumor.

Molecular Pathways Regulating GCSC

Identifying the unique properties of CSC might allow for development and formulation of therapeutic strategies that are more effective and durable. Considerable interest has been directed to better understand the expression of markers specific for CSC. Such a strategy may lead to development of targeted therapies using antibodies or active immunotherapy. It may also be important to investigate signaling mechanisms employed by CSC for survival and proliferation because: (1) CSC appear to be more reliant on signaling networks active during development compared with differentiated cancer cells; (2) surface marker may not always correlate with tumorigenicity.

EGF–EGFR Pathway and Downstream Signaling

Activation of the EGFR pathway is a common occurrence in gliomas, a feature not necessarily unique to CSC. EGFR signaling is a critical driver of tumorigenesis in animal models and gene amplification is seen in as many as 50% of malignant gliomas (Bachoo et al. 2002; Smith et al. 2001). GCSC appear to be highly dependent on EGFR signaling for maintenance of the undifferentiated state and expansion of the CD133 fraction (Soeda et al. 2008). Not surprisingly in vitro propagation of GCSC requires supplementation with EGF ligand. Yet, clinical trials with EGF receptor tyrosine kinase inhibitors have for the most part been disappointing (van den Bent et al. 2009). This may be due to poor in vivo activity of the drugs in attenuating EGFR signaling (Lassman et al. 2005), downstream signaling activating events, and concomitant activation of multiple other receptor tyrosine kinases providing redundant growth signals (Stommel et al. 2007). The gene for tumor suppressor, phosphatase and tensin homolog (PTEN), is frequently deleted in GBM, leading to downstream activation of the pathway (Mellinghoff et al. 2005). Observation that GCSC show preferential sensitivity to Akt inhibition provides potential therapeutic opportunities as small molecule inhibitors are currently in early phase trials (Eyler et al. 2008).

STAT3

Persistent activation of the signal transducer and activator of transcription 3 (STAT3) is seen in many cancers. EGF along with a variety of cytokines that signal through gp130 complex can trigger STAT3 activation at the tyrosine-705 position through recruitment of janus kinase-2 (JAK2) (Zhong et al. 1994; Boulton et al. 1995). Although STAT3 has long been a target of interest in cancer, the observation that NSC are characterized by STAT3 activation at the serine-727 residue makes this molecule particularly relevant for GCSC (Androutsellis-Theotokis et al. 2006).

Basic Fibroblast Growth Factor

bFGF has been implicated in a broad scope of biological processes including limb development, wound healing, and tumorigenesis (Johnson and Tabin 1997). This ligand is also a critical component in supporting in vitro growth of human embryonic stem cells and NSC (Gritti et al. 1996). Although the exact contribution in gliomagenesis is unclear, bFGF is found in high concentrations in the brain and contributes to angiogenesis, a role that is likely relevant to glioma growth (Takahashi et al. 1992; Cao et al. 2003).

Bone Morphogenetic Protein

Bone morphogenetic proteins (BMPs) are growth factors and cytokines with a wide ranging spectrum of activities from embryonic patterning to regulation of skeletal development. BMP in concert with FGF can regulate development of neural progenitors (Lillien and Raphael 2000). BMP4 has been reported to be a potent inhibitor of GCSC (Piccirillo et al. 2006).

Bmi1

Bmi1, a polycomb ringer finger oncogene is a negative regulator of *INF4a* locus (Itahana et al. 2003). It has been shown to be essential in maintenance of self-renewal capacity of NSC (Molofsky et al. 2003). Therefore, the critical role of bmi1 in GCSC self-renewal is not a surprise (Abdouh et al. 2009). However, the report that bmi1 can regulate tumor development in *INK4a* independent manner suggest interaction with other pathways that will be of interest to determine (Bruggeman et al. 2007).

Sonic Hedgehog

Sonic hedgehog (Shh) is a member of the hedgehog family of morphogens. Medulloblastoma, a common childhood brain tumor that often shows activation of the Shh pathway responds favorably to inhibition of Shh (Berman et al. 2002). Recent reports that GBM CSC are also sensitive to Shh inhibition has led to clinical trials that are currently on-going (Bar et al. 2007).

Notch

The notch pathway, a highly conserved signaling network present in all metazoans, regulates cell fate decisions via cell–cell interaction (Artavanis-Tsakonas et al. 1983, 1999). Notch signaling has been shown to be key player in regulating the number of NSC (Androutsellis-Theotokis et al. 2006). Because notch signaling is involved in cell fate by direct contact and regulates NSC, it is a logical candidate for study in GCSC. Activation of the signaling cascade requires two distinct cleavages within the membranous region of the notch protein in the signal receiving cell, prior to liberation of the active notch intracellular domain. One such enzymatic reaction involves the γ-secretase protein, a complex for which inhibitors are available. Inhibitors of the γ-secretase enzyme seem to reduce formation of CD133+ GCSC neurospheres in vitro and attenuate tumorigenicity in mice models (Purow et al. 2005; Fan et al. 2009). Clinical trials in GBM using notch inhibitors are currently ongoing.

Hypoxia Inducible Factors

Regional tumor tissue hypoxia is seen in many cancers including GBM. A poorly developed intratumoral vascular network and resulting low oxygen environment interfere with adequate delivery of drugs and limits the therapeutic effectiveness of irradiation. This is in consonance with the observation that high hypoxia inducible factor (HIF) expression correlates with poor outcome for a variety of cancers (Aebersold et al. 2001; Birner et al. 2001; Shimogai et al. 2008). Two recent reports show that hypoxia by activating HIF leads to enhanced growth of GCSC (Li et al. 2009; Soeda et al. 2009). There is much interest in developing therapeutic approaches that target hypoxia. Inhibitors said to have specific activity against HIF-1α are currently in early phase trials. Semenza and colleagues reported that cardiac glycosides are inhibitors of HIF (Zhang et al. 2008). We found that in addition to HIF inhibition, cardiac glycosides disrupt growth of GCSC (Lee et al. 2009).

Clinical Implications of GCSC

Significance of GCSC in Neuro-Oncology

The possibility that treatment resistance and subsequent disease relapse of malignant gliomas may in part be dependent on activation of developmental-stem cell programs presents an occasion to recognize the importance of developmental biology in cancer. Gliomagenesis, progression to higher grade, and recurrence can be construed as a failed histogenesis. Better understanding the reasons for such failure may lead to unexpected insight into the disease process. CSC model remains a hypothesis, and there is no uniformly agreed-upon definition or laboratory assay to identify GCSC. Yet, the observation that dissociated cells from GBM can be enriched for tumorigenicity by prior selection has been repeatedly demonstrated by multiple investigators. GCSC also appear to play an important role in recruitment of blood vessels, a dynamic process required for subsequent growth of the tumor (Bao et al. 2006b). Gene signature study of several cancer types shows that expression of stem cell program genes is correlated with aggressive grade and poor outcome (Ben-Porath et al. 2008). Clearly, it is a field that merits further investigation. This is particularly applicable to neuro-oncology, a field that has witnessed frustratingly slow advancement. In clinical neuro-oncology the observation that temozolomide, an oral alkylating chemotherapeutic agent, may extend survival by additional 2–3 months for patients with GBM was considered to be a major therapeutic breakthrough (Stupp et al. 2005). Currently, rationally designed clinical approaches to target the GCSC are being conducted. These studies should offer further insight into the disease pathogenesis and point to new areas of investigation.

GCSC in Therapeutic Resistance

The CSC hypothesis provides a potential explanation for failure of conventional therapies for malignant gliomas. The extensive infiltration of tumor cells into surrounding normal brain precludes a complete removal of all tumor cells as there is no physical margin separating tumor cells from normal tissue. According to the model, the remaining CSC offer greater resistance to irradiation and chemotherapy (Bao et al. 2006a). Soon after adjuvant therapy, recapitulation of the tumor from remaining cells occurs as seen in xenograft orthotopic models. This explanation requires that CSC are left behind even after extensive resection and perhaps after hemispherectomy (Dandy 1928).

For a disease that offers few options at relapse, recurrent GBM has recently received United States FDA's approval for bevacizumab, a neutralizing antibody against VEGF (Vredenburgh et al. 2007a; Kreisl et al. 2009). With the recognition that GCSC might reside in perivascular niche much like their normal neural stem cell relatives (Palmer et al. 2000; Shen et al. 2004; Gilbertson and Rich 2007), it was hoped that anti-angiogenic therapy may offer added protection against GCSC

(Eyler and Rich 2008). It was hoped that the clinical effectiveness of bevacizumab in patients with recurrent GBM may involve attenuation of GCSC activity within the niche. However, unsuspected outcomes with this class of agents have been observed, as even short-term use led to increased metastatic potential and local invasiveness, including mouse models of GBM (Paez-Ribes et al. 2009; Ebos et al. 2009). Use of bevacizumab in patients with GBM has been associated with widespread increase in non-contrast enhancing lesions indicative of augmented invasiveness of the tumor cells (Iwamoto et al. 2009; Verhoeff et al. 2009). Immunohistochemical analysis showed increase in expression of HIF-1α in tumors treated with bevacizumab (Iwamoto et al. 2009). We reported that hypoxia (1% oxygen) confers expansion of the GCSC and maintenance of the undifferentiated phenotype through a mechanism in part dependent on HIF-1α induction (Soeda et al. 2009). We also found that the low oxygen environment promoted GCSC invasiveness (unpublished). It is conceivable that disease relapse after bevacizumab treatment involves activation of GCSC. A therapeutic strategy involving a combination of anti-angiogenic agent with a drug targeting hypoxia may be worth considering.

Conclusion

Since the formal declaration of "War on Cancer" brought on by President Nixon's signing of the "National Cancer Act of 1971," considerable progress has been witnessed for a variety of hematopoietic malignancies and solid tumors. Much of the improved cancer prognosis and the occasional cures have in origin, insights from laboratory investigations. Knowledge of brain tumor biology has expanded a great deal since 1971. There are several large text books filled with detailed information on brain tumor genetics, histopathology, signaling pathways, mouse models, and other biological processes involved with gliomagenesis. Yet, prognosis for patients with GBM has changed little over the same period. The CSC hypothesis, by emphasizing the presence of cellular heterogeneity, has generated much attention (both positive and negative) in neuro-oncology, and proposes an alternative treatment strategy. Does the presence of cellular diversity require invoking CSC hypothesis? Such requirement does not exist. Presence of intratumoral heterogeneity within a presumably clonally derived tumor cell population does not necessarily imply CSC are at work, although the CSC hypothesis offers at least an additional model to study this refractory disease. It therefore remains to be determined how successful we will be by targeting that element of tumor heterogeneity that is represented by its self-renewing CSC component.

References

Abdouh M, Facchino S, Chatoo W, Balasingam V, Ferreira J, Bernier G (2009) BMI1 sustains human glioblastoma multiforme stem cell renewal. J Neurosci 29 (28):8884–8896

Aebersold DM, Burri P, Beer KT, Laissue J, Djonov V, Greiner RH, Semenza GL (2001) Expression of hypoxia-inducible factor-1alpha: a novel predictive and prognostic parameter in the radiotherapy of oropharyngeal cancer. Cancer research 61 (7):2911–2916

Al-Hajj M, Wicha MS, Benito-Hernandez A, Morrison SJ, Clarke MF (2003) Prospective identification of tumorigenic breast cancer cells. Proceedings of the National Academy of Sciences of the United States of America 100 (7):3983–3988

Androutsellis-Theotokis A, Leker RR, Soldner F, Hoeppner DJ, Ravin R, Poser SW, Rueger MA, Bae SK, Kittappa R, McKay RD (2006) Notch signalling regulates stem cell numbers in vitro and in vivo. Nature 442 (7104):823–826

Androutsellis-Theotokis A, Rueger MA, Park DM, Mkhikian H, Korb E, Poser SW, Walbridge S, Munasinghe J, Koretsky AP, Lonser RR, McKay RD (2009) Targeting neural precursors in the adult brain rescues injured dopamine neurons. Proceedings of the National Academy of Sciences of the United States of America 106 (32):13570–13575

Artavanis-Tsakonas S, Muskavitch MA, Yedvobnick B (1983) Molecular cloning of Notch, a locus affecting neurogenesis in Drosophila melanogaster. Proceedings of the National Academy of Sciences of the United States of America 80 (7):1977–1981

Artavanis-Tsakonas S, Rand MD, Lake RJ (1999) Notch signaling: cell fate control and signal integration in development. Science (New York, NY) 284 (5415):770–776

Bachoo RM, Maher EA, Ligon KL, Sharpless NE, Chan SS, You MJ, Tang Y, DeFrances J, Stover E, Weissleder R, Rowitch DH, Louis DN, DePinho RA (2002) Epidermal growth factor receptor and Ink4a/Arf: convergent mechanisms governing terminal differentiation and transformation along the neural stem cell to astrocyte axis. Cancer cell 1 (3):269–277

Bailey P, Cushing H. (1926) A Classification of the Tumors of the Glioma Group on a Histogenetic Basis With a Correlated Study of Prognosis. Lippincott, Philadelphia

Bao S, Wu Q, McLendon RE, Hao Y, Shi Q, Hjelmeland AB, Dewhirst MW, Bigner DD, Rich JN (2006a) Glioma stem cells promote radioresistance by preferential activation of the DNA damage response. Nature 444 (7120):756–760

Bao S, Wu Q, Sathornsumetee S, Hao Y, Li Z, Hjelmeland AB, Shi Q, McLendon RE, Bigner DD, Rich JN (2006b) Stem cell-like glioma cells promote tumor angiogenesis through vascular endothelial growth factor. Cancer research 66 (16):7843–7848

Bar EE, Chaudhry A, Lin A, Fan X, Schreck K, Matsui W, Piccirillo S, Vescovi AL, DiMeco F, Olivi A, Eberhart CG (2007) Cyclopamine-mediated hedgehog pathway inhibition depletes stem-like cancer cells in glioblastoma. Stem cells (Dayton, Ohio) 25 (10):2524–2533

Beier D, Hau P, Proescholdt M, Lohmeier A, Wischhusen J, Oefner PJ, Aigner L, Brawanski A, Bogdahn U, Beier CP (2007) CD133(+) and CD133(−) glioblastoma-derived cancer stem cells show differential growth characteristics and molecular profiles. Cancer research 67 (9):4010–4015

Ben-Porath I, Thomson MW, Carey VJ, Ge R, Bell GW, Regev A, Weinberg RA (2008) An embryonic stem cell-like gene expression signature in poorly differentiated aggressive human tumors. Nature genetics 40 (5):499–507

Berman DM, Karhadkar SS, Hallahan AR, Pritchard JI, Eberhart CG, Watkins DN, Chen JK, Cooper MK, Taipale J, Olson JM, Beachy PA (2002) Medulloblastoma growth inhibition by hedgehog pathway blockade. Science (New York, NY) 297 (5586):1559–1561

Birner P, Schindl M, Obermair A, Breitenecker G, Oberhuber G (2001) Expression of hypoxia-inducible factor 1alpha in epithelial ovarian tumors: its impact on prognosis and on response to chemotherapy. Clin Cancer Res 7 (6):1661–1668

Boulton TG, Zhong Z, Wen Z, Darnell JE, Jr., Stahl N, Yancopoulos GD (1995) STAT3 activation by cytokines utilizing gp130 and related transducers involves a secondary modification requiring an H7-sensitive kinase. Proceedings of the National Academy of Sciences of the United States of America 92 (15):6915–6919

Bruggeman SW, Hulsman D, Tanger E, Buckle T, Blom M, Zevenhoven J, van Tellingen O, van Lohuizen M (2007) Bmi1 controls tumor development in an Ink4a/Arf-independent manner in a mouse model for glioma. Cancer cell 12 (4):328–341

Cao R, Brakenhielm E, Pawliuk R, Wariaro D, Post MJ, Wahlberg E, Leboulch P, Cao Y (2003) Angiogenic synergism, vascular stability and improvement of hind-limb ischemia by a combination of PDGF-BB and FGF-2. Nature medicine 9 (5):604–613

Capela A, Temple S (2002) LeX/ssea-1 is expressed by adult mouse CNS stem cells, identifying them as nonependymal. Neuron 35 (5):865–875

Collins AT, Berry PA, Hyde C, Stower MJ, Maitland NJ (2005) Prospective identification of tumorigenic prostate cancer stem cells. Cancer research 65 (23):10946–10951

Conheim V (1875) Congenitales, quergestreiftes muskelsarkom der nieren. Virchows Arch Pathol Anat Physiol Klin Med 65:64–69

Dalerba P, Cho RW, Clarke MF (2007) Cancer stem cells: models and concepts. Annual review of medicine 58:267–284

Dandy WE (1928) Removal of right cerebral hemisphere for certain tumors with hemiplegia. JAMA 90 (11):823–825

DeAngelis LM (2001) Brain tumors. The New England journal of medicine 344 (2):114–123

Doetsch F, Caille I, Lim DA, Garcia-Verdugo JM, Alvarez-Buylla A (1999) Subventricular zone astrocytes are neural stem cells in the adult mammalian brain. Cell 97 (6):703–716

Doetsch F, Petreanu L, Caille I, Garcia-Verdugo JM, Alvarez-Buylla A (2002) EGF converts transit-amplifying neurogenic precursors in the adult brain into multipotent stem cells. Neuron 36 (6):1021–1034

Ebos JM, Lee CR, Cruz-Munoz W, Bjarnason GA, Christensen JG, Kerbel RS (2009) Accelerated metastasis after short-term treatment with a potent inhibitor of tumor angiogenesis. Cancer cell 15 (3):232–239

Eyler CE, Foo WC, LaFiura KM, McLendon RE, Hjelmeland AB, Rich JN (2008) Brain cancer stem cells display preferential sensitivity to Akt inhibition. Stem cells (Dayton, Ohio) 26 (12): 3027–3036

Eyler CE, Rich JN (2008) Survival of the fittest: cancer stem cells in therapeutic resistance and angiogenesis. J Clin Oncol 26 (17):2839–2845

Fan X, Khaki L, Zhu TS, Soules ME, Talsma CE, Gul N, Koh C, Zhang J, Li YM, Maciaczyk J, Nikkhah G, Dimeco F, Piccirillo S, Vescovi AL, Eberhart CG (2009) Notch Pathway Blockade Depletes CD133-Positive Glioblastoma Cells and Inhibits Growth of Tumor Neurospheres and Xenografts. Stem Cells. doi:10.1002/stem.254

Fidler IJ, Kripke ML (1977) Metastasis results from preexisting variant cells within a malignant tumor. Science (New York, NY) 197 (4306):893–895

Galli R, Binda E, Orfanelli U, Cipelletti B, Gritti A, De Vitis S, Fiocco R, Foroni C, Dimeco F, Vescovi A (2004) Isolation and characterization of tumorigenic, stem-like neural precursors from human glioblastoma. Cancer research 64 (19):7011–7021

Gilbertson RJ, Rich JN (2007) Making a tumour's bed: glioblastoma stem cells and the vascular niche. Nature reviews 7 (10):733–736

Gritti A, Parati EA, Cova L, Frolichsthal P, Galli R, Wanke E, Faravelli L, Morassutti DJ, Roisen F, Nickel DD, Vescovi AL (1996) Multipotential stem cells from the adult mouse brain proliferate and self-renew in response to basic fibroblast growth factor. J Neurosci 16 (3):1091–1100

Hanahan D, Weinberg RA (2000) The hallmarks of cancer. Cell 100 (1):57–70

Holland EC, Celestino J, Dai C, Schaefer L, Sawaya RE, Fuller GN (2000) Combined activation of Ras and Akt in neural progenitors induces glioblastoma formation in mice. Nature genetics 25 (1):55–57

Ignatova TN, Kukekov VG, Laywell ED, Suslov ON, Vrionis FD, Steindler DA (2002) Human cortical glial tumors contain neural stem-like cells expressing astroglial and neuronal markers in vitro. Glia 39 (3):193–206

Itahana K, Zou Y, Itahana Y, Martinez JL, Beausejour C, Jacobs JJ, Van Lohuizen M, Band V, Campisi J, Dimri GP (2003) Control of the replicative life span of human fibroblasts by p16 and the polycomb protein Bmi-1. Molecular and cellular biology 23 (1):389–401

Iwamoto FM, Abrey LE, Beal K, Gutin PH, Rosenblum MK, Reuter VE, DeAngelis LM, Lassman AB (2009) Patterns of relapse and prognosis after bevacizumab failure in recurrent glioblastoma. Neurology 73 (15):1200–1206

Jackson EL, Garcia-Verdugo JM, Gil-Perotin S, Roy M, Quinones-Hinojosa A, VandenBerg S, Alvarez-Buylla A (2006) PDGFR alpha-positive B cells are neural stem cells in the adult SVZ that form glioma-like growths in response to increased PDGF signaling. Neuron 51 (2):187–199

Johe KK, Hazel TG, Muller T, Dugich-Djordjevic MM, McKay RD (1996) Single factors direct the differentiation of stem cells from the fetal and adult central nervous system. Genes & development 10 (24):3129–3140

Johnson RL, Tabin CJ (1997) Molecular models for vertebrate limb development. Cell 90 (6): 979–990

Joo KM, Kim SY, Jin X, Song SY, Kong DS, Lee JI, Jeon JW, Kim MH, Kang BG, Jung Y, Jin J, Hong SC, Park WY, Lee DS, Kim H, Nam DH (2008) Clinical and biological implications of CD133-positive and CD133-negative cells in glioblastomas. Laboratory investigation; a journal of technical methods and pathology 88 (8):808–815

Kim CF, Jackson EL, Woolfenden AE, Lawrence S, Babar I, Vogel S, Crowley D, Bronson RT, Jacks T (2005) Identification of bronchioalveolar stem cells in normal lung and lung cancer. Cell 121 (6):823–835

Kreisl TN, Kim L, Moore K, Duic P, Royce C, Stroud I, Garren N, Mackey M, Butman JA, Camphausen K, Park J, Albert PS, Fine HA (2009) Phase II trial of single-agent bevacizumab followed by bevacizumab plus irinotecan at tumor progression in recurrent glioblastoma. J Clin Oncol 27 (5):740–745

Lacroix M, Abi-Said D, Fourney DR, Gokaslan ZL, Shi W, DeMonte F, Lang FF, McCutcheon IE, Hassenbusch SJ, Holland E, Hess K, Michael C, Miller D, Sawaya R (2001) A multivariate analysis of 416 patients with glioblastoma multiforme: prognosis, extent of resection, and survival. Journal of neurosurgery 95 (2):190–198

Lagasse E (2008) Cancer stem cells with genetic instability: the best vehicle with the best engine for cancer. Gene therapy 15 (2):136–142

Lapidot T, Sirard C, Vormoor J, Murdoch B, Hoang T, Caceres-Cortes J, Minden M, Paterson B, Caligiuri MA, Dick JE (1994) A cell initiating human acute myeloid leukaemia after transplantation into SCID mice. Nature 367 (6464):645–648

Lassman AB, Rossi MR, Raizer JJ, Abrey LE, Lieberman FS, Grefe CN, Lamborn K, Pao W, Shih AH, Kuhn JG, Wilson R, Nowak NJ, Cowell JK, DeAngelis LM, Wen P, Gilbert MR, Chang S, Yung WA, Prados M, Holland EC (2005) Molecular study of malignant gliomas treated with epidermal growth factor receptor inhibitors: tissue analysis from North American Brain Tumor Consortium Trials 01-03 and 00-01. Clin Cancer Res 11 (21):7841–7850

Lee DH, Soeda A, Mintz A, Engh J, Egorin M, Pollack IF, Kassam A, Park DM (2009) Clinically achievable concentrations of digitoxin inhibit HIF-1alpha and induces apoptosis of human glioma stem cells. Neuro-oncology 11 (5):595

Lendahl U, Zimmerman LB, McKay RD (1990) CNS stem cells express a new class of intermediate filament protein. Cell 60 (4):585–595

Li Z, Bao S, Wu Q, Wang H, Eyler C, Sathornsumetee S, Shi Q, Cao Y, Lathia J, McLendon RE, Hjelmeland AB, Rich JN (2009) Hypoxia-inducible factors regulate tumorigenic capacity of glioma stem cells. Cancer cell 15 (6):501–513

Lillien L, Raphael H (2000) BMP and FGF regulate the development of EGF-responsive neural progenitor cells. Development (Cambridge, England) 127 (22):4993–5005

Louis DN, Ohgaki H, Wiestler OD, Cavenee WK (eds) (2007) WHO Classification of Tumours of the Central Nervous System. World Health Organization Classification of Tumours, 4th edn. International Agency for Research on Cancer (IARC), Lyon

Lubensky IA, Vortmeyer AO, Kim S, Lonser RR, Park DM, Ikejiri B, Li J, Okamoto H, Walbridge S, Ryschkewitsch C, Major E, Oldfield EH, Zhuang Z (2006) Identification of tumor precursor cells in the brains of primates with radiation-induced de novo glioblastoma multiforme. Cell cycle (Georgetown, Tex 5 (4):452–456

Mellinghoff IK, Wang MY, Vivanco I, Haas-Kogan DA, Zhu S, Dia EQ, Lu KV, Yoshimoto K, Huang JH, Chute DJ, Riggs BL, Horvath S, Liau LM, Cavenee WK, Rao PN, Beroukhim R, Peck TC, Lee JC, Sellers WR, Stokoe D, Prados M, Cloughesy TF, Sawyers CL, Mischel PS (2005) Molecular determinants of the response of glioblastomas to EGFR kinase inhibitors. The New England journal of medicine 353 (19):2012–2024

Molofsky AV, Pardal R, Iwashita T, Park IK, Clarke MF, Morrison SJ (2003) Bmi-1 dependence distinguishes neural stem cell self-renewal from progenitor proliferation. Nature 425 (6961): 962–967

O'Brien CA, Pollett A, Gallinger S, Dick JE (2007) A human colon cancer cell capable of initiating tumour growth in immunodeficient mice. Nature 445 (7123):106–110

Ogden AT, Waziri AE, Lochhead RA, Fusco D, Lopez K, Ellis JA, Kang J, Assanah M, McKhann GM, Sisti MB, McCormick PC, Canoll P, Bruce JN (2008) Identification of A2B5+CD133-tumor-initiating cells in adult human gliomas. Neurosurgery 62 (2):505–514; discussion 514–505

Osawa M, Hanada K, Hamada H, Nakauchi H (1996) Long-term lymphohematopoietic reconstitution by a single CD34-low/negative hematopoietic stem cell. Science 273 (5272):242–245

Paez-Ribes M, Allen E, Hudock J, Takeda T, Okuyama H, Vinals F, Inoue M, Bergers G, Hanahan D, Casanovas O (2009) Antiangiogenic therapy elicits malignant progression of tumors to increased local invasion and distant metastasis. Cancer cell 15 (3):220–231

Palmer TD, Willhoite AR, Gage FH (2000) Vascular niche for adult hippocampal neurogenesis. The Journal of comparative neurology 425 (4):479–494

Park DM, Li J, Okamoto H, Akeju O, Kim SH, Lubensky I, Vortmeyer A, Dambrosia J, Weil RJ, Oldfield EH, Park JK, Zhuang Z (2007a) N-CoR pathway targeting induces glioblastoma derived cancer stem cell differentiation. Cell cycle (Georgetown, Tex 6 (4):467–470

Park DM, Rich JN (2009) Biology of glioma cancer stem cells. Molecules and cells 28 (1):7–12

Park DM, Zhuang Z, Chen L, Szerlip N, Maric I, Li J, Sohn T, Kim SH, Lubensky IA, Vortmeyer AO, Rodgers GP, Oldfield EH, Lonser RR (2007b) von Hippel-Lindau disease-associated hemangioblastomas are derived from embryologic multipotent cells. PLoS medicine 4 (2):e60

Peiffer J, Kleihues P (1999) Hans-Joachim Scherer (1906–1945), pioneer in glioma research. Brain pathology (Zurich, Switzerland) 9 (2):241–245

Piccirillo SG, Reynolds BA, Zanetti N, Lamorte G, Binda E, Broggi G, Brem H, Olivi A, Dimeco F, Vescovi AL (2006) Bone morphogenetic proteins inhibit the tumorigenic potential of human brain tumour-initiating cells. Nature 444 (7120):761–765

Purow BW, Haque RM, Noel MW, Su Q, Burdick MJ, Lee J, Sundaresan T, Pastorino S, Park JK, Mikolaenko I, Maric D, Eberhart CG, Fine HA (2005) Expression of Notch-1 and its ligands, Delta-like-1 and Jagged-1, is critical for glioma cell survival and proliferation. Cancer research 65 (6):2353–2363

Quintana E, Shackleton M, Sabel MS, Fullen DR, Johnson TM, Morrison SJ (2008) Efficient tumour formation by single human melanoma cells. Nature 456 (7222):593–598

Ravin R, Hoeppner DJ, Munno DM, Carmel L, Sullivan J, Levitt DL, Miller JL, Athaide C, Panchision DM, McKay RD (2008) Potency and fate specification in CNS stem cell populations in vitro. Cell stem cell 3 (6):670–680

Renfranz PJ, Cunningham MG, McKay RD (1991) Region-specific differentiation of the hippocampal stem cell line HiB5 upon implantation into the developing mammalian brain. Cell 66 (4):713–729

Reya T, Morrison SJ, Clarke MF, Weissman IL (2001) Stem cells, cancer, and cancer stem cells. Nature 414 (6859):105–111

Reynolds BA, Tetzlaff W, Weiss S (1992) A multipotent EGF-responsive striatal embryonic progenitor cell produces neurons and astrocytes. J Neurosci 12 (11):4565–4574

Reynolds BA, Weiss S (1992) Generation of neurons and astrocytes from isolated cells of the adult mammalian central nervous system. Science (New York, NY) 255 (5052):1707–1710

Rich JN, Eyler CE (2008) Cancer stem cells in brain tumor biology. Cold Spring Harbor symposia on quantitative biology 73:411–420

Shen Q, Goderie SK, Jin L, Karanth N, Sun Y, Abramova N, Vincent P, Pumiglia K, Temple S (2004) Endothelial cells stimulate self-renewal and expand neurogenesis of neural stem cells. Science (New York, NY) 304 (5675):1338–1340

Shimogai R, Kigawa J, Itamochi H, Iba T, Kanamori Y, Oishi T, Shimada M, Sato S, Kawaguchi W, Sato S, Terakawa N (2008) Expression of hypoxia-inducible factor 1alpha gene affects the outcome in patients with ovarian cancer. Int J Gynecol Cancer 18 (3):499–505

Singh SK, Clarke ID, Terasaki M, Bonn VE, Hawkins C, Squire J, Dirks PB (2003) Identification of a cancer stem cell in human brain tumors. Cancer research 63 (18):5821–5828

Singh SK, Hawkins C, Clarke ID, Squire JA, Bayani J, Hide T, Henkelman RM, Cusimano MD, Dirks PB (2004) Identification of human brain tumour initiating cells. Nature 432 (7015): 396–401

Smith JS, Tachibana I, Passe SM, Huntley BK, Borell TJ, Iturria N, O'Fallon JR, Schaefer PL, Scheithauer BW, James CD, Buckner JC, Jenkins RB (2001) PTEN mutation, EGFR amplification, and outcome in patients with anaplastic astrocytoma and glioblastoma multiforme. Journal of the National Cancer Institute 93 (16):1246–1256

Soeda A, Inagaki A, Oka N, Ikegame Y, Aoki H, Yoshimura S, Nakashima S, Kunisada T, Iwama T (2008) Epidermal growth factor plays a crucial role in mitogenic regulation of human brain tumor stem cells. The Journal of biological chemistry 283 (16):10958–10966

Soeda A, Park M, Lee D, Mintz A, Androutsellis-Theotokis A, McKay RD, Engh J, Iwama T, Kunisada T, Kassam AB, Pollack IF, Park DM (2009) Hypoxia promotes expansion of the CD133-positive glioma stem cells through activation of HIF-1alpha. Oncogene 28 (45): 3949–3959

Stommel JM, Kimmelman AC, Ying H, Nabioullin R, Ponugoti AH, Wiedemeyer R, Stegh AH, Bradner JE, Ligon KL, Brennan C, Chin L, DePinho RA (2007) Coactivation of receptor tyrosine kinases affects the response of tumor cells to targeted therapies. Science (New York, NY) 318 (5848):287–290

Stupp R, Mason WP, van den Bent MJ, Weller M, Fisher B, Taphoorn MJ, Belanger K, Brandes AA, Marosi C, Bogdahn U, Curschmann J, Janzer RC, Ludwin SK, Gorlia T, Allgeier A, Lacombe D, Cairncross JG, Eisenhauer E, Mirimanoff RO (2005) Radiotherapy plus concomitant and adjuvant temozolomide for glioblastoma. The New England journal of medicine 352 (10):987–996

Takahashi JA, Fukumoto M, Igarashi K, Oda Y, Kikuchi H, Hatanaka M (1992) Correlation of basic fibroblast growth factor expression levels with the degree of malignancy and vascularity in human gliomas. Journal of neurosurgery 76 (5):792–798

Tohyama T, Lee VM, Rorke LB, Marvin M, McKay RD, Trojanowski JQ (1992) Nestin expression in embryonic human neuroepithelium and in human neuroepithelial tumor cells. Laboratory investigation; a journal of technical methods and pathology 66 (3):303–313

Uchida N, Buck DW, He D, Reitsma MJ, Masek M, Phan TV, Tsukamoto AS, Gage FH, Weissman IL (2000) Direct isolation of human central nervous system stem cells. Proceedings of the National Academy of Sciences of the United States of America 97 (26):14720–14725

Uhrbom L, Dai C, Celestino JC, Rosenblum MK, Fuller GN, Holland EC (2002) Ink4a-Arf loss cooperates with KRas activation in astrocytes and neural progenitors to generate glioblastomas of various morphologies depending on activated Akt. Cancer research 62 (19):5551–5558

Valtz NL, Hayes TE, Norregaard T, Liu SM, McKay RD (1991) An embryonic origin for medulloblastoma. The New biologist 3 (4):364–371

van den Bent MJ, Brandes AA, Rampling R, Kouwenhoven MC, Kros JM, Carpentier AF, Clement PM, Frenay M, Campone M, Baurain JF, Armand JP, Taphoorn MJ, Tosoni A, Kletzl H, Klughammer B, Lacombe D, Gorlia T (2009) Randomized phase II trial of erlotinib versus temozolomide or carmustine in recurrent glioblastoma: EORTC brain tumor group study 26034. J Clin Oncol 27 (8):1268–1274

Verhoeff JJ, van Tellingen O, Claes A, Stalpers LJ, van Linde ME, Richel DJ, Leenders WP, van Furth WR (2009) Concerns about anti-angiogenic treatment in patients with glioblastoma multiforme. BMC cancer 9 (1):444

Vescovi AL, Galli R, Reynolds BA (2006) Brain tumour stem cells. Nat Rev Cancer 6 (6):425–436. doi:nrc1889 [pii] 10.1038/nrc1889

Virchow R (1858) Cellular Pathology. Berlin

Vredenburgh JJ, Desjardins A, Herndon JE, 2nd, Dowell JM, Reardon DA, Quinn JA, Rich JN, Sathornsumetee S, Gururangan S, Wagner M, Bigner DD, Friedman AH, Friedman HS (2007a) Phase II trial of bevacizumab and irinotecan in recurrent malignant glioma. Clin Cancer Res 13 (4):1253–1259

Vredenburgh JJ, Desjardins A, Herndon JE, 2nd, Marcello J, Reardon DA, Quinn JA, Rich JN, Sathornsumetee S, Gururangan S, Sampson J, Wagner M, Bailey L, Bigner DD, Friedman AH, Friedman HS (2007b) Bevacizumab plus irinotecan in recurrent glioblastoma multiforme. J Clin Oncol 25 (30):4722–4729

Wang J, Sakariassen PO, Tsinkalovsky O, Immervoll H, Boe SO, Svendsen A, Prestegarden L, Rosland G, Thorsen F, Stuhr L, Molven A, Bjerkvig R, Enger PO (2008) CD133 negative glioma cells form tumors in nude rats and give rise to CD133 positive cells. International journal of cancer 122 (4):761–768

Zhang H, Qian DZ, Tan YS, Lee K, Gao P, Ren YR, Rey S, Hammers H, Chang D, Pili R, Dang CV, Liu JO, Semenza GL (2008) Digoxin and other cardiac glycosides inhibit HIF-1alpha synthesis and block tumor growth. Proceedings of the National Academy of Sciences of the United States of America 105 (50):19579–19586

Zhong Z, Wen Z, Darnell JE, Jr. (1994) Stat3: a STAT family member activated by tyrosine phosphorylation in response to epidermal growth factor and interleukin-6. Science (New York, NY) 264 (5155):95–98

Zhu Y, Guignard F, Zhao D, Liu L, Burns DK, Mason RP, Messing A, Parada LF (2005) Early inactivation of p53 tumor suppressor gene cooperating with NF1 loss induces malignant astrocytoma. Cancer cell 8 (2):119–130

Chapter 9
Breast Cancer Stem Cells

Nuria Rodríguez Salas, Enrique González González,
and Carlos Gamallo Amat

Introduction

We now know that some solid neoplasms, such as breast cancer, contain a subpopulation of cells with stem cell properties. This subpopulation, also known as cancer stem cells (CSC), could be responsible for the malignant transformation and the progression of the disease (Wicha et al. 2006). This hypothesis could be useful in clinical practice, not only explaining a lot of the remaining questions about the disease behavior, solving the frequent failure to conventional therapies, and defining the future therapeutic approach with the development of novel targeted therapies.

Breast cancer is one of the most common malignancies in women nowadays. Despite advances in early detection and adjuvant therapy, a substantial proportion of patients are diagnosed as advanced or metastatic disease at initial presentation or suffer a disease relapse. Metastatic breast cancer is incurable, chemotherapy obtain palliative effects, but only have a short benefit in terms of overall survival. This therapeutic limitation is associated with intrinsic neoplastic heterogeneity. The identification of tumor heterogeneity has highlighted the need to appropriately define different phenotypes for individual patients to enable more tailored therapies. The molecular profiling studies in breast cancer divided it in six phenotypes: Luminal-A, Luminal-B, Basal-like, Normal-breast-like, Her-2 enriched, and Claudin-low (Prat and Perou 2011); these studies finally show that breast cancer is a heterogeneous disease in terms of histology, therapeutic response, dissemination patterns to distant

N.R. Salas (✉)
Medical Oncology Unit, Hospital Universitario Infanta Leonor,
C/ Gran Vía del Este nº 80, 28031 Madrid, Spain
e-mail: nuria.rodriguez@salud.madrid.org

E.G. González
Surgery Department, Hospital del Henares, Madrid, Spain

C.G. Amat
Pathology Department, Medical School, Autónoma University, Madrid, Spain

sites, and patient outcome. Cancer stem cell hypothesis could explain not only this tumour heterogeneity, but also the intrinsic or acquired resistance to conventional therapy in breast cancer, like chemotherapy, radiotherapy, and hormonal maneuvers.

Solid Tissue Stem Cell: Definition

The term stem cell is referred to cells that have two basic properties: the capacity to self-renew and the capacity to generate daughter cells that can differentiate in different cell lineages (also called progenitor cells or transit-amplifying cells). The self-renewal program could be symmetric, in which one stem cell generates two identical daughter stem cells, or asymmetric in which one of the daughter cells become a stem cell like its mother, and the other daughter cell differentiates and loses the ability to divide again (this cell is committed to enter a differentiation pathway but not yet in end-stage differentiation) (Cicalese et al. 2009). This ability of the cells to divide asymmetrically is essential for generating diverse cell types during normal development. In this process, localized phosphorylation is responsible for asymmetric segregation on cell fate, and finally asymmetric mitosis occurs because of the exquisite functional control of centrosomes and microtubules dynamics. The relevance in tumor biology of this process and the pathways that controls it, such as Numb and Notch, is of increasing interest (Knoblich 2010).

The mechanisms that govern self-renewal are essential for the physiological remodeling and repairing in normal tissues. The pathways that regulate the self-renewal mechanisms are similar under physiological and pathological conditions. These pathways in mammary gland are Wnt pathway, Notch pathway, Hedgehog, and others alike: Prl/GH (*Prolactine/Growth Hormone*), EGF (*Epidermal Growth Factor*), TGFβ (*Transforming Growth Factor β*), and ER (*Estrogen Receptor*) (Dontu et al. 2003).

Normal Mammary Architecture: Epithelial Cell Hierarchy

The human mammary gland is a compound tubuloalveolar gland that consists of two lineages of epithelial cells: luminal cells (that differentiates into alveolar and ductal cells) and myoepithelial cells. A small number of ductal basally positioned small undifferentiated cells (also called electron-lucent cells when observed by electron microscopy) represents the normal mammary stem cells. These normal mammary stem cells provide the capacity for extensive cellular expansion associated with pregnancy and also generate differentiated cells that support lactation (Stingl et al. 2006).

The primitive breast stem cells are estrogen receptor negative. These cells generate progenitor cells that finally differentiate into luminal and myoepithelial lineages which are defined by specific sets of markers. Luminal lineages are positive to Keratins 7,8,18, and 19 and positive to Epithelial Specific Antigen (ESA). Myoepithelial cells in contrast are positive to Keratins 5, 14, and 19 and positive to Smooth Muscle Actin (SMA) (Villadsen et al. 2007).

The origin of mammary gland based in stem cells has been demonstrated in several experiments that show how one single stem cell can generate the entire mammary gland (Dontu et al. 2003).

The study of breast stem cells has come about through a variety of observations and experiments validated in vivo and in xenotransplant assays. Stem cells have the ability to repopulate mouse adult mammary glands upon serial transplantation (Shackleton et al. 2006).

A single cell characterized as either cluster of differentiation (CD) $CD29^{high}$/$CD24^+$ or $CD49f^{high}$/$CD24^+$ was able to reconstitute a functional mammary gland, when this cell was transplanted into a cleared mouse mammary fat pad. The murine mammary stem cell does not express estrogen receptors (ER) or progesterone receptors (PR) but it is able to give rise to ER and PR expressing cells (Vaillant et al. 2007).

In human tissues, stem cells could display anchorage-independent growth. Experiments using normal breast tissue from mammoplasties identificates cells that can grow in non-adherent substrata in serum-free conditions, and growth in spherical colonies called mammospheres. Mammosphere-initiating cells are capable of generating human mammary structures when transplanted into the fat pads of NOD/SCID mice (*immunosuppressed non-obese diabetic/severe combined immunodeficiency mice*) that had been "humanized" by the introduction of human mammary fibroblasts (Dontu et al. 2003; Liu et al. 2006).

Breast Cancer Stem Cells: Breast Cancer Cellular Origins and Tumorigenesis

The evidence of the normal stem cells in solid tissues forced investigators to reconsider how multistep tumor progression occurs. In the classical random or stochastic theory, a cell in an organ, such as the breast, can be transformed by the right combination of mutations. As a result, all or most of the cells in a fully developed cancer are equally malignant. Malignancies then progress through further mutation and clonal selection.

The cancer stem cell hypothesis proposes a different model based on a hierarchical organization (Wicha et al. 2006). According to this hypothesis, a neoplasia originates from the malignant transformation of an adult stem cell through the deregulation of the normally tightly regulated self-renewal program (Cobaleda et al. 2008). This model holds that a breast carcinoma may contain genetically and morphologically diverse populations of cells, including primitive stem cells, luminal or basal progenitor cells (also called sometimes transient amplifying cells), and terminally differentiated cells (Fig. 9.1).

Perhaps, a neoplasia arises from a tumorigenic CSC rather than from the much larger population of neoplastic progenitor cells. This means that mutations in one stem cell could be transmitted to descendant cells, which can then launch new clonal successions. Conversely, mutation then strikes the genomes of transit-amplifying cells cannot be transmitted further, because these cells only have a limited replicative ability. Therefore, the CSC represent a minority of the neoplastic cells in tumor

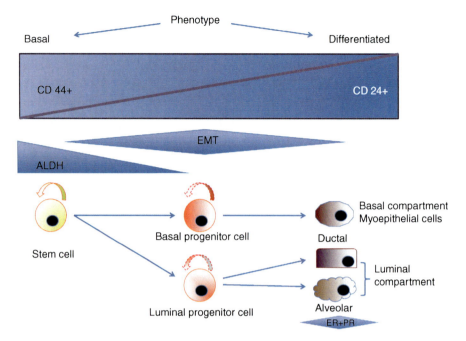

Fig. 9.1 Markers and schematic model of cellular hierarchy in the mammary gland. EMT: Epithelial-to-mesenchymal transition. Through this complex process epithelial cells lose cell-to-cell contacts and cell polarity, down-regulate epithelial associated genes, and acquire mesenchymal gene expression and undergo major changes in their cytoskeleton. ALDH1: enzyme responsible for the oxidation of intracellular aldehydes. Plays a role in early differentiation of stem cells. CD44: encodes by alternative splicing two variants: CD44H mainly expressed on cells of the lymphohematopoietic origin and plays an important role in adhesion and cell migration. CD44E is preferentially expressed on epithelial cells and is involved in promoting homotypic cell aggregation. CD24: encodes a small, heavily glycosylated cell-surface adhesion protein. ER: estrogen receptor PR: progesterone receptor

masses, while the progenitor and differentiated neoplastic cells represent the majority of the bulky of the tumour. Most cancer cells have only limited proliferative potential, but CSC have self-renewal capacity that could drive the tumorigenesis process. The CSC are probably responsible for the repopulation of tumor mass reminding normal mammary glands.

The cancer stem cell biology need also be understood in the context of tumor-stroma interactions. Just as normal stem cells are maintained in niches that provide specialized microenvironment. These niches contain stromal cells, fibroblasts, and immune cells and maintain and permit the growth of neoplastic cells. There is a complex and dynamic interplay breast cancer cells and stroma that permit invasion and metastasis inducing process such as epithelial-to-mesenchymal transition, interaction with cytokines such as TGF-β and IL-6, IL-8, SDF-1, and others that can govern cancer cell homing to sites of distant metastases (Fig. 9.2).

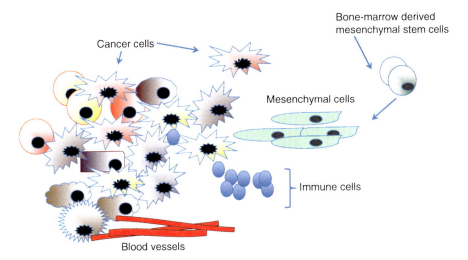

Fig. 9.2 Breast tumoral niche. *Yellow*: normal and tumoral stem cells. *Orange*: normal and tumoral progenitor cells. *Red*: normal and tumoral basal differentiated cells. *Purple*: normal and tumoral ductal cells. *Brown*: normal and tumoral alveolar cells. *Green*: mesenchymal cells and bone-marrow derived mesenchymal stem cells. *Blue*: immune cells

Recently the mesenchymal stem cells (MSC) have been implicated in the breast CSC niches. This heterogeneous and multipotent subset of mesenchymal stroma cells have fibroblast-like morphology, form colonies that can differentiate into adypocytes, osteocytes, and chondrocytes; are important in the control of niches through its recruitment from bone-marrow to this niches by the signals of IL-6 and IL-8 and its receptors in the stem cells (CXCL7, CXCR1, respectively). The interaction between MSC and CSC have been demonstrated both in vitro and in in vivo mouse models. The cytokine network involving CSC and the microenvironment stimulates self-renewal of breast CSC and accelerate the growth of human breast cancer, and have focused the attention of investigators to target this novel pathway (Liu et al. 2011).

In summary, the cancer stem cell hypothesis has gained considerable interest in the recent years. This theory states that cells in a cancer are maintained by a small subset of cells, defined as CSC. These cells possess properties of normal tissue stem cells, including indefinite self-renewal, slow replication, resistant to xenobiotics (including chemotherapeutics), high DNA-repair capacity, and the ability to give rise to daughter cells that differentiate. These daughter cells are arrested in various stages of differentiation and mutational status, resulting in tumor heterogeneity and mixed responses to standard and investigational therapies. By dividing asymmetrically, CSC maintain the stem cell pool and simultaneously generate committed progenitor cells and finally the tumor cells that are the bulky of the neoplasia.

This hypothesis provides a possible explanation to why cancer may be so difficult to eradicate (Stingl and Caldas 2007). If this model is correct, the therapeutic eradication of cancer requires elimination of the CSC. Chemotherapeutic strategies using antimitotic agents, DNA-damaging agents, antimetabolites or even growth factor receptor-kinase inhibitors often are aimed at actively proliferating cells. These treatments are likely to be ineffective against CSC, which can remain quiescent for extended periods of time. Effective therapies for CSC, with deregulated pathways that govern self-renewal, may have to target symmetric division. However, potential difficulties lie in the narrow therapeutic index, since normal stem cells have the same self-renewal signaling pathway. A cytotoxic chemotherapy combination approach may be useful for the elimination of the bulk of the tumor and prime for stem cell proliferation followed by a cancer stem cell-targeted therapy.

Breast Cancer Stem Cells Experimental Models

The MCF-10F cells are non-transforming ER-negative cells line, because of the malignant transformation of this cell line using 17β-estradiol investigators could produce poorly differentiated tumors with a basal-like phenotype. The genomic alteration of these transformed cell lines shows stem cell characteristics, such as epithelial-to-mesenchymal phenotype, CD44+/CD24- cell surface markers, show asymmetric division and alterations in expression of Numb and Notch pathways (Russo et al. 2010).

Mouse models of breast carcinogenesis using the mammary specific mouse mammary tumor virus (MMTV) promoter, have suggested that different oncogene targets mammary stem cells or progenitor cells. MMTV-Wnt1 transgenic mice developed tumors that expressed both epithelial and myoepithelial markers (Li et al. 2003). This data suggests that Wnt pathway, among others, may affect primitive stem or progenitor cells perhaps by involving deregulation of self-renewal pathways.

Experiments in rats with chemical carcinogens and in mouse infected with MMTV show that breast tumor arise only if the "aggression" occurs earlier in the life of the animal. This data suggest that breast cancer initiation occurs in a period between puberty and first pregnancy, period named by Russo as "*susceptibility window*" (Russo et al. 1982). The normal breast stem cells are target for oncogenic events, for example, ionizing radiation and other events at time unknown. Many years later these cells suffer the stimuli of endogenous (estrogen stimuli) or exogenous agents developing breast cancer.

In human breast cancer different reports try to prove how the stem cells are targets for malignant transformation, by the demonstration of mutational changes in genes or in pathways essential for the self-renewal process. BRCA1 gene (*Breast Cancer tumor suppressor gene 1*), implicated in inherited breast cancer, plays an important role in stem cell self-renewal and in differentiation of a progenitor cell. Because of the BRCA1 gene function in DNA repair and in maintaining chromosome stability, researchers have proposed that the loss of BRCA1 function may produce genetically unstable stem or progenitor cells that serve as prime target for further carcinogenic events (Liu et al. 2008).

9 Breast Cancer Stem Cells

It was proposed that breast carcinogenesis may be initiated by epigenetic changes such as silencing of p16^{INK4a}. Since p16^{INK4a} is known to be a downstream target of the polycomb gene BMI1 which regulates stem cell self-renewal (Holst et al. 2003).

Isolation and Characterization of Breast Cancer Stem Cells

The isolation and characterization of CSC remains a challenge. In order to validate the method selected as an appropriate technique to isolate CSC, it is crucial to use assays that can assess the stem cell properties of its self-renewal and its differentiation.

Xenograft

The xenograft model is based on the orthotopic injection of human cancer cells into the humanized cleared fat pad of immunodeficient mice. It can initiate and maintain the tumor growth upon serial passages. It is presently the most robust model for demonstrating stem cell properties. In addition to self-renewal, CSC also retain the ability to differentiate, albeit abnormally, also generating non-self-renewing cell population that constitutes the bulk of the tumor (Polyak 2007).

In Vitro assays

The cell culture technique adapted from normal breast tissue is based on the mammosphere technique: Tumorosphere-initiating cells have stem cell properties including the ability to survive and grow in suspension in serum-free conditions. In contrast, more differentiated tumor cells are anchorage-dependent and undergo anoikis in these conditions (Ponti et al. 2005). The tumorosphere culture has also been used in different studies to screen for drugs capable of targeting the cancer stem cell populations.

CD44$^+$/CD24$^{-/low}$/lin$^-$ Phenotype

By using cell surface markers and flow cytometry we can identify a population of cells in human breast cancer that display cancer stem cell properties. This population was defined by the expression of cell surface markers (CD44$^+$/CD24$^{-/low}$/lin$^-$). As few as 200 of these cells were able to form tumors in NOD/SCID mice, whereas 20,000 cells that did not display this phenotype failed to generate tumors (Dontu et al. 2003).

Side Population Technique

This method is useful to identify stem cell population in breast cancer cell lines. This method is based on the overexpression of transmembrane transporters, such as the adenosine triphosphate (ATP)-binding cassettes molecule ABCG2/BCRP1 in stem cells. These molecules actively exclude vital dyes such as Hoechst 33342 or Rhodamine 123, a property not found in differentiated cells that retain the dye (Kim et al. 2002). A side population was isolated from the MCF7 breast cancer cell line utilizing Hoechst dye exclusion. This population, representing 2% of the total cells, contained the tumorigenic fraction, as demonstrated by transplantation in NOD/SCID mice.

Aldehyde Dehydrogenase 1

Ginestier et al. (2007) first described the expression of Aldehyde Dehydrogenase 1 (ALDH1) as a stem cell marker that can be utilized to isolate human mammary stem cells. This ALDH1 expression can be detected utilizing an enzymatic assay (ALDEFLUOR; Aldagen, Durham, North Carolina). ALDH1 is a detoxifying enzyme responsible for the oxidation of intracellular aldehydes. This enzyme plays a role in early differentiation of stem cells through its function in oxidizing retinol into retinoic acid. The researches have demonstrated that ALDEFLUOR-positive cells isolated from human breast cancer display properties of CSC, through the ability of these cells, but not ALDEFLUOR-negative cells, to generate tumors in NOD/SCID mice. Serial passage of the ALDEFLUOR-positive cells generates tumors that recapitulated the phenotypic heterogeneity of the initial tumor. Interesting enough, the ALDEFLUOR-positive cell population detected in breast tumors has a small overlap with the previously described cancer stem cell, $CD44^+/CD24^-/lin^-$ phenotype (Al-Hajj et al. 2003). In this report analyzing ALDH1 expression in 577 human breast carcinomas, the authors have shown that this stem or progenitor cell marker is a powerful predictor of poor clinical outcome and correlates with tumor histological grade, ER and PR negativity, proliferation index as assessed by Ki-67 expression, and Her2 overexpression. Other authors study the different isoforms of ALDH in breast CSC, characterized 19 isoforms of this enzyme in patients' breast tumors by genome microarray expression analysis and quantitative PCR. They show that the ALDH1A3 isoforms have the best correlation (better that the ALDH1A1 isoform more frequently studied in breast specimens by immunohistochemistry), with the ALDH activity in vivo, and correlates with tumor grade, disease stage and is predictive of the tumor metastatic spread. ALDH1A3 isoform could be a novel marker with clinical applicability (Marcato et al. 2011).

Clinical Outcome

Breast Cancer Heterogeneity

In a recent study published by Pece et al., the authors report the purification and molecular characterization of normal human mammary stem cells from cultured mammospheres, using a fluorescent marker, PKH26, which labels quiescent cells (Pece et al. 2010). PKH26-positive cells formed both basal and luminal cells in two-dimensional differentiation assay. These PKH26-positive cells were able to re-establish mammary development in the fat pad of immunosuppressed mice. The researchers performed microarray expression profiles on these PKH26-positive cells, and the signature obtained was used as a marker of normal and breast CSC. The data in breast cancer shows a correlation between higher levels of stem cells gene signature and poorly differentiation grade cancers. The author has also demonstrated that the stem cells isolated from poorly differentiated breast tumors had significantly a higher number of stem cells than well-differentiated tumors.

Metastasis and Tumor Dormancy

Approximately half of the women with early breast cancer suffer relapse of the illness, sometimes long after the primary treatment and remission. This relapse can be explained based on the persistence of dormant CSC. The mechanisms through which these cells reawake have not yet been identified. The study of these processes may be essential for the complete eradication of these CSC (Blau et al. 2001).

The dissemination of breast cancer is the main cause of death in breast cancer patients. Using the stem cell hypothesis we can conclude that only CSC are capable of giving rise to a tumor metastasis, although the tumor sheds millions of cells into the blood, only a few of them can generate secondary tumors (Gonzalez-Sarmiento and Perez-Losada 2008).

Metastatic cascade consists of a series of processes that move tumor cells from the primary tumor to distant location. Various factors are involved in intravasation, extravasation, and survival in bloodstream and in the target organ. The induction of epithelial-to-mesenchymal transition in breast cancer cells results in the acquisition of stem-cell properties, including the ability to form mammospheres, resistance to apoptotic signals, facilitates the blood intravasation, and generation of circulating tumor cells. Different studies show that a significant proportion of circulating tumor cells shows stem cell phenotype, such as expression of NOTCH1, ALDH1, and are typically triple negative (estrogen and progesterone receptor-negative and HER2-negative) (Mego et al. 2010).

Detection and monitoring circulating cancer cells in blood samples, some of them with stem cell properties, could be an interesting predictive test useful in monitoring the treatment and outcome of breast cancer patients, and perhaps also investigate novel targeted therapies and allows in the future personalized therapy.

Treatment Response

Like normal stem cells, CSC are predominantly quiescent cells in G0-phase. The current cancer therapies are targeted to proliferating cells. Stem cells have membrane proteins, such as ATP-binding cassettes that can pump out chemotherapeutic agents (Li et al. 2008). Enzymes such as ALDH, which are highly expressed in stem cells, are able to metabolize chemotherapeutic agents such as cyclophosphamide (Bunting et al. 1994). CSC may contribute to radioresistance through preferential activation of the DNA damage checkpoint response and an increase in DNA repair capacity (Phillips et al. 2006).

Putting these facts together, the stem cell hypothesis explains how difficult it is to completely eradicate all breast cancer cells. Through this hypothesis we only fully eradicate all cancer cells if we are able to target CSC with self-renewal capacity.

Identification of Breast Cancer Stem Cells: Clinical Feasibility and Clinical Utility

The ALDH1 expression analysis in 577 human breast carcinomas show that this stem cell marker is a poor prognostic predictive marker in breast cancer and it is correlated with histological grade, hormonal receptors negativity, and elevated expression of the proliferation index measured by Ki67 expression and with Her2 positive status. Other studies using this technique corroborate these results in relation to the prognostic impact in human breast carcinomas (Marcato et al. 2011; Morimoto et al. 2009; Resetkova et al. 2010; Tanei et al. 2009; Charafe-Jauffret et al. 2009).

The efficiency of the Her2-targeted therapies may be explained by the role of Her2 in the regulation of the cancer stem cell population. Interestingly enough, in the series of 577 breast carcinomas analyzed by Ginestier et al. (2007), a significant correlation between expression of the stem cell marker ALDH1 and Her2 was found. Furthermore, Korkaya et al. (2008) have recently shown that Her2 overexpression in normal human mammary epithelial cells as well as mammary carcinomas increases the proportion of stem cells as indicated by ALDH1 expression. The clinical relevance of this was demonstrated in a recent neoadjuvant breast cancer trial. Tumor regression induced by neoadjuvant chemotherapy was associated with an increase in CD44+/CD24− CSC in residual tumors. In contrast, breast cancers with Her2 amplification had an increased proportion of CD44+/CD24− cells before treatment that was reduced by the administration of the Her1 and Her2 dual oral inhibitor Lapatinib (Li et al. 2008).

9 Breast Cancer Stem Cells

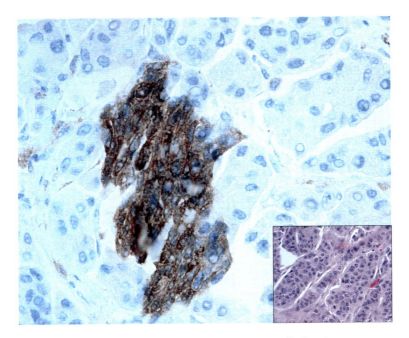

Fig. 9.3 ALDH1 immunoexpression in a group of breast cancer cells (*inset*)

In Fig. 9.3 we show the ALDH1 immunoexpression in a group of breast cancer cells in a clinical specimen.

Future Perspectives in Therapy: Novel Stem Cells-Targeted Therapies

Nowadays we have the possibility to design rationale strategies for targeted therapies that reverses the mechanisms that are used by the CSC to establish the metastases niche, blocking the mechanisms that allow this cell to resist conventional chemo-, hormone-, and radiotherapies, and finally block the cancer stem cell survival. Different targeted therapies are under clinical trials: Notch pathways inhibitors such as γ-secretase inhibitor (this pathway is essential for the asymmetric division of CSC) (Nickoloff et al. 2003). Hedgehog inhibitors, such as cyclopamide analogs (this pathway is responsible for normal mammary gland development and is implicated in stem cell self-renewal) (Hatsell and Frost 2007). Oral hedgehog inhibitor are in phase II trials in combination with chemotherapy and are relatively non-toxic. Other strategies are (1) the blockage of PTEN (*phosphatase and tensin homolog on chromosome 10*) and therefore the survival pathway mediated by PI3K/mTOR (*lipid kinase phosphoinositide 3-kinase/mamalian target of rapamicine*) with the mTOR inhibitors: everolimus and temsirolimus (Saal et al. 2008), and (2) the replacement of the function of p53 pathway with Mdm-2 antagonists due to the importance of PI3K and p53 pathways that are deregulated in CSC and are responsible for the deregulation of the self-renewal mechanism and the chemotherapy resistance (Wang and El-Deiry 2008).

Another targeted therapy approach is to target the network between Her2 signaling and Notch pathway. Magnifico and cols using breast cancer cell lines demonstrates the important role of Her2 in maintaining CSC population, this is the explanation of the efficacy of Trastuzumab in those breast cancer that have amplification of Her2 and, also in a small proportion of non-Her2-amplified tumors (Korkaya and Wicha 2009; Magnifico et al. 2009). A relationship between Her2 and Notch pathway has been suggested by the demonstration that the Her2 promoter contains Notch-binding sequences, so that Her2-overexpression cells display activated Notch signaling; in contrast, inhibition of Notch using small interfering RNA or γ-secretase inhibitors results in down-regulation of Her2. Targeting Her2 with the dual oral agent Lapatinib in addition to chemotherapy reduces the CSC population (Liu and Wicha 2010).

Notch are a family of four types of transmembrane receptors with five different ligands, that regulate in the stem cells the self-renewal pathways and cell-fate determination. There are different strategies to target Notch: γ-secretase inhibitors, ligands antibodies and interfering with the cytoplasmic nuclear mediators ADAM, and MAML (Harrison et al. 2010a). Notch4 are the most important in cancer stem cell, targeting this receptor in in vivo and in vitro models produces the more robust effect with a complete inhibition of tumor initiation (Harrison et al. 2010b).

Another development strategy to target breast cancer stem cell is through blockade IL-8 receptor, CXCR1, using specific antibodies or repertaxin, a small molecule CXRC1 inhibitor. In mouse breast cancer xenografts repertaxin reduce the development of systemic metastasis. In cells lines Ginestier y cols, demonstrates that chemotherapy affect only at the bulk of the tumor that are sensitive, for example, to docetaxel, but is this model breast CSC are stimulated via IL-8 bystander effect and increases their number and still more, these stem cells are resistant to apoptosis via FASL. Repertaxin treatment blocks IL-8 CXCR1 signaling and inhibits breast CSC self-renewal and survival. When repertaxin treatment is combined with chemotherapy the CSC are sensitized to the bystander killing effect mediated by FASL (Ginestier et al. 2010).

Currently there are multiple potential anti-CSC agents in preclinical and clinical trials. While these are promising agents the likelihood of clinical success will depend on many aspects including safety, trial design, and rational endpoints (McDermott and Wicha 2010). The emerging technologies employing automated screening of compounds are exploiting traditional and novel molecules. Other novel treatment modalities such as oncolytic viral therapy, differentiation therapy and nanotechnology are on relevant interest (Patel et al. 2010). These clinical trials will provide a direct test of the cancer stem cell hypothesis.

References

Al-Hajj M, Wicha MS, Benito-Hernandez A, et al. (2003)Prospective identification of tumorigenic breast cancer cells. Proc Natl Acad Sci USA 100:3983–3988

Blau, H. M., Brazelton, T. R., & Weimann, J. M. (2001) The evolving concept of a stem cell: entity or function? Cell 105: 829–841

Bunting KD, Lindahl R, Townsend AJ. (1994). Oxazaphosphorine-specific resistance in human MCF-7 breast carcinoma cell lines expressing transfected rat class 3 aldehyde dehydrogenase. J Biol Chem 269:23197–23203

Charafe-Jauffret E, Ginestier C, Iovino F, et al. (2009) Breast cancer cells lines contain functional cancer stem cells with Metastatic Capacity and a Distinct Molecular signature. Cancer Res 69:1302–1313

Cicalese, A., Bonizzi, G., Pasi, C.E., et al (2009). The tumor suppressor p53 regulates polarity of self-renewing divisions in mammary stem cells. Cell 20:1083–1095

Cobaleda C, Cruz JJ, González-Sarmiento R, Sánchez-García I, Pérez-Losada J (2008). The Emerging Picture of Human Breast Cancer: as a Stem Cell-based Disease. Stem Cell Rev 4:67–79

Dontu G, Abdallah WM, Foley JM, et al. (2003) In vitro propagation and transcriptional profiling of human mammary stem/progenitor cells. Genes Dev 17:1253–1270

Ginestier C, Hur MH, Charafe-Jauffret E, et al. (2007) ALDH1 is a marker of normal and malignant human mammary stem cells and a predictor of poor clinical outcome. Cell Stem Cell 1:555–567

Ginestier C, Liu S, Diebel ME, Korkaya H, Luo M, et al. (2010) CXCR1 blockade selectively targets human breast cancer stem cells in vitro and in xenografts. J Clin Invest 120 (2): 485–497

Gonzalez-Sarmiento, R. and Perez-Losada, J. (2008) Breast Cancer as a Stem Cell Disease. Current Stem Cell Research and Therapy 3, 55–65

Harrison H, Farmie G, Brennan KR, Clarke RB. (2010a) Breast Cancer Stem Cells: something out of notching?. Cancer Res 2010; 70 (22): 8973–8976

Harrison H, Farnie, G, Howell SJ, et al. (2010b) Regulation of breast cancer stem cell activity by signalling through the Notch4 receptor. Cancer Res 70 (2): 709–718

Hatsell S, Frost AR. (2007)Hedgehog signaling in mammary gland development and breast cancer. J Mammary Gland Biol Neoplasia 12:163–173

Holst CR, Nuovo GJ, Esteller M, et al. (2003) Methylation of p16(INK4a) promoters occurs in vivo in histologically normal human mammary epithelia. Cancer Res 63: 1596–1601

Kim M, Turnquist H, Jackson J, et al. (2002) The multidrug resistance transporter ABCG2 (breast cancer resistance protein 1) effluxes Hoechst 33342 and is overexpressed in hematopoietic stem cells. Clin Cancer Res 8:22–28

Knoblich JA (2010). Asymmetric cell division: recent developments and their implications for tumour biology. Nat Rev Mol Cell Biol 11: 849–860

Korkaya H and Wicha M. (2009) Her-2, Notch and breast cancer stem cells. Clin Cancer Res 15: 1845–46

Korkaya H, Paulson A, Iovino F, et al. (2008) HER2 regulates the mammary stem/progenitor cell population driving tumorigenesis and invasion. Oncogene 27:6120–6130

Li X, Lewis MT, Huang J, et al. (2008) Intrinsic resistance of tumorigenic breast cancer cells to chemotherapy. J Natl Cancer Inst 100(9):672

Li Y, Welm B, Podsypanina K, et al. (2003) Evidence that transgenes encoding components of the Wnt signaling pathway preferentially induce mammary cancers from progenitor cells. Proc Natl Acad Sci USA 100:15853–15858

Liu S and Wicha M. (2010) Targeting breast cancer stem cells. JCO 28; 25: 4006–4012

Liu S, Dontu G, Mantle ID, et al. (2006). Hedgehog signaling and BMI-1 regulate self-renewal of normal and malignant human mammary stem cells. Cancer Res 66:6063–6071

Liu S, GinestierC , Ou SJ, Clouthier SG, Patel S , et al. (2011) Breast Cancer Stem Cells Are Regulated by Mesenchymal Stem Cells through Cytokine Networks. Cancer Res 7 (2): 814–824

Liu S, Ginestier C, Charafe-Jauffret E, et al. (2008) BRCA1 regulates human mammary stem/progenitor cell fate. Proc Natl Acad Sci USA 105:1680–1685

Magnifico A, Albano L, Campaner S, et al. (2009) Tumor-initiating cells of Her2-positive carcinoma cell lines express the highest oncoprotein levels and are trastuzumab sensitive. Clin Cancer Res 15: 2010–21

Marcato P, Dean CA, Araslanova R et al. (2011) Aldehyde Dehydrogenase Activity of Breast Cancer Stem Cells is Primarily Due to Isoform ALDH1A3 and Its Expression is Predictive of Metastasis. Stem Cells 1; 29: 32–45

McDermott SP, Wicha M. (2010)Targeting breast cancer stem cells. Mol Oncol 4: 404–419

Mego M, Mani SA and Cristofanilli M. (2010) Molecular mechanisms of metastasis in breast cancer – clinical applications. Nat Rev Clin Oncol 7: 693–701

Morimoto K, Kim S, Tanei T, et al. (2009) Stem cell marker aldehyde dehydrogenase 1-positive breast cancers are characterized by negative estrogen receptor, positive human epidermal growth factor receptor type 2, and high Ki67 expression. Cancer Sci 100: 1062–1068

Nickoloff BJ, Osborne BA, Miele L. (2003) Notch signaling as a therapeutic target in cancer: a new approach to the development of cell fate modifying agents. Oncogene 22:6598–6608

Patel SA, Ndabahaline A, Lim PK, Milton R, Rameshwar P. (2010) Challenges in the development of future for breast cancer stem cells. Breast Cancer 2: 1–11

Pece S, Tosoni D, Confalonieri S, et al (2010). Biological and Molecular Heterogeneity of Breast Cancers Correlates with Their Cancer Stem Cell Content. Cell 140: 62–73

Phillips TM, McBride WH, Pajonk F. (2006) The response of CD24(−/low)/CD44+ breast cancer-initiating cells to radiation. J Natl Cancer Inst 98:1777–1785

Polyak K (2007). Breast cancer stem cells: a case of mistaken identity?. Stem Cell Rev 3 (2):107–9

Ponti D, Costa A, Zaffaroni N, et al. (2005) Isolation and in vitro propagation of tumorigenic breast cancer cells with stem/progenitor cell properties. Cancer Res 65:5506–5511

Prat A, Perou CM (2011). Deconstructing the molecular portraits of breast cancer. Mol Oncol. 5(1):5–23

Resetkova E, Reis-Filho J, Jain R., et al. (2010) Prognostic impact of ALDH1 in breast cancer: a story of stem cells and tumor microenvironment. Breast Cancer Res Treat 123(1):97–108

Russo J, Snider K, Pereira JS, Russo IH (2010). Estrogen induced breast cancer is the result in the disruption of the asymmetric cell division of the stem cell. Horm Mol Biol Clin INvestig 1 (2): 53–65

Russo J, Tay LK, Russo IH (1982). Differentiation of the mammary gland and susceptibility to carcinogenesis. Breast Cancer Research and Treatment 2: 5–73

Saal LH, Gruvberger-Saal SK, Persson C, et al. (2008) Recurrent gross mutations of the PTEN tumor suppressor gene in breast cancers with deficient DSB repair. Nat Genet 40:102–107

Shackleton M, Vaillant F, Simpson KJ, et al. (2006) Generation of a functional mammary gland from a single stem cell. Nature 439:84–88

Stingl J and Caldas C (2007). Molecular heterogeneity of breast carcinomas and the cancer stem cell hypothesis. Nat Rev Cancer 7: 791–799

Stingl J, Eirew P, Ricketson I, et al. (2006) Purification and unique properties of mammary epithelial stem cells. Nature 439:993–997

Tanei T, Morimoto K, Shimazu K, et al. (2009) Association of Breast Cancer Stem Cells Identified by Aldehyde Dehydrogenase 1 Expression with Resistance to Sequential Paclitaxel and Epirubicin-Based Chemotherapy for Breast Cancers. Clin Cancer Res 15(12): 4234–4241

Vaillant F, Asselin-Labat ML, Shackleton M, et al. (2007) The emerging picture of the mouse mammary stem cell. Stem Cell Rev 3: 114–123

Villadsen R, Fridriksdottir AJ, Ronnov-Jessen L, et al. (2007). Evidence for a stem cell hierarchy in the adult human breast. J Cell Biol 177:87–101

Wang W, El-Deiry WS. (2008) Restoration of p53 to limit tumor growth. Curr Opin Oncol 20:90–96

Wicha MS, Liu S, Dontu G (2006). Cancer stem cells: an old idea – a paradigm shift. Cancer Res 66:1883–1890

Chapter 10
Colon Cancer Stem Cells

Ugo Testa

Introduction

Stem cells are a unique long-lived cell population endowed with the peculiar biologic property of self-renewal (i.e. the capacity to generate daughter cells with an identical developmental potential) and of differentiation (i.e. the capacity to generate multiple cell types). Stem cells may undergo three different types of cell divisions: (a) An asymmetric stem cell division, in which a stem cell generates two daughters, one remaining in the niche as a stem cell and the other committed for differentiation; if a stem cell undergoes always asymmetric divisions remains immortal. (b) A symmetric stem cell division producing two stem cells. (c) A symmetric stem cell division generating two cells destined to differentiate. The asymmetric divisions are more frequent, while the symmetric divisions occur less frequently.

The best characterized multipotent stem cell is the hematopoietic stem cell and until few years ago, a very limited number of other adult stem cell populations outside the bone marrow have been characterized. One of these is represented by intestinal stem cell. The existence of intestinal cells was proposed many years ago (Leblond et al. 1948) and subsequently supported through various types of evidences.

Tissue-restricted stem cells have some general biological properties. Although they are not easily distinguishable from other epithelial cells, they possess some membrane-specific markers consistently used for their identification and characterization. Tissue stem cells are thought to be quiescent and to undergo division only rarely: this conception is supported by the observation that these cells usually do not express proliferation-associated markers. Usually, typical proliferation markers such as proliferating cell nuclear antigen (PCNA), Ki67 or 5-bromo-2-deoxyuridine (BrdU) are able to label the compartment of progenitor (and precursor) cells, which

U. Testa (✉)
Department of Hematology, Oncology and Molecular Medicine,
Istituto Superiore di Sanità, Viale Regina Elena 299, 00161 Rome, Italy
e-mail: ugo.testa@iss.it

represents the direct progeny of the differentiation of stem cells, but not the stem cell compartment. Tissue stem cells are located in peculiar structures called niches, peculiar areas delimited by extracellular substrates that provide an optimal microenvironment for the survival and differentiation of stem cells. Particularly, the stem cell niche represents the microenvironment that lodges the stem cell and controls its activity of self-renewal and differentiation. The stem cell niche is typically comprised of epithelial and mesenchymal cells and extracellular substrates. Therefore, the microenvironment present in the stem cell niche may change according to the physiologic demand and plays a key role in determining and controlling the activity of stem cells.

The gastrointestinal stem cell niche plays an essential role in maintaining the integrity of the intestinal epithelium. This niche is made up of proliferating and differentiating epithelial cells surrounded by mesenchymal cells. These mesenchymal cells play an essential role, promoting the epithelial–mesenchymal crosstalk required to maintain the integrity of the niche (Yen and Wright 2006). A peculiar feature of the intestinal stem cell niche is given by the presence of myofibroblasts adjacent to crypt base, which are believed to elaborate paracrine signals regulating the neighbouring intestinal stem cells (Crosnier et al. 2006). Within the intestinal stem cell niche Wnt and Notch signals are absolutely required for stem cell maintenance and differentiation (Pinto et al. 2003; Fre et al. 2005).

Interestingly, a recent report showed the existence in *Drosophila* of a transient niche playing a role in stem cell fate, i.e. in establishing intestinal stem cells starting from progenitors of intestinal stem cells: this niche allows proliferation and differentiation of these progenitors into intestinal stem cells (Mathur et al. 2010).

In normal homeostatic conditions, the number of intestinal stem cells remained nearly constant, thus imposing an absolute need for stem cell asymmetric cell division, generating half of daughter cells that retain stem cell properties. Fate asymmetry can be obtained either through a genetic intrinsically determined mechanism (*intrinsic asymmetry*) or through a more complex mechanism generated by the whole cell population, where stem cell fate following cell division is specified up only to some probability (*population asymmetry*). Some studies supported more the mechanism of intrinsic asymmetry. At the level of each intestinal crypt, cell homeostasis can be maintained by stem cells through two different stem cell dynamics: (a) crypts can be maintained by a hierarchy in which a single stem cell generates, through asymmetric cell divisions, a progeny of stem cells with a more limited stemness and proliferative potential; (b) crypts can be maintained by a relatively homogeneous population of equipotent stem cells, in which stem cell loss is adequately compensated through the multiplication of other stem cells. Recent studies based on cell-labelling procedures (cell tracking studies) and analysis of cellular dynamics do not support a hierarchical arrangement of intestinal stem cells, but identify a pool of relatively equipotent stem cells that is regulated by the behaviour of neighbours (Lopez-Garcia et al. 2010). Particularly, it was shown that the death of a stem cell is compensated by the multiplication of a neighbour, leading to a neutral drift dynamics, where different clones either contract or expand at random, until they take over the crypt or they are lost (Lopez-Garcia et al. 2010). This conclusion is confirmed by an additional study based on the same methodology (Snippert et al. 2010). Interestingly, this additional study showed that most intestinal stem cells divide symmetrically, generating two identical daughter cells with similar cell fates. According to these findings, the cellular dynamics of intestinal crypts are consistent with a model where they double their number each day and stochastically adopt a stemness or a differentiating cell fate (Snippert et al. 2010).

Wnt/β-Catenin Signalling Pathway

Given the key role of Wnt/β-catenin signalling in intestinal stem cell physiology and in development of colon cancer, it seems necessary to provide an outline of this important signalling pathway. This pathway uses an unusual mechanism for transmitting information to the cell nucleus, using a control of the stability of two proteins, axin and β-catenin. Particularly, it was shown that in the absence of Wnt activation, β-catenin is degraded through the action of a "destruction complex" composed by a scaffold protein, axin and its numerous patterns, including the tumour suppressor *adenomatous polyposis coli* (APC), *glycogen synthase kinase 3* (GSK3) and *casein kinase 1* (CK1). GSK3 and CK1 present in this complex phosphorylate the amino terminal region of β-catenin, thus favouring its recognition by an E3 ubiquitin ligase, with subsequent ubiquitination and degradation by the proteasome (reviewed in MacDonald et al. 2009). This continual degradation of β-catenin totally prevents the possibility that this protein could reach the nucleus and activate Wnt target genes, whose expression is repressed by the transcriptional repressor TCF/LEF. The Wnt/β-catenin signalling is activated when a Wnt ligand binds to one of the Wnt receptors, such as the Frizzled receptor and its co-receptor, LRP6 (*low-density related protein 6*) or LRP5. The activated receptor results in phosphorylation of LRP6 with its capacity to bind the Axin degradation complex at the level of the activated receptor. The binding of the Axin complex at the level of the Wnt receptor had the consequence to inhibit the axin-dependent phosphorylation of β-catenin, with its consequent stabilization (MacDonald et al. 2009).

19 Wnt ligands have been identified and they are cysteine-rich proteins composed by 350–400 amino acids, containing an N-terminal signal peptide for secretion. Drosophila Wingless is the Wnt ligand most investigated in vivo and in vitro. Several secreted proteins antagonize or modulate Wnt/β catenin signalling. Secreted frizzled related proteins (sFRPs) and Wnt inhibitory protein (WIF) bind to Wnt and to Fz, and, through this mechanism, act as Wnt antagonists for β-catenin signalling (Bovolenta et al. 2008).

Following its stabilization, β-catenin is shuttled to and retained in the nucleus through a mechanism that remains still to be elucidated. However, it is evident that β-catenin stabilization is not sufficient to allow its nuclear accumulation; in fact, recent studies have shown that Wnt activation of the Rac1 GTPase is required for β-catenin nuclear localization (Wu et al. 2008). The effects of β-catenin on gene regulation are mediated through the binding to the TCF/LEF family of transcription factors. TCF acts as a repressor of gene transcription through the binding with the repressor TLE1. Following its nuclear accumulation, β-catenin complexes with TCF, displacing TLE1 and recruiting coactivators of gene activation. An important co-activator of β-catenin is telomerase: the telomerase protein component TERT (telomerase reversed transcriptase) interacts with gene promoters of Wnt-dependent genes and activates their transcription (Park et al. 2009). In the absence of TLE1 binding, TCF acts as an activator of gene transcription. TCF proteins are transcription factors and bind to a DNA-binding consensus sequence CCTTTGWW (W identifies either T or A), known as the Wnt responsive element (WRE), altering chromatin conformation.

APC acts on WRE antagonizing β-catenin-mediated gene activation through the replacement of coactivators with corepressors; APC mutants observed in colon cancer cells are unable to act as β-catenin repressors (Sierra et al. 2006). GSK3 also associates with the WRE in a cyclic fashion coordinated with APC, thus suggesting that it may have together with APC a negative impact on β-catenin-mediated activation of transcription (Sierra et al. 2006).

Since Wnt/β-catenin signalling regulates various important cellular functions, such as proliferation, commitment and differentiation during development and adult tissue homeostasis, it is not surprising that the number of Wnt target genes is very wide and tissue and developmentally or physiologically controlled (MacDonald et al. 2009). The stimulatory effect of Wnt signalling on cell proliferation is exerted through a stimulation of cyclinD1 and c-myc in G_1/S phase, but also during mitosis through unknown targets (Davidson et al. 2009).

Deregulated Wnt signalling was observed in many cancers and, particularly, in colon cancer. In colon cancer cells, a constitutively activated β-catenin signalling may result from three different events: APC deficiency or β-catenin mutations or autocrine Wnt signalling. The main effect of this constitutive Wnt signalling at the level of intestinal stem cells, leading to an activation of these cells (Reya and Clevers 2005).

NOTCH signalling is triggered through the binding of a ligand (*Jagged, Delta, Delta-like, Serrate*) present on the membrane of one cell to a receptor (*NOTCH1→ NOTCH4*) present on the membrane of the contacting cell. Therefore, the NOTCH signalling pathway is a complex cell signalling system mediated through cell to cell contact. Following the binding of a NTCH ligand to a NOTCH receptor, a proteolytic cleavage of the NOTCH receptor, with consequent release of the cytoplasmic tail (*NICD*) of a NOTCH receptor is observed; the released NICD translocates to the nucleus and associated with CSL transcription factors and subsequently affects the expression of a wide number of target genes. Among them, the most important are represented by the HES (hairy/enhancer of split) family of transcription factors. Experiments of modulation of NOTCH activity in normal mouse intestine showed that: (a) inhibition of NOTCH signalling results in exit from the proliferative compartment and differentiation in postmitotic goblet cells (Van Es et al. 2005); (b) transgenic expression of NCID in the intestine leads to expansion of enterocyte progenitor cells (Fre et al. 2005).

Normal Intestinal Stem Cells

The intestinal epithelium is renewed about every 5 days and therefore requires the continuous replacement with new cellular elements. As in other tissues at rapid cell renewal, the tissue integrity must be maintained by a population of quiescent stem cells. In order to maintain the intestinal epithelium that need the production of billions of intestinal cells daily, these quiescent stem cells must be periodically forced to proliferate and differentiate giving rise to transit amplifying (TA) cells. These TA cells are believed to be short-lived and if this is true one must conclude that quiescent stem cells have frequently to proliferate and differentiate. However, an alternative mechanism could spare quiescent stem cells from the dangers deriving from their frequent cycling. In fact, recent studies have identified a population of intestinal stem cells that is long-lived in spite its constant cycling activity (Li and Clevers 2010). Emerging evidence indicated that also in other tissues at rapid renewal, such as the hair follicle, there is the coexistence of both quiescent, out of the cell cycle, metabolically scarcely active and able to retain DNA labels and active, cycling, not able to retain DNA labels, stem cells (Li and Clevers 2010).

The existence of intestinal stem cells has been postulated 60 years ago. The epithelial layer of human colon is made up of a single layer of columnar epithelial cells, which originates finger-like invaginations, the crypts, into the underlying connective tissue of the lamina propria. The crypts of Lieberkühn represent the basic functional units of the intestine. These crypts have peculiar cellular organization with stem cells located at the base of the crypts at the level of the so-called stem-cell niches formed by the stem cells themselves and the mesenchymal cells located around the crypt base. On the contrary, the terminally differentiated cells are located at the level of the top of the crypts; they pertain to four epithelial cell types: colonocytes that represent the absorptive enterocytes; the mucus-secreting goblet cells; the peptide hormone-secreting enteroendocrine cells; the Paneth cells usually scattered at the bottom of the crypts.

In 1974 Cheng and Leblond formulated the concept that all these four cell types originate from a single multipotent intestinal stem cell (*Unitarian Hypothesis*) through a number of committed progenitors (Cheng and Leblond 1974). These progenitors and transit differentiating intestinal precursors, originated from the differentiation of intestinal stem cells, occupy the lower two-thirds of the crypt. Given this location within the crypt of stem cells, it is not surprising that proliferation occurs at the base of crypts. The large majority of cells migrate up from the crypts to the villi, while few cells migrate below the stem cells to originate Paneth cells, usually present at the bottom of the crypts.

Intestinal crypts both in animals and in humans are of clonal origin, thus indicating that all the cells composing a crypt are derived from the proliferation and differentiation of a single stem cell. This important conclusion is based in the case of mice on the analysis of allophonic, teraparental mice and mice heterozygous for a defective glucose 6 phosphate dehydrogenase (G6PD) allele (Ponder et al. 1985; Schmidt et al. 1988). Using mitochondrial DNA mutations as a marker of clonal expansion of intestinal stem cell progeny, it was provided clear evidence that all cells within a small human intestinal crypt are derived from one common stem cell (Gutierrez-Gonzalez et al. 2009). It is of interest to note that in neonatal mouse intestinal crypts are polyclonal and, through a peculiar process, crypts become monoclonal by 2 weeks of age and remain monoclonal throughout all adult life (Schmidt et al. 1988).

Direct evidence that all crypt-forming cells derive from crypt basal columnar cells (CBCCs) comes from lineage tracking experiments. These experiments provided evidence that some Lgr5 (Leucine-rich-repeat containing G-protein-coupled receptor 5) near at the base of the crypt possess the important property to generate all intestinal cells (multilineage differentiation) and therefore are putative stem cells (Barker et al. 2007; Barker and Clevers 2007). LGR5 is a member of the G-protein-coupled receptor (GPCR) family comprising proteins with seven transmembrane domains and is a target of Wnt signalling. GPCRs function as receptors for various classes of ligand, including peptide hormones and chemokines. To date, the ligand for, and function of, LGR5-related signalling remains largely unknown. More recently, it was provided additional and more convincing evidence that Lgr5$^+$ crypt intestinal cells exhibit stem cell properties: single isolated Lgr5$^+$ cells can be grown in culture and, under appropriate conditions, undergo proliferation and differentiation giving rise to organoids containing several crypt like structures (Sato et al. 2009). Lgr5 is uniquely expressed in stem cells and is switched off in their immediate daughters, the transit amplifying cells (Van der Flier et al. 2009a). It is important to note that Lgr5$^+$ cells represent a long-lived and cycling multipotent stem cell population (Barker et al. 2007). Lgr5$^+$ stem cells are distinct from position +4 label retaining cells (LRCs) in that Lgr5 stem cells do not retain DNA labels and are sensitive to CDC25 inactivation, supporting their proliferating features (Lee et al. 2009). Lgr5 was also identified as a marker of stem cells in the stomach: Lgr5 positive cells are found at the base of mature pyloric glands (Barker et al. 2010). The physiological function as well as the signalling pathway(s) involved upon Lgr5 activation, is still poorly understood due to the lack of identified natural ligand. Recently, studying Lgr5 gene knock-out mice it was shown that Lgr5 deficiency induces premature differentiation of Paneth cells with concomitant upregulation of Wnt signalling (Garcia et al. 2009). These observations suggest that Lgr5 could act as a negative regulator of Wnt pathway in progenitor cells of the developing intestinal epithelium.

An additional marker expressed on intestinal stem cells is represented by the membrane antigen CD133. In fact, using CD133-knockin mice, Zhu et al. (2009) have shown that CD133 (a pentaspan transmembrane glycoprotein that localizes at the level of membrane protrusions) positive cells are present at the bottom of crypts and co-express Lgr5. Like Lgr5 cells, CD133$^+$ cells can generate the entire intestinal epithelium, thus establishing CD133 as an additional marker for CBC-type intestinal stem cells. However, the analysis of the expression patterns and use of CD133 knock-in mice showed that CD133 mRNA was expressed throughout the lower half of the crypt and was not specifically associated with the Lgr5 cells, but may mark stem cells as well as early transit amplifying cells (Snippert et al. 2009).

Olfactomedin 4 (OLFM4), which was identified in a differential gene expression profile for Lgr5-positive cells, has been shown to be highly expressed in CBCs by in situ hybridization in human small intestine and colon and may therefore be a marker for human intestinal and colon stem cells (Van der Flier et al. 2009b). Human OLFM4 is highly expressed in human colon crypts as demonstrated by microarray analysis (Kosinski et al. 2007). OLFM4 encodes a secreted molecule with unknown function, originally cloned from human myeloblasts (Zhang et al. 2002).

BMI-1, a polycomb group protein involved in self-renewal of stem cells, is another potential marker of intestinal stem cells. Using a tamoxifen-inducible CRE from the Bmi-1 locus, it has been shown that BMI-1 is expressed at the level of a small number of quiescent stem cells located near the bottom of the crypts in the small intestine at a position corresponding at about cell position +4 (Sangiorgi and Capecchi 2008). BMI-1-positive cells populate all epithelial intestinal lineages (Sangiorgi and Capecchi 2008). Interestingly, BMI-1 was found to be a marker also for quiescent pancreatic stem cells (Sangiorgi and Capecchi 2009).

Another potential marker of intestinal stem cells is represented by the protein Mushashi-1, a RNA-binding protein initially found to be associated with early asymmetric divisions in *Drosophila* sensory organ precursor cells. An antibody specific to this protein stains a small number of cells distributed at cell position 4–5 in adult small intestine and few cells at the base of the crypts in the large intestine (Potten et al. 2003). Importantly, cells at the +4 cell position expressing the putative stem cell marker Musashi-1 are not sensitive to the inactivation of the cell cycle protein CDC25, thus supporting their quiescent features (Lee et al. 2009). The function of Musashi-1 at the level of intestinal stem cell biology is largely unknown. However, a recent study based on the enforced expression of Musashi-1 in a human intestinal cell line showed an inhibitory effect of this protein on Paneth cell differentiation; according to these observations it was suggested that Musashi-1 could contribute to maintain the undifferentiated phenotype of intestinal stem cells (Murayama et al. 2009).

Sox9, a transcription factor that plays a key role in embryogenic formation of several tissues, is expressed by intestinal stem cells and also by transient amplifying cells and terminally differentiated Paneth cells at the crypt base. Recently, using a Sox9 (EGFP) model, it was provided evidence that Sox9 expression marks intestine stem cells that form organoids in vitro (Gracz et al. 2010). Interestingly, a prospective search revealed that CD24 is expressed in the Sox9 population and marks intestinal stem cells (Gracz et al. 2010). This observation provides an indication about a membrane marker that could considerably facilitate FACS-enrichment of intestinal cells. A recent study showed that Sox9-expressing cells act as progenitors of intestinal, adult liver, and exocrine pancreas (Furuyama et al. 2011).

A new promising putative stem cell marker is represented by doublecortin CaM kinase-like-1 (DCAMLK-1), a microtubule-associated kinase initially described in nervous tissue and, more recently, in gut epithelial progenitor cells (Giannakis et al. 2006). A recent study identified DCAMLK-1-positive cells in the intestinal stem cell zone (+4) and found mitotic DCAMLK-1-expressing intestinal stem cells 24 h following radiation injury, thus indicating the important role of these cells for tissue reparation (May et al. 2008). A more recent study showed that DCAMLK-1 is predominantly expressed in quiescent, label retaining cells in the lower two-thirds of intestinal crypt epithelium and in occasional crypt-based columnar cells (May et al. 2009). Interestingly, it was shown that DCAMLK-1 is located also at the level of cell

Table 10.1 Markers of the normal intestinal stem cells

Marker	Characteristics of positive cells and biologic properties of the marker	Reference
BMI1	Quiescent stem cells located around position 4+ that generate all intestinal epithelial lineages (lineage tracing). The proto-oncogene BMI1 controls stem cell division	Sangiorgi and Capecchi (2008)
Label retaining (BrdU)	Quiescent stem cells located around position 4+ (no lineage tracing)	Potten et al. (1974)
DCAMKL-1 (Doublecortin and CAM kinase-like-1)	Quiescent stem cells located around position 4+ (no lineage tracing). Microtubule-associated kinase	Giannakis et al. (2006) and May et al. (2008, 2009)
Musashi-1	Quiescent stem cells located around position 4+ (no lineage tracing). RNA-binding protein	Potten et al. (2003), Lee et al. (2009), and Samuel et al. (2009)
LGR5	Active cycling crypt base columnar cells that generate all intestinal epithelial lineages (lineage tracing). In vitro LGR5-positive cells give rise to organoids. LGR5-positive stem cells do not retain DNA labels. LGR5 deficiency deregulates Wnt signalling	Barker et al. (2007), Sato et al. (2009), and Garcia et al. (2009)
CD133 (Prominin-1)	Active cycling crypt base columnar cells that generate all intestinal epithelial lineages (lineage tracing). CD133-positive cells overlap with LGR5-positive cells. CD133 could inhibit stem cell differentiation	Vermeulen et al. (2008), Zhu et al. (2009), and Snippert et al. (2009)
ALDH1 (Aldehyde dehydrogenase)	Crypt base columnar cells in human small intestine and colon	Huang et al. (2009a, b)
OLFM4 (Olfactomedin 4)	Crypt base columnar cells in human small intestine and colon. Its expression overlaps with that of LGR5. The OLFM4 gene encodes a secreted molecule with unknown function, cloned from myeloblasts	Van der Flier et al. (2009a, b)
CCK-2R (Cholecystokinin 2 receptor)	Predominant expression on proliferating progenitors. CCK-2R expression on these cells is upregulated by progastrin. Deletion of CCK-2R in mice abrogates progastrin-dependent increase in colonic proliferation and in progenitors expressing DCAMKL-1 and stem cells expressing LGR5. CCK-2R is the primary receptor for cholecystokinin (CCK) and amidated gastrin	Jin et al. (2009)
CD166 (Activated leukocyte cell adhesion molecule)	Predominant expression at the level of Paneth cells and intervening crypt-based Columnar cells (putative stem cells). The function of CD166 in stem cells and the stem cell niche remains to be demonstrated	Levin et al. (2010)

surface, in addition to its cytoplasmic location, and be therefore used as a marker for intestinal stem cell isolation using specific antibodies (May et al. 2009) (Table 10.1).

Other studies suggest that cholecystokinin 2 receptor (CCK-BR) could be an additional marker of colonic stem and progenitor cells. In fact, CCK-BR was found to be expressed on colon crypt cells near to the proliferative zone; furthermore, increased levels of progastrin induce an expansion of CCK-BR positive cells (Jin et al. 2009). Inactivation of CCK-BR reduced the number and the proliferation of Lgr5-positive or DCLK-1-positive cells in progastrin-overexpressing mice, thus suggesting that CCK-BR expression is present at the level of colonic stem and progenitor cells (Jin et al. 2009).

A promising new marker for colon stem cells is aldehyde dehydrogenase 1 (ALDH1). ALDH1 is a detoxifying enzyme that oxidizes intracellular aldehydes and thereby confers resistance to alkylating agents and to oxidative stress, thus contributing to the longevity of stem cells. ALDH also converts retinol to retinoic acid, a modulator of cell proliferation and, particularly, of stem cell proliferation and differentiation. Immunostaining analysis of normal crypts showed that ALDH1-positive cells are sparse and limited to the normal crypt bottom (Huang et al. 2009a).

CD166, also known as activated leukocyte cell adhesion molecule (ALCAM) was recently described as a new potential maker identifying all the staminal region of the human and murine crypts (Levin et al. 2010). In fact, immunohistochemical studies with anti-CD166 mAbs provided evidence about marked CD166 expression in epithelial cells at the base of the crypts (both Paneth cells and intervening crypt-based columnar cells) both in small intestine and colon (Levin et al. 2010). Isolated CD166⁺ cells coexpress other markers previously reported to be expressed on intestinal stem cells. However, only a small fraction of CD166⁺ cells express the stem cell marker Lgr5 (Levin et al. 2010).

Eph receptors of the B class, which bind the transmembrane Ephrin-B ligands, have been explored as potential markers of intestinal stem cells. The EphB2, EphB3, and Eph B4 receptors and the Ephrin-B1 and Ephrin-B2 ligands are expressed in complementary gradients along the intestinal crypts: EphB receptors are expressed, like Lgr5⁺, at the bottom of the crypts at the level of proliferating progenitors and their expression is progressively lost during differentiation of these progenitor cells; in contrast, Ephrin-B ligands expression progressively increases following differentiation of intestinal cryptal cells (Holmberg et al. 2006). Eph B/Ephrin-B ligands expression in intestinal crypts is controlled by Wnt/β-catenin signalling. Inhibition of EphB2/EphB3 signalling has been shown to reduce the number of proliferating cells, without altering the stem cell number, thus suggesting that is unlikely that these receptors are a biomarker of intestinal stem cells.

The organization and position of different cell types composing the intestinal crypts and particularly of stem cells have been extensively studied in the mouse. It was suggested that the exact location of stem cells in the niche is different between the colon and the small intestine, with the putative stem cell compartment present at the base in the colon crypt, but at the position 4–5 in the small intestinal crypts, above the basal Paneth cells (Marsham et al. 2002). Recent studies in mice have shed some doubts about the exact location of the niche in the small intestine crypt. Barker et al. (2007) showed that Lgr5⁺ putative intestinal stem cells are present at the base of the crypt mixed with Paneth cells; however, Sangiorgi and Capecchi (2008) showed that Bmi 1 positive intestinal stem cells are located above the Paneth cells at cell position +4; Fellous et al. (2009), exploiting a technique for detecting the expansion of a single cell's progeny that contains mitochondrial DNA mutation, provided evidence that the stem cell niche is located at the base of colon crypts and above the Paneth cell region in the small intestine.

Recent studies have provided evidence about a close physical association of Lgr5 stem cells with Paneth cells; importantly, CD24⁺ Paneth cells express EGF, Wnt3 and NOTCH Ligand DLL4, all acting as essential growth factor signals for stem cell maintenance (Sato et al. 2011). Co-culturing of sorted Lgr5⁺ stem cells with Paneth cells induces a marked improvement of in vitro organoid formation (Sato et al. 2011). Genetic removal of Paneth cells in vivo determines the concomitant depletion of intestinal Lgr5⁺ stem cells (Sato et al. 2011). These studies strongly support the concept that Paneth cells constitute the niche for Lgr5 stem cells in intestinal crypts.

Taking into account all these evidences, a model of two types of intestinal stem cells was proposed: quiescent stem cells at the traditional +4 locations in a prolonged quiescent state, due to their inhibitory microenvironment, and the active cycling stem cells, representing a cell population able to respond to stimulatory signals by adjacent mesenchymal cells (Scoville et al. 2008).

As above mentioned, asymmetric stem cell divisions preserve stem cell number, while generating a differentiated cell progeny. Orienting the mitotic spindle relative to surrounding tissue is a cellular strategy used by stem cells to divide asymmetrically. In a recent study, Quyn et al. (2010)examined the mitotic spindle orientation of intestinal cells within the first seven cell region from the bottom of the crypt (1–7 cells), compared to that of cells distributed in the upper region (>7) of the crypt. These authors have observed that spindle orientation is different in 1–7 cells compared to >7 cells: in the former ones the spindle orientation was perpendicular, while in the latter ones was parallel to the apical lumen. Importantly, this stereotypical mitotic spindle orientation correlates with cell fates and, particularly, with the symmetry of cell divisions. Particularly, it was shown that 1–7 cells undergo asymmetric cell division and the stem cell population generated at each cell division retains the "immortal strand". The "immortal DNA strand" corresponds to the "original template DNA" and is retained in the stem cell, while the newly replicated DNA is retained by the differentiating progenitor cells originated during each asymmetric division of a stem cell. Therefore, in murine intestinal stem cells there is a complex mechanism that co-ordinately regulates asymmetric DNA segregation, cell position in the intestinal crypts and cell fate. Interestingly, both mitotic spindle orientation and asymmetric cell divisions are lost in the stem cell compartment of APC mutants (Quyn et al. 2010).

Stem Cell Origin of Colon Cancer

Colorectal Carcinogenesis

Cancer development is commonly regarded as a multistep process involving an initial mutagenic event called *tumour initiation*: in this initial event a genomic mutation leads to a malignant phenotype, associated with only a limited growth advantage on the normal counterpart. This initial event is followed by additional mutagenic events and/or epigenetic events, collectively known as *tumour promotion*, involving the growth of a mutated cell clone and proliferation of tumour cells. This process culminates this last process is known as *tumour progression*. Colon cancer represents a unique model to explore these different stages of tumour development. Fearon and Vogelstein (1990) initially proposed a model, called *adenoma → carcinoma sequence model*, in which certain mutations were directly related to different stages of tumour development. In line with this model, tumour initiation was triggered by mutations occurring at the level of the APC gene, which is responsible for adenoma formation and the development of a so-called "dysplastic crypts." After this stage, the occurrence of additional mutations at the level of K-ras, p53 and SMAD4, favour tumour promotion and progression, characterized by increased growth rate of the adenoma, the expansion of individual particularly malignant clones with consequent tumour invasion and metastasis.

As above mentioned, the current evidences indicate that mutations at the level of the APC tumour suppressor gene initiate the process of colon tumour formation. APC function in normal colon is related to a negative regulation of Wnt signalling through targeting of β-catenin for proteosomal degradation. In cells harbouring a mutated APC gene, as a consequence of the absent inhibitory effect exerted by Wnt signalling, β-catenin accumulates and, after its translocation in the nucleus, acts as a co-activator of TCF-LEF. The β-catenin/TCF-LEF complex acts in turn as a transcriptional activator of key cell-cycle regulatory genes, cyclin D1 and c-myc. Therefore, according to this model of APC function its loss induces an immediate activation of Wnt signalling and a subsequent dysregulation and nuclear accumulation of β-catenin. Recent studies carried out on human colon cells have shown that APC loss induced intestinal differentiation defects, whereas proliferation defects and nuclear accumulation of β-catenin require additional activation of K RAS (Phelps et al. 2009). The effects of APC mutation induced intestinal differentiation defects depend on the transcriptional corepressor C-terminal binding protein-1 (CtBP1) (Phelps et al. 2009). Therefore, following APC loss, CtBP1 contributes to adenoma initiation as a first step, whereas K-RAS activation and β-catenin nuclear localization promote adenoma progression to carcinomas as a second step (Phelps et al. 2009).

Therefore, the *adenoma → carcinoma sequence model* indicates that colon cancer tumour progression is dictated by a growing genomic instability. Subsequent studies have shown that mutations observed in colon cancer are associated with two types of genomic instability and harbour mutations of different sets of genes: chromosomal instability and microsatellite instability. Chromosomal instability includes the presence of different numerical or structural chromosome changes and is observed in about 70% of colon cancers and has been related to mutations of set of genes following the *adenoma → carcinoma sequence model* (Miyazaki et al. 1999). In contrast, microsatellite instability is observed in about 15% of cases and is characterized by mutations or variations in the length of microsatellite sequences, occurring as a result of defective DNA mismatch repair genes. Besides defects in DNA mismatch repair genes, microsatellite instability has been related to mutations of a peculiar set of genes involving BAX, insulin-like growth factor 2 receptor (IGF2R) and transforming growth factor receptor 2 (TGFβR2) (Walther et al. 2009). Colon cancers associated with microsatellite instability have an improved prognosis, compared to colon cancers associated with chromosomal instability.

The *adenoma → carcinoma sequence model* can be revisited taking into account the existence of cancer stem cells. These cells are regarded as the cells that initiate and maintain the tumour bulk. According to this view, it was hypothesized that the first mutational hit occurs at the level of a colonic stem cell that, being long-lived, has the opportunity in the time to accumulate additional oncogenic mutations and epigenetic changes. Once transformed, cancer stem cells are able to undergo either symmetric or asymmetric cell divisions, thus generating both other cancer stem cells and progenitors which in turn generate a cancer cell progeny.

This cancer stem cell origin of colon cancer recently received some direct experimental support in studies of tumorigenesis. Thus, it was demonstrated that transformation of stem cells through loss of APC is an extremely efficient route towards initiating intestinal adenomas (Barker et al. 2009). Furthermore, observations on Lgr5 expression suggest that a stem cell/progenitor cell hierarchy is maintained in early stem cell-derived adenomas (Barker et al. 2009). The ensemble of these observations supports the view that a colon cancer stem/progenitor cell is the cell of origin of colon cancer.

As above mentioned the initial events in colon cancer tumorigenesis, corresponding to the stage just after tumour initiation, should lead to the expansion of a clone of mutated stem cells. Thus, after tumour initiation stem cell overpopulation should be observed. The hypothesis of stem cell overpopulation was originally developed from a mathematical modelling of colon tumorigenesis (Boman et al. 2001), in which stem cell overpopulation was found to be the key event at the cellular level that links the initiating molecular event (an APC mutation) to the earliest tissue abnormality, a proliferative change in mutant colonic crypts of familial adenomatous polyposis (FAP) patients. Stem cell overpopulation not only initiates colon tumorigenesis but also drives tumour growth (Boman and Huang 2008; Boman et al. 2007). The study of the expression of markers for crypt base cells (i.e. putative stem cell markers) provided direct biological evidence in favour of the stem cell overpopulation hypothesis (Boman et al. 2004, 2008): in fact immunohistochemical studies during adenoma development in familial adenomatous polyposis provided evidence about an expansion of stem cell crypt base cell population. In line with these observations, the percentage of Lgr5-positive cells was markedly higher in adenomas than in normal colon mucosal crypts (Fan et al. 2010; Uchida et al. 2010). Lgr5 expression was still higher in colon carcinomas than in adenomas. In line with these observations, the severe polyposis phenotype caused in mouse by truncation of APC at codon 1322 is associated with an increased number of colon stem cells and increased expression of the Wnt target and stem cell marker Lgr5 (Lewis et al. 2010).

Colon Cancer Stem Cells

The theory that cancer in adults derives from aberrant stem cells represents a modern interpretation of the so-called embryonal rest theory proposed by J. Cohnheim in 1867 (mentioned in Hamburger and Salmon 1977). According to this theory cancers arise from resident tissue stem cells or progenitor cells; therefore, tumours can be considered as aberrant organs, in which only a small subset of cancer cells, the cancer stem cells, initiate and maintain the tumour and are capable of metastatic spread (Reya et al. 2001). The contribution of stem cells to tumour development was first noted in early studies of leukaemia (Bonnet and Dick 1997) and of teratocarcinoma (Sell and Pierce 1994). Cancer stem cells, like normal stem cells, give rise to a cell progeny more or less heterogeneous, following the different types of tumours that are capable of various degrees of differentiation (Lobo et al. 2007).

The research on colon cancer stem cells, as well as for other tumours, was characterized by the identification of cell membrane markers useful for the isolation, amplification in vitro and characterization of these cells and by the development of in vivo assays. Two sets of membrane markers have merged as the most useful for the identification of colon cancer stem cells: CD133 (Prominin-1) and CD144. CD133 is a five-transmembrane domain protein that is located at the level of the membrane protrusions of embryonal epithelial structures (Corbeil et al. 2000). Given its peculiar location, a role for CD133 as an "organizer" of the plasma membrane topology was hypothesized (Corbeil et al. 2001). However, to date, its function remains unknown. A role of CD133 in maintaining stem cell properties through an inhibitory action on cell differentiation was tentatively proposed (Weigmann et al. 1997) (Table 10.2).

Two different groups of investigators have identified human colon cancer initiating cells using CD133 as a marker (Ricci-Vitani et al. 2007; O'Brien et al. 2007). These studies have shown that: CD133$^+$ colon cancer cells represent about 2.5% of the bulk tumour cells, they were devoid of intestinal differentiation markers such as cytokeratin 20, while they express the epithelial adhesion molecule EpCAM; CD133$^+$ but not CD133$^-$ colon cancer cells are able to generate tumours of the same histotype when injected in nude mice; CD133$^+$ colon cancer cells can be amplified in vitro as floating aggregates called *tumour spheres*, which can be maintained in vitro and are able to form colon cancers when injected into immunodeficient SCID mice; upon growth factor deprivation, CD133$^+$ cells gradually differentiate, became adherent and express intestinal differentiation markers such as CK20 (Ricci-Vitani et al. 2007; O'Brien et al. 2007).

Table 10.2 Membrane markers of colon cancer stem cells

Marker	Main features	References
CD133 (Prominin-1)	Some reports claim that only CD133+ colon cancer cells could initiate tumorigenesis. Other reports indicate that both CD133+ and CD133− colon cancer cells could initiate tumorigenesis. The level of CD133 expression is higher in colon cancer cells than in normal colon mucosa. The level of CD133 expression in colorectal cancer is a negative prognostic factor	Ricci-Vitani et al. (2007), O'Brien et al. (2007), Shmelkov et al. (2008), Vermeulen et al. (2008), Horst et al. (2008, 2009), and Artells et al. (2010)
CD44	CD44, EpCAM and CD166-positive colon cancer cells are highly tumorigenic. CD44 is a cell surface adhesion molecule that mediates cell–extracellular matrix interaction through binding to its ligand hyaluronan. CD44 is a downstream target of the Wnt/β-catenin pathway. CD44 mediates apoptosis resistance in both normal colon and colon cancer cells and is required or enhances several growth factor/signal transduction pathways	Dalerba et al. (2007) and Chu et al. (2009)
CD26 (Dipeptidyl peptidase IV)	A sub-population of CD26+ colon cancer stem cells (CD133+ and CD44+) display a high capacity of tumour growth both in vitro and in vivo. CD26+ cells were uniformly present in both the primary and metastatic tumours in colorectal cancer patients with liver metastasis. In patients without distant metastasis at the time of presentation, CD26 positivity in the primary tumours predicted distant metastasis in the follow-up. CD26+ cells were chemoresistant and determine formation of distant metastases when injected into mice	Pang et al. (2010)

The identification of CD133 as a colon cancer stem cell marker was challenged by Shmelkov et al. (2008). In fact, these authors, using a knockin LacZ reporter mouse in which the expression of LacZ is driven by the endogenous CD133 promoter, showed that CD133 expression in the mouse colon is not restricted to stem cells and both CD133+ and CD133− colon cancer cells could initiate tumorigenesis (Shmelkov et al. 2008). More recently, it was shown that single CD133+/CD24+ colon cancer stem cells can self-renew and reconstitute a complete and differentiated carcinoma (Vermeulen et al. 2008). Importantly, spheroid cultures of these colon cancer stem cells contain expression of other stem cell markers such as Lgr5, CD44, nuclear β-catenin and CD166 (Vermeulen et al. 2008). Finally, Horst et al. have shown that the level of CD133 expression in colon cancer is a negative prognostic marker (Horst et al. 2008). Using three different monoclonal antibodies against the CD133 antigen, these same authors have shown that CD133 positivity, coupled with nuclear β-catenin positivity, identify colon cancer cases associated with low survival (Horst et al. 2009a). They showed also that CD133-positive colon cancer cells are negative for antigens associated with epithelial differentiation (Horst et al. 2009a). Other studies have confirmed that the level of CD133 expression in colon cancer is a negative prognostic factor. Thus, Artells et al. have analyzed in 64 colorectal cancer patients CD133 mRNA level in cancer tissue compared to normal colon tissue and have shown that expression levels were higher in tumour than in normal tissue (Artells et al. 2010). Furthermore, CD133 higher levels were associated with shorter overall survival and relapse-free interval (Artells et al. 2010). Finally, in a recent study carried out on 54 colon cancer patients Horst et al. associated high CD133 expression with liver metastasis (Horst et al. 2009b). However, other clinical variables, such as age, gender, tumour size and histological grade, were independent of CD133 expression levels (Horst et al. 2009b). Furthermore, in this study the authors depleted CD133 in cultured colon cancer cell lines Caco-2 and LoVo, expressing high and moderate endogenous levels of CD133, respectively. CD133 knockdown does not affect the proliferation, migration, invasiveness and colony formation capabilities of colon cancer cells (Horst et al. 2009b). These observations support the view that CD133 is a marker with high prognostic impact for colon cancer, but it seems to have no obvious functional impact as driving force of this malignancy.

Until recently, CD133 expression was regarded as restricted to undifferentiated colon cancer cells. However, a recent study showed that CD133 changes its conformation upon differentiation, but not its level of expression; particularly, the decrease of AC133 epitope reactivity was due to a change in CD133 glycosylation, thus suggesting that CD133 is exposed on both colon cancer stem cells and in their differentiated progeny (Kemper et al. 2010).

The other membrane marker used for the identification of colon cancer stem cells is CD44, a class I transmembrane glycoprotein acting as a receptor for constituents of the extracellular matrix, such as hyaluronic acid, and a downstream target of the Wnt/β-catenin pathway (Manhaba et al. 2008). CD44 proteins regulate growth, survival, differentiation and migration and may be therefore involved in tumour progression and metastasis (Orian-Rousseau 2010). In colorectal cancer, the expression of CD44 is enhanced both in adenomas and in carcinomas (Wielenga et al. 2000). Particularly, expression of total CD44 and of CD44v3, CD44v6 and CD44v8-v10 isoforms, correlates with bad prognosis (Wielenga et al. 2000). Furthermore, the invasion of colon cancer cells in Mtrigel in vitro is dependent upon CD44 binding to hyaluronic acid and on accumulation of hyaluronic acid in pericellular region (Kim et al. 2004). Colon cancer stem cells were shown to express the CD44 and the epithelial adhesion molecule EpCAM; furthermore, in some colorectal cancer, cancer stem cells were found to express also CD166 and the positivity for this antigen associated with CD44 and EpCAM positivity could be used for further enrichment of colon cancer stem cells (Dalerba et al. 2007). It is important to note that immunohistochemical analysis of normal colon crypts shows that CD44 expression is not limited only at the level of the stem cell compartment at the crypt bottom, but extends also at the level of the cells making part of the proliferative compartment.

A subsequent study has validated CD44 as a robust marker of highly tumorigenic colon cancer cells with stem cell-like properties (Chu et al. 2009). Other stem cell markers, such as ALDH1, further enrich the cancer stem cell properties of the CD44 tumour population (Chu et al. 2009).

Pang et al. (2010) have explored the expression of two membrane markers, CD44 and CD26, in colorectal cancers and investigated the role of CSC subsets expressing these markers in tumorigenesis and metastasis. Particularly, they identified a subpopulation of CD26$^+$ cells present in both the primary and metastatic tumours in colorectal cancer patients with liver metastases. Importantly, in a group of patients without distant metastasis at the time of presentation, the presence of CD26$^+$ cells in their primary tumours predicted metastasis on follow-up. Isolated CD26$^+$ cells, but not CD26$^-$ cells, led to development of distant metastasis when injected into the mouse cecal wall; furthermore, CD26$^+$ cells were also associated with enhanced invasiveness and chemoresistance (Pang et al. 2010). This study suggests that analysis of CSC subsets in the primary colon cancers according to CD26$^+$ expression may have important clinical implications as a selection criterion for adjuvant therapy.

Recently, it was reported the isolation of a monoclonal antibody, mAbCC188 that selectively targets a carbohydrate epitope expressed on the surface of both colorectal cancer stem cells and their differentiated progeny, while it does not bind normal colonic mucosa (Xu et al. 2008).

It is of interest to note that in all the studies related to the use of CD133 and CD44 as markers for the identification and isolation of colon cancer stem cells it was noted the expression on these cells of EpCAM. EpCAM is a glycosylated, 30- to 40-kDa type I membrane protein, expressed in a variety of normal and malignant epithelial tissues, described several years ago as a dominant antigen in human colon carcinoma tissue. EpCAM has a dual role as cell adhesion. EpCAM has a dual role as cell adhesion molecule and receptor involved in the regulation of gene transcription and cell proliferation (Munz et al. 2009). Some lines of evidence suggest that EpCAM is required for the proliferation of cancer stem cells. Particularly, it was suggested that cancer stem cells benefit from activated EpCAM for proliferation, self-renewal, and anchorage-independent growth and invasiveness (Gires et al. 2009).

As mentioned in the section on normal intestinal stem cells recent studies have shown that ALDH1 could represent a marker for normal stem cells. Studies during progression from normal to mutant APC epithelium to adenoma, ALDH1-positive cells increased in number and became distributed farther up the crypt (Huang et al. 2009a, b). ALH1-positive cells isolated from colon cancers form tumours when inoculated in nude mice (Huang et al. 2009a, b). Interestingly, increased numbers of ALDH1-positive cells were found in the crypts of patients with chronic ulcerative colitis, a condition that predisposes to colon cancer development through a pathway known as the *inflammation-dysplasia-cancer progression* (Itzkowitz and Yio 2004). ALDH1-positive cells isolated from these patients undergo transition to cancerous stem cells after xenografting and can be propagated in vitro as tumour spheres (Corpentino et al. 2009).

Interestingly, cancer stem cells can be isolated not only from primary tumours, but also from colon cancer cell lines. In fact, it was shown that colon cancer cell lines contain cancer stem cell populations that can be enriched by the use of an in vitro Matrigel-based differentiation assay together with the selection for the expression of CD44 and CD24 cell surface markers. These CD44$^+$/CD24$^+$ cells are the most clonogenic in vitro and can initiate tumours in vivo (Yeung et al. 2010).

Therapeutics of Colon Cancer Stem Cells

Drug resistance has been long recognised as one of the major obstacles to effective chemotherapy and radiotherapy of cancer patients. One potential major mechanism responsible for drug resistance of cancer cells is the existence of a sub-population of cells within tumours that are inherently resistant to the treatments. Resistance of cancer stem cell populations to therapy was first reported in acute myeloid leukaemia stem cells (Costello et al. 2000). Since then, resistance to chemotherapy and/or radiotherapy, has been linked to cancer stem cell sub-populations in various solid tumours, including glioblastoma (Bao et al. 2006; Liu et al. 2006; Salmaggi et al. 2006), breast (Phillips et al. 2006), lung (Eramo et al. 2008) and colon (Todaro et al. 2007; Fang et al. 2010). Induction of the differentiation of cancer stem cells was associated with a decrease of their chemoresistance (Fang et al. 2010).

The identification of colon cancer stem cells has promoted many studies attempting to improve current treatments and to realize an efficacious prevention of this disease. It is evident that a major objective of these new therapeutics will consist in the targeting of colon cancer stem cells. According to the recently developed new informations on colon cancer stem cell biology, many potential targets could be envisaged: (a) agents targeting the stem cell niche; (b) agents targeting symmetric autoreplicative tumour stem cell division; (c) agents targeting functional cancer stem cell markers; (d) agents targeting constitutively activated signalling pathways in colon cancer stem cells. In this context, various attempts have been tested and are summarized below.

Some studies have explored the possible role of the blockade of growth factor signalling. A first study explored the role of IGF-IR signalling in sustaining colon cancer stem cell growth. Initial studies have shown that IGF-IR inhibition in an orthoptic model of metastatic colon cancer in the murine liver leads to decreased tumour growth by increased apoptosis (Bauer et al. 2007). The same studies carried out at the level of chemoresistant colon cancer cell lines provided evidence that these cells are particularly sensitive to tumour inhibition mediated by blocking anti-IGF-IR mAbs (Dallas et al. 2009).

Another signalling pathway of potential interest for inhibiting colon cancer stem cells is represented by hedgehog (HH)-Gli signalling pathway. HH signalling transduction requires the binding of HH to the transmembrane receptor Patched (Ptch); this binding determines the release of the repression of Smo by Ptch. This derepression determines the activation of Gli transcription factors. Constitutive activation of the HH pathway is observed in many tumours. HH-GLI activity is increased in colon cancer and increases with tumour progression. Importantly, HH-GLI activity was shown to be required for the survival of cancer stem cells in vivo and modulate the rate of CD133⁺ stem cell growth (Varnat et al. 2009). Inhibition of HH signalling markedly reduces colon cancer stem cell growth in vivo (Varnat et al. 2009).

Eph receptors and Ephrins have been shown to affect the growth, migration and invasion of cancer cells (Pasquale 2010). EphB receptors play a peculiar role in intestinal tumorigenesis in that they promote cell proliferation in the intestinal epithelium and function as tumour suppressors by controlling cell migration and inhibiting invasive growth. Recent studies have shown that cell migration and cell proliferation are controlled through independent mechanisms by EphB2. Particularly, EphB2-regulated cell positioning is mediated by phosphatidylinositol 3-kinase, whereas EphB2 regulates cell proliferation via its tyrosine kinase activity through an Abl-cyclin D1 pathway (Genander et al. 2009). During the progression from adenoma to colon carcinoma in humans, cyclinD1 regulation becomes uncoupled from EphB signalling, allowing continued proliferation with invasive growth. The dissociation of EphB2 signalling pathways enables the selective inhibition of the mitogenic effect without affecting the tumour suppressor function and permits the identification of a pharmacological strategy to suppress tumour growth (Genander et al. 2009).

An additional potential target at the level of colon cancer stem cells is represented by the cytokine interleukin-4 (IL-4). In fact, it was shown that IL-4 is upregulated in CD133⁺ colon cancer stem cells and contributes to protect these cells from apoptosis (Todaro et al. 2007). The tumorigenic growth of colon cancer stem cells was scarcely affected by 5-fluorouracil or oxaliplatin; however, if these cells were first incubated with anti-IL-4 antibodies markedly increase their sensitivity to both 5-fluorouracil and oxaliplatin (Todaro et al. 2007).

A potentially important target is the stem cell niche. Several major signalling pathways, involving Wnt and Notch, play a key role in maintaining the intestinal stem cell microenvironment. The stem cell niche plays a very important role in the control of the proliferation, migration and invasiveness of colonic stem cells. Therefore, various types of strategies targeting the intestinal cancer stem cell niche represent in their complex a potentially attractive option for developing new therapeutical approaches. In this context, the targeting of the Wnt pathway seems to be particularly important not only for its role in the maintenance of the intestinal stem cell niche but also for its very frequent constitutive activation due to mutations. In fact, the mutations acting on Wnt pathway have been found in over 90% of sporadic colorectal carcinomas (Thorstensen et al. 2005). Unfortunately, no Wnt pathway-specific pharmaceutical has entered clinical testing to date, a fact largely related to the lack of suitable enzyme targets of this signalling pathway. However, some recent reports have lead to the discovery of new small-molecule inhibitors of the Wnt pathway, which will enter clinical testing soon (Garber 2009). A recent study suggested an alternative strategy for an indirect targeting of Wnt signalling in colon cancer stem cells. In fact, Vermeulen et al. (2010) found that in colon cancer cells harbouring APC and K-RAS mutations, the subfraction of cells that displayed Wnt activation were highly enriched for stem cell properties. Surprisingly, they found that Wnt activation and the resulting cancer stem cell state were not a constitutive, cell autonomous process, but required the presence of stromal myofibroblasts responsible for the production of hepatocyte growth factor (HGF) that triggers activation of survival pathways and β-catenin phosphorylation. These findings indicate that HGF targeting using c-Met inhibitors may represent an alternative strategy to inhibit Wnt signalling in colon cancer stem cells (Vermeulen et al. 2010).

Previous studies have shown that some anti-inflammatory drugs, such as COX inhibitors, have shown to inhibit Wnt signalling, albeit by poorly understood mechanisms (Maier et al. 2005). Particularly, COX inhibitors have been shown to be capable of reversing the growth of colorectal polyps, thus validating the idea that Wnt signalling could represent an important anticancer target. Widely used non-steroidal anti-inflammatory drugs, such as aspirin and sulindac, effectively prevent colon cancer both in rodent and human models of colon carcinogenesis. The cellular targets of the chemopreventive effect of these drugs seem to be intestinal stem cells. In fact, studies in murine models have shown that dietary aspirin or sulindac promoted apoptosis of intestinal stem cells with aberrant Wnt signalling (Qiu et al. 2010).

In this context, particularly interesting are two recent reports. Using a TCF/β-catenin-dependent reporter assay, Chen et al. (2009a) performed a high-throughput screening of synthetic compound libraries and identified small compounds, including IWR-1, that inhibit Wnt signalling. On the other hand, Huang et al. (2009b) identified another compound, XAV939, structurally distinct from IWR-1, that similarly acts as a potent inhibitor of Wnt signalling. These two compounds exhibit several interesting analogies: both compounds result in a dramatic stabilization of Axin protein and, through this mechanism, induce degradation of β-catenin. Furthermore, both these compounds are able to inhibit Wnt signalling both in cells that have a normal or a constitutively activated Wnt signalling pathway. The analysis of the mechanism through which these compounds stabilize Axin provided some very interesting findings. Particularly, the study carried out by Huang et al. (2009b) has lead to the identification of tankyrase enzymes as components of the Wnt signalling pathway. The tankyrases destabilize axin through a biochemical modification called PARsylation [poly(ADP-ribosyl)ation]. The Wnt inhibitor XAV939 seems to block tankyrase-mediated destabilization of axin; there is preliminary evidence that also the other inhibitor, IWR-1, could act as a tankyrase inhibitor (Huang et al. 2009b).

More recently, using yeast cell-based phenotypic drug system specific for tankyrase I, it was reported that flavone acts as a potent inhibitor of this enzyme and could represent another Wnt signalling inhibitor (Yashiroda et al. 2010).

Other recent studies have lead to the identification of 2,4-diamino-quinazoline derivatives that inhibit the β-catenin/Tcf-4 pathway (Chen et al. 2009b; Dehnhardt et al. 2010). One of these compounds, compound 9, exhibited a good profile of biological and pharmacological properties, suitable for a possible development as an anticancer drug.

Kahn et al. screened for TCF/β-catenin inhibitors and found the leading compound ICG-001 that specifically targets and inhibits the co-activator CBP (Emami et al. 2004). Treatment of colon cancer cell lines bearing APC or β-catenin mutations with this compound induces dose-dependent cell death, while normal colonic epithelial cells are resistant. The effect is also seen in APCmin mouse model and in tumour xenografts. ICG-001 should enter in clinical phase I trials.

In addition to the Wnt signalling pathway, the NOTCH pathway too may represent an important pathway involved in the maintenance of colon cancer stem cells. Particularly, delta-like 4 ligand (DLL4) is an important component of the NOTCH-mediated cancer stem cell self-renewal. Initial studies have shown that inhibition of DLL4 directly acts on tumour cells and reduces cancer stem cell frequency in colon and breast tumours (Hoey et al. 2009). In a subsequent study, the efficacy of anti-DLL4 antibodies in K-RAS mutant tumours in a panel of early passage colon tumour xenograft models derived from patients was explored. Anti-DLL4 was efficacious against both wild-type and mutant K-RAS colon cancers as a single agent and in combination with irinotecan. Further analysis of mutant K-RAS tumours indicated that the anti-DLL4/irinotecan combination resulted in a significant decrease in colon cancer stem cell frequency, while promoting apoptosis in tumour cells (Fischer et al. 2011). These observations suggest that inhibition of NOTCH signalling may represent a promising strategy to target colon cancer stem cells.

Another interesting therapeutic approach would consist in the targeting of cancer stem cells. This approach takes advantage on the identification of specific membrane markers expressed on cancer stem cells. However, to date, the studies carried out have indicated that the membrane antigens expressed on cancer stem cells are shared with normal intestinal stem cells. However, the proportion of cells positive for these markers is usually markedly higher in malignant colon tissue than in its normal counterpart. Furthermore, the antigen density could be higher on the membrane of cancer stem cells than on normal intestinal stem cells. As above mentioned, several recent studies have provided evidence that some membrane stem cell markers, including Lgr5, are markedly more expressed in adenoma and colon cancer than in normal tissues. Thus, some monoclonal antibodies targeting membrane stem cell markers could be used for the development of new therapeutical approaches anti-colorectal cancer. In this context, a recent study reported the isolation of a monoclonal antibody against Lgr5 (Sasaki et al. 2010). This monoclonal antibody has potent complement-dependent cytotoxicity activity in vitro and shows strong anti-tumour activity in vivo against xenograft model by transplanting Lgr5 expressing CHO transfectants into SCID mice (Sasaki et al. 2010). It remains to be proved whether this type of mAb may be suitable for anti-colorectal therapy.

References

Leblond CP, Stevens CE, Begoroch R. (1948) Histological localization of newly-formed desoxyribonucleic acid. Science 108: 531–533.
Yen TH, Wright NA. (2006) The gastrointestinal tract stem cell niche. Stem Cell Rev 2: 203-212.
Crosnier C, Stamataki D, Lewis J. (2006) Organizing cell renewal in the intestine: stem cells, signals and combinatorial control. Nat Rev Genet 7: 349–359.
Pinto D, Gregorieff A, Begthel H, et al (2003) Canonical Wnt signals are essential for homeostasis of the intestinal epithelium. Genes Dev 17: 1709–1713.

Fre S, Huyghe M, Mourikis P, et al (2005) Notch signals control the fate of immature progenitor cells in the intestine. Nature 435: 959–963.

Mathur D, Bost A, Driven I, et al (2010) A transient niche regulates the specification of Drosophila intestinal stem cells. Science 327: 210–213.

Lopez-Garcia C, Klein G, Simons BD et al (2010) Intestinal stem cell replacement follows a pattern of neutral drift. Science 330: 822–825.

Snippert HJ, van der Flier L, Sato T et al (2010) Intestinal crypt homeostasis results from neutral competition between symmetrically dividing Lgr5 stem cells. Cell 145: 134–144.

MacDonald BT, Tamai K, He X. (2009) Wnt/β-catenin signalling: components, mechanisms, and diseases. Dev Cell 17: 9–29.

Bovolenta P, Esteve P, Ruiz JM, et al (2008) Beyond Wnt inhibition: new functions of secreted Frizzled-related proteins in development and disease. J Cell Sci 121: 737–746.

Wu X, Tu X, Joeng KS, et al (2008) Rac1 activation controls nuclear localization of beta-catenin during canonical Wnt signalling. Cell 133: 340–353.

Park J, Venteicher AS, Hong Y, et al (2009) Telomerase modulates Wnt signalling by association with target gene chromatin. Nature 460: 66–72.

Sierra J, Yoshida T, Joazeiro CA et al (2006) The APC tumor suppressor counteracts beta-catenin activation and H3K4 methylation at Wnt target genes. Genes Dev 20: 586–600.

Davidson G, Shen J, Huang YL, et al (2009) Cell cycle control of Wnt receptor activation. Dev cell 17: 788–799.

Reya T, Clevers H. (2005) Wnt signalling in stem cells and cancer. Nature 434: 843–850.

Van Es JH, van Gijn ME, Riccio D, et al (2005) Notch/γ-secretase inhibition turns proliferative cells in intestinal crypts and adenomas into goblet cells. Nature 435: 959–963.

Li L, Clevers H. (2010) Coexistence of quiescent and active adult stem cells in mammals. Science 327: 542–545.

Cheng H, Leblond CP. (1974) Origin, differentiation and renewal of the four main epithelial cell types in the mouse small intestine. V. Unitarian theory of the origin of the four epithelial cell types. Am J Anat 141: 537–561.

Ponder BA, Schmidt GH, Wilkinson MM, et al (1985) Derivation of mouse intestinal crypts from single progenitor cells. Nature 313: 689–691.

Schmidt GH, Winton DJ, Ponder BA (1988) Development of the pattern of cell renewal in the crypt-villus unit of chimaeric mouse small intestine. Development 103: 785–790.

Gutierrez-Gonzalez L, Deheragoda M, Novelli M et al (2009) Analysis of the clonal architecture of the human small intestine epithelium establishes a common stem cell for all lineages and reveals a mechanism for the fixation and spread of mutations. J Pathol 217: 489–496.

Barker N, van Es JH, Kuipers J et al (2007) Identification of stem cells in small intestine and colon by marker gene Lgr5. Nature 449: 1003–1007.

Barker N, Clevers H (2007) Tracking down the stem cells of the intestine: strategies to identify adult stem cells. Gastroenterology 133: 1755–1760.

Sato T, Vries RG, Snippert HJ et al (2009) Single Lgr stem cells build crypt-villus structures in vitro without a mesenchymal niche. Nature 459: 262–265.

Van der Flier L, van Gijn ME, Hatzis P et al (2009a) Transcription factor Achaete Suite-Like 2 controls intestinal stem cell fate. Cell 136: 903–912.

Lee G, White LS, Hurov KE, et al (2009) Response of small intestinal epithelial cells to acute disruption of cell division through CDC25 deletion. Proc Natl Acad Sci USA 106: 4701–4706.

Barker N, Huch M, Kujala P, et al (2010) Lgr5+ve stem cells drive self-renewal in the stomach and build long-lived gastric units in vitro. Cell Stem Cells 6: 25–36.

Garcia MI, Ghiani M, Lefort A, et al (2009) LGR5 deficiency deregulates Wnt signalling and leads to precocious Paneth cell differentiation in the fetal intestine. Dev Biology 331: 58–67.

Zhu L, Gibson P, Currle DS et al (2009) Prominin 1 marks intestinal stem cells that are susceptible to neoplastic transformation. Nature 457: 603–607.

Snippert HJ, van Es JH, van den Born M, et al (2009) Prominin-1/CD133 marks stem cells and early progenitors in mouse small intestine. Gastroenterology 136: 2187–2194.

Van der Flier LG, Haegebarth A, Stauge DE, et al (2009b) OLFM4 is a robust marker for stem cells in human intestine and marks a subset of colorectal cancer cells. Gastroenterology 137: 15–17.

Kosinski C, Li VS, Chan AS, et al (2007) Gene expression patterns of human colon tops and basal crypts and BMP antagonists as intestinal stem cell niche factors. Proc Natl Acad Sci USA 104: 15418–15423.

Zhang J, Liu WL, Thang DC, et al (2002) Identification and characterization of a novel member of olfactomedin-related protein family, hGC-1, expressed during myeloid lineage development. Gene 283: 83–93.

Sangiorgi E, Capecchi MR. (2008) Bmi1 is expressed in vivo in intestinal stem cells. Nature Genet 40: 915–920.

Sangiorgi E, Capecchi MR. (2009) Bmi1 lineage tracing identifies a self-renewing pancreatic acinar cell subpopulation capable of maintaining pancreatic organ homeostasis. Proc Natl Acad Sci USA 106: 7101–7106.

Potten CS, Booth C, Tudor GL et al (2003) Identification of a putative intestinal stem cell and early lineage marker, musashi-1. Differentiation 71: 28–41.

Murayama M, Okamoto R, Tsuchiya K, et al (2009) Musashi-1 suppresses expression of Paneth cell-specific genes in human intestinal epithelial cells. J Gastroenterol 44: 173–182.

Gracz AD, Ramalingam S, Magness ST. (2010) Sox9-expression marks a subset of CD24-expressing small intestine epithelial cells that form organoids in vitro. Am J Physiol Gastrointest Liver Physiol, 298: 4590–4600.

Furuyama K, Kawaguchi Y, Akiyama H et al (2011) Continuous cell supply from Sox9-expressing progenitor zone in adult liver, exocrine pancreas and intestine. Nature Genet 43: 34–41.

Giannakis M, Stappenbeck TS, Mills JC, et al (2006) Molecular properties of adult mouse gastric and intestinal epithelial progenitors in their niches. J Biol Chem 281: 11292–11300.

May R, Riehl TE, Hunt C, et al (2008) Identification of a novel putative gastrointestinal stem cell and adenoma stem cell marker, doublecortin and CaM kinase-like-1, following radiation injury and in adenomatous coli/multiple intestinal neoplasia mice. Stem Cells 26: 630–637.

May R, Sureban SM, Hoang N, et al (2009) Doublecortin and CaM Kinase-like-1 and Leucine-Rich-Repeat-Containing G-protein-coupled receptor mark quiescent and cycling intestinal stem cells, respectively. Stem Cells 27: 2571–2579.

Jin G, Ramanathan V, Quanta M, et al (2009) Inactivating cholecystokinin-2 receptor inhibits progastrin-dependent colonic crypt fission, proliferation, and colorectal cancer in mice. J Clin Invest 119: 2691–2701.

Huang EH, Hynes MJ, Zhang T, et al (2009a) Aldehyde dehydrogenase 1 is a marker for normal and malignant human colonic stem cells (SC) and tracks SC overpopulation during colon tumorigenesis. Cancer Res 69: 3382–3389.

Levin TG, Powell AE, DavesPS, et al (2010) Characterization of the intestinal cancer stem cell marker CD166 in the human and mouse gastrointestinal tract. Gstroenterology 139: 2072–2082.

Holmberg J, Genander M, Halford MM et al (2006) EphB receptors coordinate migration and proliferation in the intestinal stem cell niche. Cell 125: 1151–1163.

Marsham E, Booth C, Potten CS. (2002) The intestinal epithelial stem cell. Bioessays 24: 91–98.

Fellous TG, McDonald S, Burkert J, et al (2009) A methodological approach to tracing cell lineage in human epithelial tissues. Stem Cells 27: 1410–1420.

Sato T, Van Es J, Snippert HJ et al (2011) Paneth cells constitute the niche for Lgr5 stem cells in intestinal crypts. Nature, 469: 415–418.

Scoville DH, Sato T, He XC, et al (2008) Current view: intestinal stem cells and signalling. Gastroenterology 134: 849–864.

Quyn AJ, Appleton PL, Carey FA, et al (2010) Spindle orientation bias in gut epithelial stem cell compartments is lost in precancerous tissues. Cell Stem Cell 5: 175–181.

Fearon ER, Vogelstein B. (1990) A genetic model for colorectal tumorigenesis. Cell 61: 759–767.

Phelps RA, Chidester S, Dehghanizadeh S, et al (2009) A two-step model for colon adenoma initiation and progression caused by APC loss. Cell 137: 623–634.

Miyazaki M, Furuya T, Shiraki A, et al (1999) The relationship of DNA ploidy to chromosomal instability in primary human colorectal cancers. Cancer Res 59: 5283–5285.

Walther A, Johnstone E, Swanton C et al (2009) Genetic prognostic and predictive markers in colorectal cancer. Nat Rev Cancer 9: 489–499.

Barker N, Ridgway RA, van Es JH, et al (2009) Crypt stem cells as the cells-of-origin of intestinal cancer. Nature 457: 608–611.

Boman BM, Fields JZ, Bohnham-Carter O et al (2001) Computer modelling implicates stem cell overproduction in colon cancer initiation. Cancer Res 61: 8408–8411.

Boman BM, Huang E. (2008) Human colon cancer stem cells: a new paradigm in gastrointestinal oncology. J Clin Oncol 26: 2828–2838.

Boman BM, Wicha MS, Fields JZ, et al (2007) Symmetric division of human cancer stem cells- a key mechanism in tumor growth that should be targeted in future therapeutic approaches. Clin Pharmacol Ther 81: 893–898.

Boman BM, Walters R, Fields JZ, et al (2004) Colonic crypt changes during adenoma development in familial adenomatous polyposis: immunohistochemical evidence for expansion of the crypt base cell population. Am J Pathol 165: 1489–1498.

Boman BM, Fields JZ, Cavanaugh KL, et al (2008) How dysregulated colonic crypt dynamics cause stem cell overpopulation and initiate colon cancer. Cancer Res 6: 3304–3313.

Fan XS, Wu HY, Yu HP, et al (2010) Expression of Lgr5 in human colorectal carcinogenesis and its potential correlation with β-catenin. Int J Colorect Dis 25: 583–590.

Uchida H, Yamazaki K, Fukuma M, et al (2010) Overexpression of leucin-rich repeat-containing G protein-coupled receptor 5 in colorectal cancer. Cancer Sci, in press.

Lewis A, Segditsas S, Deheragoda M, et al (2010) Severe polyposis in Apc^{1322T} mice is associated with submaximal Wnt signaling and increased expression of the stem cell marker Lgr5. Gut 59: 1680–1686.

Hamburger AW, Salmon SE. (1977) Primary bioassay of human tumor stem cells. Science 197: 461–463.

Reya T, Morrison SJ, Clarke MF, et al (2001) Stem cells, cancer and cancer stem cells. Nature 414: 105–111.

Bonnet D, Dick JE. (1997) Human acute myeloid leukemia is organized as a hierarchy that originates from a primitive hematopoietic cell. Nat Med 3: 730–737.

Sell S, Pierce GB. (1994) Maturation arrest of stem cell differentiation is a common pathway for the cellular origin of teratocarcinomas and epithelial cancers. Lab Invest 70: 6–22.

Lobo NA, Shimono Y, Qian D, et al (2007) The biology of cancer stem cells. Annu Rev Cell Dev Biol 23: 675–699.

Corbeil D, Roper K, Hellwig A, et al (2000) The human AC133 hematopoietic stem cell antigen is also expressed in epithelial cells and targeted to plasma membrane protrusions. J Biol Chem 275: 5512–5520.

Corbeil D, Roper K, Fargeas CA, et al (2001) Prominin: a story of cholesterol, plasma membrane protrusions and human pathology. Traffic 2: 82–91.

Weigmann A, Corbeil D, Hellwig A, et al (1997) Prominin, a novel microvilli-specific polytopic membrane protein of the apical surface of epithelial cells, is targeted to plasmalemmal protrusions of non-epithelial cells. Proc Natl Acad Sci USA 94: 12425–12430.

Ricci-Vitani L, Lombardi D, Pilozzi E, et al (2007) Identification and expansion of human colon-cancer-initiating cells. Nature 445: 111–115.

O'Brien CA, Pollett A, Gallinger S, et al (2007) A human colon cancer cell capable of initiating tumor growth in immunodeficient mice. Nature 445: 106–110.

Shmelkov SV, Butler JM,Hooper AT, et al (2008) CD133 expression is not restricted to stem cells, and both CD133⁺ and CD133⁻ metastatic colon cancer cells initiate tumors. J Clin Invest 118: 2111–2120.

Vermeulen L, Todaro M, de Sousa Mello, et al (2008) Single-cell cloning of colon cancer stem cells reveals a multi-lineage differentiation capacity. Proc Natl Acad Sci USA 105: 13427–13432.

Horst D, Kriegl L, Engel J, et al (2008) CD133 expression is an independent prognostic marker for low survival in colorectal cancer. Br J Cancer 99: 1285–1289.

Horst D, Kriegl L, Engel J, et al (2009a) CD133 and nuclear beta-catenin: the marker combination to detect high risk cases of low stage colorectal cancer. Eur J Cancer 45: 2034–2040.

Artells R, Moreno I, Diaz T, et al (2010) Tumor CD133 mRNA expression and clinical outcome in surgically resected colorectal cancer patients. Eur J Cancer 46: 642–649.

Horst D, Scheel SK, Liebmann S, et al (2009b) The cancer stem cell marker CD133 has high prognostic impact but unknown functional relevance for the metastasis of human colon cancer. J Pathol 219: 427–434.

Kemper K, Sprick MR, de Bree M, et al (2010) The AC133 epitope, but not the CD133 protein, is lost upon cancer stem cell differentiation. Cancer Res 70: 719–729.

Manhaba R, Klingbeil P, Nuebel T, et al (2008) CD44 and EpCAM cancer-initiating cell markers. Curr Mol Med 8: 784–804.

Orian-Rousseau V. (2010) CD44, a therapeutic target for metastasising tumours. Eur J Cancer 46: 1271–1277.

Wielenga VJ, van der Neut R, Offerhaus GJ, et al (2000) CD44 glycoproteins in colorectal cancer: expression, function, and prognostic value. Adv Cancer Res 77: 169–187.

Kim HR, Wheeler MA, Wilson CM et al (2004) Hyaluronan facilitates invasion of colon carcinoma cells in vitro via interaction with CD44. Cancer Res 64: 4569–4576.

Dalerba P, Dylla SJ, Park IK, et al (2007) Phenotypic characterization of human colorectal cancer stem cells. Proc Natl Acad Sci USA 104: 10158–10163.

Chu P, Clanton DJ, Snipas TS, et al (2009) Characterization of a subpopulation of colon cancer cells with stem cell-like properties. Int J Cancer 124: 1312–1321.

Pang R, Law WL, Chu A, et al (2010) A subpopulation of CD26+ cancer stem cells with metastatic capacity in human colorectal cancer. Cell Stem Cell 6: 603–615.

Xu M, Yuan Y, Xia Y, et al (2008) Monoclonal antibody CC188 binds a carbohydrate epitope expressed on the surface of both colorectal cancer stem cells and their differentiated progeny. Clin Cancer Res 14: 7461–7469.

Munz M, Baeuerle PA, Gires O (2009) The emerging role of EpCAM in cancer and stem cell signalling. Cancer Res 69: 5627–5629.

Gires O, Klein CA, Baeuerle PA. (2009) On the abundance of EpCAM on cancer stem cells. Nature Rev Cancer 9: 143–150.

Itzkowitz SH, Yio X. (2004) Inflammation and cancer IV. Colorectal cancer in inflammatory bowel disease: the role of inflammation. Am J Physiol Gastrointest Liver Physiol 287: G7–17.

Corpentino JE, Hynes MJ, Appelman HD, et al (2009). Aldehyde dehydrogenase-expression colon stem cells contribute to tumorigenesis in the transition from colitis to cancer. Cancer Res 69: 8208–8215.

Yeung TM, Gandhi SC, Wilding JL, et al (2010) Cancer stem cells from colorectal cancer-derived cell lines. Proc Natl Acad Sci USA 107: 3722–3727.

Costello RT, Mallet F, Gaugler B, et al (2000) Human acute myeloid leukemia CD34+/CD38- progenitor cells have decreased sensitivity to chemotherapy and Fas-induced apoptosis, reduced immunogenicity, and impaired dendritic cell transformation capacities. Cancer Res 60: 4403–4411.

Bao S, Wu Q, McLendon RE, et al (2006) Glioma stem cells promote radioresistance by preferential activation of the DNA damage response. Nature 444: 756–760.

Liu G, Yuan X, Zeng Z, et al (2006) Analysis of gene expression and chemoresistance of CD133+ cancer stem cells in glioblastoma. Mol Cancer 5: 67–77.

Salmaggi A, Boiardi A, Gelati M, et al (2006) Glioblastoma-derived tumospheres identify a population of tumor stem-like cells with angiogenic potential and enhanced multidrug resistance phenotype. Glia 54: 850–860.

Phillips TM, McBride WH, Pajonk F. (2006) The response of CD24 (-/low)/CD44 breast cancer-initiating cells to radiation J Natl Cancer Inst 98: 1777–1785.

Eramo A, Lotti F, Sette G, et al (2008) Identification and expansion of the tumorigenic lung cancer stem cell population. Cell death Differ 15: 504–514.

Todaro M, Alea MP, Di Stefano AB, et al (2007) Colon cancer stem cells dictate tumor growth and resist cell death by production of interleukin-4. Cell Stem Cell 1: 389–402.

Fang DD, Kim YI, Lee CN, et al (2010) Expansion of CD133+ colon cancer cultures retaining stem cell properties to enable cancer stem cell target discovery. Brit J Cancer, 102: 1265–1275.

Bauer TW, Fan F, Liu W, et al (2007) Targeting of insulin-like growth factor-I receptor with a monoclonal antibody inhibits growth of hepatic metastases from human colon carcinoma in mice. Ann Surg Oncol 14: 2838–2846.

Dallas NA, Xia L, Fan F, et al (2009) Chemoresistant colorectal cancer cells, the cancer stem cell phenotype, and increased sensitivity to insulin-like growth factor-I receptor inhibition. Cancer Res 69: 1951–1957.

Varnat F, Duquet A, Malerba M, et al (2009) Human colon cancer epithelial cells harbour active HEDGEHOG-GLI signalling that is essential for tumor growth, recurrence, metastasis and stem cell survival and expansion. EMBO Mol Med 1: 338–351.

Pasquale EB. (2010) Eph receptors and ephrins in cancer: bidirectional signalling and beyond. Nature Rev Cancer 10: 165–180.

Thorstensen L, Lind GE, Lovig T et al (2005) Genetic and epigenetic changes of components affecting the WNT pathway in colorectal carcinomas stratified by microsatellite instability. Neoplasia 7: 99–108.

Garber K. (2009) Drugging the Wnt pathway: problems and progress. J Natl Cancer Inst 101: 548–550.

Vermeulen L, Melo F, van der Heijden M, et al (2010) Wnt activity defines colon cancer stem cells and is regulated by the microenvironment. Nature Cell Biol 12: 468–476.

Maier TJ, Janssen A, Geisslinger A, et al (2005) Targeting the beta catenin/APC pathway: a novel mechanism explain the cyclooxygenase-2-independent anticarcinogenic effect of celecoxib in human colon carcinoma cells. FASEB J 19: 1353–1355.

Qiu W, Wang X, Leibowitz B et al (2010) Chemoprevention by nonsteroidal anti-inflammatory drugs eliminates oncogenic intestinal cells via SMAC-dependent apoptosis. Proc Natl Acad Sci USA 107: 2027–2032.

Chen B, Dodge ME, Tang W, et al (2009a) Small molecule-mediated disruption of Wnt-dependent signalling in tissue regeneration and cancer. Nature Chem Biol 5: 100-107.

Huang SM, Mishina YM, Liu S, et al (2009b) Tankyrase inhibition stabilizes axin and antagonizes Wnt signalling. Nature 462: 614–620.

Yashiroda Y, Okamoto R, Hatsugai K, et al (2010) A novel yeast cell-based screen identifies flavone as a tankyrase inhibitor. Biochem Biophys Res Commun 394: 569–573.

Chen Z, Venkatesan AM, Dehnhardt CM, et al (2009b) 2,4-diamino-quinazolines as inhibitors of β-catenin/Tcf-4 pathway: potential treatment for colorectal cancer. Biorg Med Chem Letters 19: 4980–4983.

Dehnhardt CM, Venkatesan AM, Chen Z, et al (2010) Design and synthesis of novel diaminoquinazolines with in vivo efficacy for β-catenin/T-cell transcriptional factor 4 pathway inhibition. J Med Chem 53: 897–910.

Emami KH, Nguyen C, Ma H et al (2004) A small molecule inhibitor of beta-catenin/CREB-binding protein transcription. Proc Natl Acad Sci USA 101: 12682–12687.

Hoey T, Yen WC, Axelrod F et al (2009) DLL4 blockade inhibits tumor growth and reduces tumor-initiating cell frequency. Cell Stem Cell 5: 168–177.

Fischer M, Yen WC, Kapoun AM, et al (2011) Anti-DLL4 inhibits growth and reduces tumor initiating cell frequency in colorectal tumors with oncogenic KRAS mutations. Cancer Res, 71: 1520–1525.

Sasaki Y, Kosaka H, Usami K, et al (2010) Establishment of a novel monoclonal antibody against LGR5. Biochem Biophys Res Commun 394: 498–502.

Potten CS, Kovacs L, Hamilton E. (1974) Continuous labelling studies on mouse skin and intestine. Cell Tissue Kinet 7: 271–283.

Genander M, Halford MM, Xu NJ et al. (2009) Dissociation of EphB2 signalling pathways mediating progenitor cell proliferation and tumor suppression. Cell 139: 679–692.

Chapter 11
Liver Tumor-Initiating Cells/Cancer Stem Cells: Past Studies, Current Status, and Future Perspectives[*]

Kwan Ho Tang, Stephanie Ma, and Xin-Yuan Guan

Introduction

Hepatocellular carcinoma (HCC) is one of the most prevalent malignancies worldwide. Although surgical interference is available for patients with early-stage HCC, only 25% of patients are amendable to surgery since most patients are diagnosed at such an advanced stage when these therapies are no longer an option. Treatment of the disease is also further complicated by a high rate of recurrence and its strong resistance to traditional anticancer therapies including those of chemotherapy and radiotherapy. Therefore, understanding the roots and mechanisms underlying hepatocarcinogensis is essential for the management of the disease. Recently, a minor population with tumor and stem cell-like properties has been detected in a number of established HCC cell lines, as well as freshly resected HCC clinical specimens. A number of studies have also elucidated molecular mechanisms underlying hepatocarcinogenesis in these tumor-initiating cells (TICs) or cancer stem cells (CSCs). A better understanding of the cellular organization of HCC will allow us to establish novel therapies targeting specific cell types like CSCs.

---

[*]Kwan Ho Tang and Stephanie Ma contributed equally to this work.

K. Ho Tang • S. Ma
Department of Pathology, Li Ka Shing Faculty of Medicine, Queen Mary Hospital,
The University of Hong Kong, Pok Fu Lam, Hong Kong

X.-Y. Guan (✉)
Department of Clinical Oncology, Li Ka Shing Faculty of Medicine, Queen Mary Hospital,
The University of Hong Kong, Pok Fu Lam, Hong Kong
e-mail: xyguan@hkucc.hku.hk

Markers of Liver CSCs

Side Population

The side population (SP) phenotype, first introduced by Goodell et al. in the context of bone marrow hematopoietic cells, is determined by the cell's ability to efflux the DNA interacting Hoechst 33342 dye through adenosine triphosphate (ATP)-binding cassette (ABC) membrane transporters (Goodell et al. 1996). The technique is now extensively applied for the enrichment of normal stem cells in a wide array of tissue types (Challen and Little 2006); as well as in the enrichment of CSCs in hematological and solid tumors (Moserle et al. 2010), including HCC (Haraguchi et al. 2006; Chiba et al. 2006).

In 2006, Chiba et al. first reported the identification of a SP in a proportion of several established HCC cell lines – 0.25% SP and 0.8% SP in Huh7 and PLC/PRF/5 cells, respectively (Chiba et al. 2006). In the same study, the research group also tested two other liver cell lines, HepG2 and Huh6, but failed to identify such SP from these cells. Compared to non-SP cells, SP cells isolated from both Huh7 and PLC/PRF/5 displayed an enhanced proliferative and anti-apoptotic potential and exhibited bi-potentiality to differentiate into both hepatocyte and cholangiocyte lineages, as evident by its expression of hepatocyte-specific marker alpha-fetoprotein (AFP) and cholangiocyte-specific marker cytokeratin 19 (CK19). Further, in vivo experiments found SP subpopulation to possess a greater ability to initiate tumors in immunodeficient mice. As little as 1×10^3 SP cells isolated from Huh7 or PLC/PRF/5 cells were able to initiate tumor formation, while injection of 1×10^6 non-SP cells failed to generate a tumor in the same model. More importantly, these tumors exhibited the ability to self-renew as evident by its ability to serially propagate themselves in secondary animal recipients. Microarray analysis on SP and non-SP cells isolated from both Huh7 and PLC/PRF/5 identified a number of "stemness genes" to be preferentially upregulated in SP, including ABC transporters and the polycomb-group (PcG) gene product, Bmi-1 (Chiba et al. 2006, 2008). Subsequent studies by the same group defined a vital role for Bmi-1 in the maintenance of tumor-initiating SP cells (Chiba et al. 2008; see section "Bmi-1").

Similarly, work by Haraguchi et al. (2006) in the same year also identified a SP in HCC cell lines Huh7 (0.9%) and Hep3B (1.8%). Also consistent with studies by Chiba et al., their studies failed to identify a SP in HepG2 cells. Using a human whole genome oligo microarray, the authors determined differentially expressed genes between SP and non-SP lineages of Huh7 and found an increase in expression of genes involved in ABC transporters/multidrug resistance (BCRP1, MDR1), signaling pathways of normal stem cells (BMP2, JAG1), as well as chemoresistance (CEACAM6). SP cells isolated from Huh7 cells displayed an enhanced survival against chemotherapeutic drugs doxorubicin, 5-fluorouracil and gemcitabine. Most interestingly, CD133 was found to stain strongly positive in SP cells but not in non-SP cells (Table 11.1).

11 Liver Tumor-Initiating Cells/Cancer Stem Cells: Past Studies, Current Status...

Table 11.1 Commonly used markers to identify liver CSCs

Marker	Frequency	Origin	Cell line(s) studied	Minimum number of cells required for tumor imitation in vivo (mouse strain)	Reference
SP	0–0.8%	Cell lines	HepG2, Huh6, Huh7, PLC/PRF/5	1×10^3 (NOD-SCID)	Chiba et al. (2006)
SP	0–1.8%	Cell lines	Huh7, Hep3B, HepG2	–	Haraguchi et al. (2006)
CD133+	0.05–46.79%	Cell lines	Huh7, HepG2, Hc	– (SCID)	Suetsugu et al. (2006)
CD133+	0.1–2%	Cell lines	SMMC-7721	1×10^2 (NOD-SCID)	Yin et al. (2007)
CD133+	0–90%	Cell lines	MiHA, H2P, H2M, H4M, HepG2, Huh7, PLC8024, Hep3B	1×10^3 (SCID)	Ma et al. (2007)
CD133+	1.3–13.6%	Clinical samples	–	2×10^4 (SCID)	Ma et al. (2010)
CD133+	0.1–93.18%	Cell lines	SMMC-7721, MHCC-LM3, HepG2, MHCC-97L, Huh7, Hep3B	1×10^2 (NOD-SCID)	Zhu et al. (2010)
CD133+CD44+	0.09–1.88%	Cell lines	Huh7, SMMC-7721, MHCC-LM3, HepG2	1×10^2 (NOD-SCID)	Zhu et al. (2010)
CD133+ALDH+	0–55.71%	Cell lines	MiHA, H2P, H2M, H4M, HepG2, Huh7, PLC8024, Hep3B	5×10^2 (SCID)	Ma et al. (2008b)
EpCAM+	–	Cell lines	Huh1, Huh7, Hep3B, SK-Hep-1, HLE, HLF	2×10^2 (NOD-SCID)	Yamashita et al. (2009)
EpCAM+	1.4–5.2%	Clinical samples	–	1×10^4 (NOD-SCID)	Yamashita et al. (2009)
OV6+	0.2–3%	Cell lines	Huh7, PLC, SMMC-7721, Hep3B, HepG2	5×10^3 (NOD-SCID)	Yang et al. (2008a)
CD90+	0–1.85%	Cell lines	MiHA, HepG2, Hep3B, PLC, Huh7, MHCC-97L, MHCC-97H	2×10^3 (Nude)	Yang et al. (2008b)
CD90+	0.42–8.57%	Clinical samples	–	1×10^3 (SCID)	Yang et al. (2008b)
CD90+	0.04–2.34%	Cell lines	MiHA, HepG2, Hep3B, PLC, Huh7, MHCC-97L, MHCC-97H	5×10^2 (Nude)	Yang et al. (2008c)
CD90+	0.03–6.2%	Clinical samples	–	2.5×10^3 (SCID)	Yang et al. (2008c)
CD90+CD44+	0–2.53%	Cell lines	MiHA, HepG2, Hep3B, PLC, Huh7, MHCC-97L, MHCC-97H	5×10^2 (Nude)	Yang et al. (2008c)

SP side population, *ALDH* aldehyde dehydrogenase

Markers

CD133[+]

Since 2006, work from a number of laboratories has pointed to CD133 as a CSC marker of HCC. Suetsugu et al. (2006) provided the first evidence suggesting CD133 to be a novel marker of CSC in established HCC cell lines. CD133 expression was detected in all three HCC cell lines tested (Huh7, HepG2, and fetal hepatocyte cell line Hc), with expression ranging from 0.05% (Hc) to 46.79% (Huh7). Functional studies on sorted CD133 cells from Huh7 found CD133[+] cells to exhibit higher tumorigenic potential both in vitro and in vivo. CD133[+] cells were able to self-renew as evident by their ability to generate CD133[−] cells in vivo. In addition, CD133[+] cells also expressed higher expression of AFP and lower mRNA expression of mature hepatocyte markers, glutamine synthetase (GS), and cytochrome P450 3A4 (CYP3A4). In 2007, Yin et al. likewise found CD133[+] cells isolated from HCC cell line SMMC-7721 to display a higher tumorigenicity and clonogenicity ability as compared with CD133[−] cells (Yin et al. 2007). CD133 expression in SMMC-7721 ranged from 0.1 to 2% in. In vivo, sorted CD133[+] cells were also able to induce tumor formation with fewer numbers of cells and in a shorter period of time when injected into immunodeficient mice via either intrahepatic or intraperitoneal inoculation, than compared with CD133[−] cells. In addition to HCC cell lines, Yin et al. also further studied CD133 expression levels in 85 human HCC specimens by immunohistochemistry (IHC) technique. CD133[+] cells were found in most HCC tissue samples tested, though they only represented a very small subpopulation of the total cancer cells (0.1–1%). In contrast, CD133 expression was absent in normal hepatocytes or biliary epithelial structures in portal area; while only minimal CD133 expression was occasionally detected in adjacent non-tumorous liver tissues in HCC patients as well as liver tissues from patients with liver cirrhosis.

In the same year as when the former two research groups published their findings, our research team has also similarly identified CD133 to be a CSC marker in HCC (Ma et al. 2007). Unlike the work from the previous two groups, the basis for our study on CD133 stemmed from a genome-wide microarray analysis comparing RNA collected from different time points of a mouse partial hepatectomy model where over 70% of the mouse liver mass was removed. Liver regeneration following partial hepatectomy has been documented to rely on a subset of stem cells. Since normal stem cells and CSCs share common properties, we believe that identification of normal liver stem cells will lend insight into the understanding of the events that regulate liver cell self-renewal and differentiation. Using this platform, we found prominin-1 (the mouse homologue of human CD133) to be significantly involved in the early events of liver regeneration, with its expression rapidly declining immediately following restoration of the liver. CD133 expression was subsequently analyzed by flow cytometry in a series of human liver cell lines including the normal, immortalized liver cell line MiHA, hepatoblastoma cell line HepG2 and HCC cell lines H2P, H2M, H4M, Huh7, PLC8024, and Hep3B. Expression of CD133 in liver cell lines positively correlated with their ability to develop tumors when injected subcutaneously in nude mice. Functional studies of sorted CD133 from liver cell lines Huh7, PLC8024, HepG2, and xenograft tumors, found CD133⁺ cells to possess a greater colon-forming efficiency as well as a greater ability to form tumors when injected either subcutaneously or intrahepatically in immunodeficient mice. As little as 1,000 CD133⁺ cells were able to initiate tumors in SCID/beige mice, while at least 50× as many CD133⁻ cells was needed to generate similar tumors in the same model. In addition, compared with CD133⁻ counterparts, CD133⁺ cells were endowed with characteristics similar to those of stem cells including the preferential expression of stem cell-associated genes (β-catenin, Notch, Smo, Bmi, and Oct3/4), the ability to self-renew (serial-transplantation in secondary animals) and the ability to differentiate into non-hepatocyte-like, angiomyogenic-like cells. Following cell-directed differentiation of CD133⁺ cells in vitro, a significant decrease in hepatocyte-expressing genes including AFP, cytokeratin 18 (CK18), transthyretin (TTR) and albumin (ALB) was observed, concomitant with a dramatic increase in muscle and cardiac-specific markers including MEF2C and MYOD1. Subsequent studies by our group also found CD133 to confer chemoresistance in HCC through the preferential activation of Akt/PKB and Bcl-2 pathway (Ma et al. 2008a; see section "Akt/PKB and Bcl-2 Pathway (CD133)").

In addition to cell lines and xenografts, our group also recently extended our studies of CD133 in human primary HCC clinical samples (Ma et al. 2010). Flow cytometry analysis of 35 human HCC specimens found CD133 to account for approximately 1.3–13.6% of the cells in the bulk tumor and increased CD133 expression to be associated with higher histological tumor grade and larger tumor size. When compared with CD133⁻ counterparts, CD133⁺ cells isolated from these HCC clinical samples not only possess the preferential ability to form undifferentiated tumor spheroids in vitro, but also express an enhanced level of stem cell-associated genes, a greater ability to form tumors when implanted orthotopically in immunodeficient mice as well as capability of being serially passaged into secondary animal recipients. Xenografts resemble the original human tumor and maintain a similar percentage of tumorigenic CD133⁺ cells. Further, quantitative PCR (qPCR) analysis on a separate cohort of HCC tissue specimens with follow-up data found CD133⁺ tumor cells to be frequently detected in low quantity in HCC and that their presence was also associated with worst overall survival and higher recurrence rates.

Song et al. (2008) also examined expression of CD133 in human HCC specimen ($n=63$) by IHC staining and in line with our findings; they also found CD133⁺ tumor cells to be frequently detected in HCC and increased CD133 expression levels to be correlated with increased tumor grade, advanced disease stage and elevated serum AFP levels. Kaplan–Meier analysis indicated that patients with increased CD133 levels had shorter overall survival and higher recurrence rates compared with patients with low CD133 expression. In addition, multivariate analyses revealed that increased CD133 expression was an independent prognostic factor for survival and tumor recurrence in HCC patients.

CD133+ Aldehyde Dehydrogenase+

Using a two-dimensional (2D) PAGE approach to compare the protein profiles between sorted CD133 subpopulations in HCC cell line Huh7, our group subsequently identified aldehyde dehydrogenase (ALDH) to be an additional marker to CD133 for the more precise identification of liver CSCs (Ma et al. 2008b). Unlike other cell surface markers, ALDH is a cytosolic enzyme. It was first found to function to oxidize intracellular aldehydes and to be highly expressed in human hematopoietic normal stem/progenitor cells (Pearce et al. 2005; Hess et al. 2006). We found the expression of several different isoforms of ALDH, including ALDH1A1, ALDH1A2, and ALDH3A1, as well as ALDH enzymatic activity, to positively correlate with CD133 expression across a panel of HCC cell lines (HepG2, Huh7, PLC8024, Hep3B, H2P, H2M, 7701, 7703, 7402). Dual-color flow cytometry for both CD133 and ALDH found ALDH to be exclusively expressed in the CD133+ subpopulation in a number of HCC cell lines. Subsequent functional studies on dually sorted CD133 and ALDH subpopulations from HCC cells PLC8024 revealed the existence of a hierarchical organization bearing tumorigenic potential in the order of CD133+ALDH+ > CD133+ALDH− > CD133−ALDH− (Ma et al. 2008b).

CD133+CD44+

Succeeding their work in 2007, Li J and his team in 2009 found HCC CSCs can be more precisely defined by the co-expression of CD133 and CD44 (Zhu et al. 2010). CD44 was found to be preferentially expressed in the CD133+ subpopulation in several HCC cell lines. For instance, they found more than 60% of Huh7 cells to be CD133 positive, but only 1.88% of the cells to be both positive for CD133 and CD44. CD133+CD44+ cells showed both cancer and stem cell-like properties, including the ability to form colonies, self-renew and differentiate. The authors claim that in vivo xenograft experiments found that the highly tumorigenic capacity of CD133+ cells previously described (Yin et al. 2007) was primarily attributed to CD133+CD44+ cell subpopulation, instead of the CD133+CD44− subpopulation. As few as 100 CD133+CD44+ cells were sufficient to consistently initiate tumors in NOD-SCID mice, while 2,500 corresponding CD133+CD44− cells resulted in either no tumor formation or tumor formation with a significantly lower efficiency than the same number of CD133+CD44+ cells. This phenomenon was repeatedly observed in sorted subpopulations from HCC cells SMMC-7721 (0.1% CD133+; 0.09% CD133+CD44+), MHCC-LM3 (0.12% CD133+; 0.11% CD133+CD44+) as well as MHCC-97L (0.29% CD133+; 0.26% CD133+CD44+). In addition, CD133+CD44+ cells exhibited a preferential exhibition of stem cell-associated genes (β-catenin and Bmi-1), as well as ABC membrane transporters (ABCB1, ABCC1, and ABCG2). CD133+CD44+ cells were also found to be more resistant to chemotherapeutic agents, doxorubicin, and vincristine.

CD90⁺ and CD90⁺CD44⁺

Apart from CD133-based identification of liver CSCs summarized above, recent work by Yang et al. (2008b, c) found CD90, a glycosylphosphatidylinositol (GPI)-anchored glycoprotein which plays a role in cell–cell and cell–matrix interactions, to be a marker of liver CSCs. Expression of CD90 in liver cell lines (MiHA, HepG2, Hep3B, PLC, Huh7, MHCC-97L, and MHCC-97H) ranged from 0 to 1.85% and positively correlated with their ability to develop tumors in vivo (Yang et al. 2008b). Sorted CD90⁺ cells from PLC and MHCC-97L cells exhibited an enhanced tumorigenic and self-renewal ability as evident by tumor inoculation experiments in nude mice and its subsequent serial transplantations. As few as 2,000 CD90⁺ cells generated tumor nodules in nude mice while 1×10^5 CD90⁻ cells still failed to do so. Based on findings in cell lines, CD90 was then used as a marker to characterize CSCs in human liver cancer specimens. Since CD90 is also expressed by leukocytes, CD45 (a common marker of leukocytes) was used in combination to CD90 to delineate leukocyte expressing CD90 and hepatic stem/progenitor cell expressing CD90. In clinical samples, trace amounts of CD90⁺CD45⁻ cells (0–0.66%) were found in normal, cirrhotic, and adjacent non-tumorous specimens, while relatively higher amounts were detected in all HCC tumor specimens examined (0.42–8.57%). The authors also claimed that CD90⁺CD45⁻ cells were detectable in 90% of blood samples from HCC patients, while absent in normal subjects or patients with cirrhotic livers. Multimarker analyses found the majority of CD90⁺CD45⁻ cells to also express CD44, CD133, epithelial surface antigen (ESA), CXCR4, CD24, and KDR. CD90⁺CD45⁻ cells from HCC tissue samples displayed significantly higher tumorigenicity as shown in vivo. As few as 1,000 cells was sufficient for tumor initiation when injected in SCID mice, while up to 1×10^5 CD90⁻CD45⁻ cells was unable to induce tumor formation in the same model. Further studies by the same group found the majority of CD90⁺ cells in HCC cell lines also concomitantly expressed CD44; and blockade of CD44 activity by a neutralizing antibody significantly induced death of CD90⁺ cells in a dose-dependent manner, thus suggesting that CD44 is pivotal for the survival of CD90⁺ cells. Similar but an extended version of this work from the same research team was published in a separate manuscript in the same year (Yang et al. 2008c). In that study, in addition to the identification of a liver CSC population marked by CD90⁺ in HCC cells and CD90⁺CD45⁻ in HCC clinical samples, the authors found that inhibition of CD44 activity by an anti-CD44 antibody selectively induced apoptosis in CD90⁺ cells and treatment of cells with a CD44 neutralizing antibody prior to tumor engraftment significantly reduced tumor initiation capability of CD90⁺ cells. Using an in vivo tumor metastatic model, CD90⁺CD44⁺ cells displayed significantly higher metastatic potential compared to their CD90⁺CD44⁻ and CD90⁺ counterparts. Lung metastasis was observed in 100% of the mice injected 4 months after intrahepatic injection with 1×10^4 CD90⁺CD44⁺ cells, while only approximately one-fifth of the mice developed lung metastasis when intrahepatically injected with CD90⁺CD44⁻ cells. No liver or lung lesions were observed in mice injected with CD90⁻ cells. Significantly higher proportion of CD90⁺CD44⁺ cells were also observed in the induced metastatic tumors than primary tumors.

Epithelial Cell Adhesion Molecule⁺ (EpCAM⁺ or CD326⁺)

In 2009, research team led by Xin-Wei Wang of the National Institute of Health found liver CSCs can also be identified by EpCAM (Yamashita et al. 2009). Earlier studies by others on EpCAM found it to represent an early biomarker for HCC (Kim et al. 2004) and to be expressed in the majority of hepatocytes in embryonic liver as well as proliferating bile ducts in cirrhotic liver (de Boer et al. 1999). Studies by Yamashita et al. found EpCAM⁺ HCC cells to be preferentially expressed in AFP⁺ cell lines (Huh1, Huh7, and Hep3B) and absent in AFP⁻ cell lines (SK-Hep-1, HLE, and HLF). This was consistent with their microarray data where they found hepatic stem cells-like HCC (HpSC-HCC) bearing EpCAM⁺AFP⁺ phenotype to have a worst prognosis than mature hepatocyte-like HCC (MH-HCC) with EpCAM⁻AFP⁻ phenotype. EpCAM⁺ cells displayed a marked ability to self-renew as demonstrated through spheroid formation assay. Spheroids retained EpCAM⁺ phenotype in all serial passages than as compared with differentiated counterparts. EpCAM⁺ cells, but not EpCAM⁻ cells also displayed a unique ability to differentiate into both EpCAM⁺ and EpCAM⁻ cells. More importantly, as little as 200 EpCAM⁺ cells were able to initiate tumors in 80% of the immunodeficient mice, while the same number of EpCAM⁻ counterparts initiated only small tumors in 10% of the mice injected over the same period duration. The same increase in tumorigenic potential was also similarly observed in sorted cells from two cases of freshly resected HCC clinical samples. 1×10^4 EpCAM⁺ cells were able to induce tumor formation in vivo while up to 1×10^6 EpCAM⁻ cells failed to do so. EpCAM is a Wnt/β-catenin signaling target and further studies by the same group found EpCAM⁺ cells to mediate tumorigenicity and self-renewal via this specific pathway. When compared with control methylated BIO (MeBIO), activation of Wnt/β-catenin signaling by GSK-3β inhibitor BIO in AFP⁺ Huh1 and Huh7 cells led to an increase in the EpCAM⁺ population, enhanced spheroid formation, induced morphological change into smaller and rounder cells and induced expression of known HpSC markers – TACSTD1, MYC, and hTERT. In addition, enrichment of EpCAM⁺ cells could be provoked further by the treatment of Wnt10B-conditioned media in Huh7 cells. Conversely, blockage of EpCAM by RNA interference dramatically decreased EpCAM⁺ cell population, as well as inhibited cellular invasion, spheroid formation and tumorigenicity in Huh1 cells.

OV6⁺

Research team led by Hong-Yang Wang found the hepatic progenitor marker, OV6, to mark CSCs of the liver (Yang et al. 2008a). In human, OV6⁺ cells were normally present in bile ductules and periportal parenchyma in non-disease human liver, but their expression surged in cirrhotic livers and in HCC. Percentage of OV6⁺ cells in HCC cell lines range from 0.2 to 3% in various HCC cell lines, including Huh7, PLC, SMMC-7721, Hep3B, and HepG2. Double staining of OV6 and CD133 antigens by flow cytometry found the majority of OV6⁺ cells to concomitantly express CD133.

Since CD133⁺ population was significantly enriched in cells positive for OV6 and that CD133 has previously been shown by other groups to mark HCC CSC populations, the authors hypothesized that OV6⁺ cells may also represent a potential CSC population. OV6⁺ cells showed a significantly higher tumorigenic potential in vivo. As few as 5,000 OV6⁺ cells was sufficient for consistent tumor formation in NOD-SCID mice while at least 50–100× more OV6⁻ cells was needed to obtain comparable results in the same model. Further, progenitor cell markers including ABCG2, AFP, albumin (ALB), c-kit, EpCAM; transcription factors expressed in early hepatic development including GATA binding protein 6 (GATA6), CAAT/enhancer binding protein alpha and beta (C/EBPα and C/EBPβ); and "stemness" genes including Notch-1, Bmi-1, Nanog, and Oct-4 were all preferentially expressed by OV6⁺ cells. The authors further investigated the involvement of Wnt/β-catenin pathway in the self-renewal of OV6⁺ cell populations. Activation of the Wnt/β-catenin pathway by BIO, a selective and potent inhibitor of GSK-3β, significantly enriched the OV6⁺ population in HCC cell lines SMMC-7721 and Huh7, whereas conversely, lentiviral transduction of OV6⁺ cells with microRNA (miRNA) targeting β-catenin substantially reduced the subpopulation percentage. OV6⁺ cells isolated from Huh7 and SMMC-7721 also showed a dramatic increase in resistance to conventional chemotherapeutic agents. Cisplatin treatment significantly enriched OV6⁺ subpopulation in a dose-dependent and time-dependent manner in both cell lines. More interestingly, this preferential resistance was found to be abolished upon β-catenin silencing by lentiviral miRNA targeted against the gene; thus indicating that β-catenin signaling was not only required for regulating self-renewal of OV6⁺ liver CSCs but also for protection of the cells from chemotherapeutics-induced cytotoxicity.

Dysregulated Self-Renewal Pathways in Liver CSCs

Bmi-1

Polycomb-group (PcG) proteins are important transcriptional repressors, contributing to epigenetic alterations during tumor development (Bracken and Helin 2009). These proteins will form multi-protein complexes, namely Polycomb Repressive Complex 1 and 2 (PRC1 and PRC2), which are able to repress transcription of a wide number of genes that are known to be vital for differentiation and cell-fate determination. It has been suggested that these complexes can through cooperation with DNA methylating enzymes, target and silence pro-differentiating and anti-proliferating genes, resulting in a blockage of differentiation and thus ultimately creating aberrant undifferentiated CSCs that bear self-renewal properties (Bracken and Helin 2009; Park et al. 2003; Molofsky et al. 2003). PcG target gene silencing has previously been reported in various cancer types; and among these, aberrant upregulation of PRC1 member Bmi-1 was found to play a particularly important role in regulating somatic stem cells (Iwama et al. 2004) as well as liver CSCs (Chiba et al. 2008). In particular, Bmi-1 expression was found to be overexpressed in liver CSCs identified by CD133[+], CD90[+], OV6[+] as well as SP (Chiba et al. 2008; Ma et al. 2007; Yang et al. 2008a, c). Chiba and colleagues performed a more detailed study on the role of Bmi-1 in the regulation of SP liver CSCs. Silencing of Bmi-1 in HCC cells Huh7 and PLC/PRF/5 by lentiviral-based approach significantly reduced the size of the SP and abolished the preferential tumorigenic potential of the SP cells, as evident by decrease in tumor size and delayed tumor onset in NOD-SCID mice (Chiba et al. 2008). Conversely, stable overexpression of Bmi-1 significantly increased the SP cells by eightfold and resulted in enhanced tumorigenicity of the SP cells. The authors went on to find that silencing Bmi-1 in HCC cell line PLC/PRF/5 SP cells can result in the de-repression of PcG target genes ARF and INK4A (Chiba et al. 2008). Subsequent studies also by their group found a positive correlation between Bmi-1 expression and the size of CD133[+] CSCs. Silencing Bmi-1 specifically reduced CD133[+] subpopulation from ~74 to ~61%. Conversely, overexpression of Bmi-1 increased the CD133[+] subpopulation from ~71 to ~84%. Results are indicative that expression level of Bmi-1 is tightly correlated with CSC phenotype represented not only by SP cells but also by CD133[+] cells.

Wnt/β-Catenin Signaling

There are now a number of studies that have found de-regulated Wnt/β-catenin signaling to be associated with liver CSCs. Xin-Wei Wang and colleagues found EpCAM[+] liver CSCs to have an activated Wnt/β-catenin signaling pathway (Yamashita et al. 2008, 2009; see section "Epithelial Cell Adhesion Molecule[+] (EpCAM[+] or CD326[+])"). Hong-Yang Wang and coworkers also found OV6[+] liver CSCs to be endowed with endogenously active Wnt/β-catenin signaling (Yang et al. 2008a; see section "OV6[+]"). More recently, Rountree et al. provided new evidence for a novel mechanism by which transforming growth factor-β (TGF-β) regulates expression of CD133[+] liver CSCs by way of epigenetic events (You et al. 2010). TGF-β1 was capable of upregulating CD133 expression in HCC cells Huh7. More importantly, TGF-β1-induced CD133[+] Huh7 cells displayed an enhanced ability to initiate tumors when injected in nude mice. Further analysis found TGF-β to induce CD133 expression, in part, via the Smad pathway since forced expression of inhibitory Smads, such as Smad6 and Smad7, attenuated TGF-β1-induced CD133 expression. CD133 expression in Huh7 cells was found to be upregulated by DNA methyltransferases (DNMT) inhibitor in both a time- and dose-dependent manner. Conversely, TGF-β1 stimulation inhibited the expression of DNMT1 and DNMT3β, which are both critical in the maintenance of regional DNA methylation. DNMT3β inhibition by TGF-β1 was partially rescued with overexpression of inhibitory Smads. Finally, the authors also found TGF-β1 treatment resulted in significant demethylation in CD133 promoter-1 in Huh7 cells.

Transforming Growth Factor-β

In 2008, Lopa Mishra and her research team reported that repression of TGF-β signaling by activation of interleukin-6 (IL-6) in hepatic stem/progenitor cells may contribute to impaired differentiation and as a result lead to HCC development (Tang et al. 2008). Hepatic stem/progenitor cells in human regenerating livers expressing stem cell-related genes like Nanog, Oct4, Stat3, as well as TGF-β signaling components including pro-differentiation proteins TGF-β receptor type II (TBRII) and embryonic liver fodrin (ELF). Using a transgenic mouse model, they found that $elf^{+/-}$ mice (heterozygous for *elf*) have a 40% greater likelihood to develop spontaneous HCC, suggesting that HCC could arise from an IL-6-driven transformed stem cell with inactivated TFG-β signaling. Likewise, suppression of IL-6 signaling by mouse knockout experiments in which the gene for IL-6 regulated protein *itih4* has been deleted resulting in reduction in HCC in $elf^{+/-}$ mice. Immunostaining of human HCC tissue specimens identified the presence of cells positive for Oct4 and Stat3 expression but absent for TGF-β signaling proteins including TBRII and ELF, thus further supporting the above claim.

miRNAs

miRNAs are an abundant class of small, non-coding RNAs that negatively regulate gene expression at the post-transcriptional level by inhibiting ribosome function, decapping the 5′cap structure, deadenylating the poly(A) tail and degrading the target mRNA. miRNAs can regulate and control a variety of biological processes including developmental timing, signal transduction, stem cell self-renewal and differentiation. In addition to regulating cell-fate decisions, some miRNAs can also function as oncogenes and tumor suppressor genes, regulating maintenance and progression of cancers and CSCs (Esquela-Kerscher and Slack 2006; deSano and Xu 2009). miRNA expression profiles have also been correlated with tumor stage, progression, and prognosis of cancer patients. These findings demonstrate that miRNAs are critical regulators of self-renewal, differentiation as well as carcinogenesis.

miR-181 in EpCAM

Following subsequent identification of EpCAM+ liver CSCs, Xin-Wei Wang and colleagues furthered their studies in 2009 and identified elevated miR-181 family members (miR-181a, miR-181b, miR-181c, and miR-181d) as critical players in regulating EpCAM+ hepatic CSCs (Ji et al. 2009). Using a global microarray-based miRNA profiling approach, the authors compared the differential miRNA profiles of 53 HpSC-HCC and 95 MH-HCC clinical samples (Budhu et al. 2008) and identified miR-181 family members to be upregulated in EpCAM⁺AFP⁺ HCC clinical samples and in EpCAM⁺ HCC cell lines that also express AFP. Further, miR-181 family members were also found to be highly expressed in embryonic livers, hepatic stem cells and CD133⁺ liver CSCs. miR-181s can promote self-renewal – inhibition of endogenous miR-181s significantly blocked the ability of EpCAM⁺ cells to form spheroids, while overexpression of miR-181s furthered their ability. Moreover, forced expression of the family members can significantly enrich the EpCAM⁺ subpopulations. miR-181s also played a role in promoting tumorigenicity since inhibition of the family members led to reduced tumor initiation ability of EpCAM⁺ cells. Interestingly, overexpression of miR-181s resulted in a concomitant activation of Wnt/β-catenin signaling and reduced expression of mature hepatocyte markers (UGT2B7 and CYP3A4). In addition, miR-181s were also found to regulate downstream mRNA targets including caudal type homeobox transcription factor 2 (CDX2), GATA6 and nemo-like kinase (NLK; an inhibitor of Wnt/β-catenin signaling). Overexpression or knockdown of miR-181s led to a decrease or increase of these target mRNAs, respectively. CDX2 and GATA6 are two transcriptional regulators activating hepatocyte differentiation and it is believed that targeting of these differentiation activations by miR-181s can maintain the CSCs in their undifferentiated state. Likewise, it is thought that targeting NLK, a Wnt/β-catenin signaling inhibitor, by miR-181s can activate Wnt/β-catenin signaling, thus enhancing the self-renewal ability of EpCAM⁺ CSCs.

miR-130b in CD133

Studies from our group also recently extended our work in the understanding of the molecular mechanism that drives CD133⁺ CSCs and their role in liver cancer progression (Ma et al. 2010). We profiled isolated CD133⁺ CSCs and CD133⁻ cells from freshly resected tumors from HCC patients and HCC cell lines using a SYBR Green-based qPCR miRNA array containing 95 well-characterized human miRNAs known to be involved specifically in stem cell self-renewal and differentiation; and identified an overexpression of miR-130b in CD133⁺ CSCs. miR-130b was also found to closely correlate with CD133 expression in a series of liver cell lines. Liver cell lines with low CD133 expression expressed relatively lower levels of miR-130b (MiHA, HepG2, H2P, H2M) while in contrast, liver cell lines with high CD133 expressed relatively higher levels of miR-130b (PLC8024, Huh7, Hep3B). Functional studies on miR-130b lentiviral-transduced Huh7 CD133⁻ or PLC8024 CD133⁻ cells demonstrated superior resistance to chemotherapeutic agents, enhanced tumorigenicity in vivo, a greater potential for self-renewal and enhanced expression of stem cell-associated markers (β-catenin, Notch-1, Sox2, Nestin, Bmi-1, and ATP-binding cassette half-transporter ABCG2). Overall, CD133⁻ cells stably expressing miR-130b displayed features more closely resembling CD133⁺ CSCs than as compared with CD133⁻ control cells. Conversely, reducing miR-130b by lentiviral knockdown in Huh7 CD133⁺ or PLC8024 CD133⁺ CSCs yield an opposing effect, leading to reduced capability to proliferate, self-renew and initiate tumor in vivo. In an effort to determine the potential downstream mRNA targets regulated by miR-130b, we performed integrative analysis combining both mRNA expression profiling and in silico predictions and identified three common putative mRNA candidates of miR-130b. Of these included the tumor suppressor gene, tumor protein p53-inducible nuclear protein 1 (TP53INP1). Luciferase reporter assay and base pairing alignment assay of the 3′-untranslated region (3′-UTR) of TP53INP1 to miR-130b further confirmed that TP53INP1 is indeed a *bona fide* target of miR-130b. An inverse TP53INP1 expression was observed following lentiviral enforced or reduced miR-130b expression in CD133⁻ and CD133⁺ cells, respectively. Expression of TP53INP1 was found to be inversely correlated with CD133 and miR-130b in both HCC clinical samples as well as liver cell lines. More importantly, silencing of TP53INP1 in Huh7 or PLC8024 CD133⁻ cells enhanced both self-renewal and tumorigenicity in vivo. Collectively, miR-130b regulates CD133⁺ liver CSCs, in part, via silencing of TP53INP1.

Pathways Mediating Therapeutic Resistance in Liver CSCs

Akt/PKB and Bcl-2 Pathway (CD133)

Many of the liver CSC populations identified by either Hoechst 33342 dye or by the various surface markers mentioned earlier in this review chapter have been shown to be more resistant to standard chemotherapeutic agents. However, the molecular mechanism by which liver CSCs escape conventional therapies remains unknown. Following the identification of CD133⁺ as liver CSCs and their superior resistance to conventional chemotherapeutic agents, doxorubicin and 5-fluorouracil, our team subsequently examined the possible mechanistic pathway by which these cells confer chemoresistance (Ma et al. 2008a). Purified CD133⁺ liver CSCs isolated from HCC cell lines and xenograft mouse models survived chemotherapy in increased proportions relative to most tumor cells which lack the CD133 phenotype; the underlying mechanism of which required the preferential expression of survival proteins involved in the Akt/PKB and Bcl-2 pathway. CD133⁺ liver CSCs showed significantly elevated levels of phosphorylated Akt (serine 473), phosphorylated Bad (serine 136) and Bcl-2 as compared to its corresponding CD133⁻ counterparts. When cultured in the presence of doxorubicin and 5-fluorouracil, the expression of each of these survival proteins in CD133⁺ cells persisted at higher concentrations of the two drugs and also for a longer period of time when exposed to a fixed concentration of the two drugs, then compared to unsorted cells or its corresponding

CD133⁻ counterparts. In addition, dual-color immunofluorescence found CD133 to co-localize with survival proteins Bcl-2 and active Akt phosphorylated at serine 473 in CD133⁺ liver CSCs from PLC8024 HCC cells. Treatment of CD133⁺ HCC cells with an AKT1 inhibitor, specific to the Akt/PKB pathway, significantly reduced the expression of the survival proteins that was normally expressed endogenously, thus confirming the importance of the Akt/PKB pathway to the increased survival of CD133⁺ liver CSCs. More interestingly, co-incubation of the AKT1 inhibitor with doxorubicin and 5-fluorouracil completely inhibited the preferential survival effect induced by CD133⁺ cells.

Therapeutic Implications

The concept of CSCs is hoped and believed to bring about important therapeutic implications. Current clinical treatment strategies, like chemotherapy and radiotherapy, are developed to target by large only the bulk rapidly proliferating tumor cells. Though these treatments seem to be initially successful, effects are often short-lived and frequently fail to provide a lasting cure for the disease. The failure to eradicate the CSC population, believed to be the roots of the disease, is believed to be the primary cause of tumor relapse. It is likely that residual CSCs, due to their highly resistant and stem cell-like abilities (self-renewal and differentiation), are able to survive in a dormant state after remission and cause tumor recurrence. As reviewed in this chapter, there is now accumulating evidences that support the existence of a CSC population in HCC. Therapeutic resistance to standard chemotherapy has also been attributed to CSCs in this cancer type. This proof-of-principle evidence provides a strong basis and rationale for the development of novel cancer therapies that specifically targets at the elimination of CSCs in addition to the bulk tumor mass. It is anticipated that in the upcoming years, translational CSC studies, against HCC, or other cancer types, will include the use of CSC-specific surface markers for antibody therapy, as well as the use of molecular targeted therapy in the specific blockage of self-renewal pathways, inhibition of survival pathways and induction of differentiation of CSCs into progenitors that do not self-renew (Frank et al. 2010; Zhou et al. 2009). In addition, further studies in the functional interactions of CSC with their microenvironment will help identify potential indirect strategies against CSCs, including those of anti-angiogenic therapy, immunotherapeutic approaches and disruption of pro-tumorigenic interactions between CSCs and their microenvironment (Frank et al. 2010; Zhou et al. 2009). Yet regardless of the mode of treatment, it is very likely that only complex combinatorial therapies targeting multiple aspects of CSCs function will provide the needed efficacy to completely eliminate CSCs and thus the roots of this disease (Fig. 11.1).

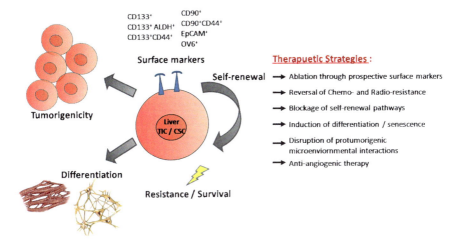

Fig. 11.1 Possible therapeutic strategies targeted against different aspects of liver CSCs. It is hoped that these approaches could potentially enhance responsiveness to current anticancer treatment protocols and may reduce the risk of tumor relapse. These strategies include, but are not limited to, blocking essential self-renewal signaling, inhibiting the survival mechanisms operative in CSCs, targeting prospective surface markers, induction of differentiation/senescence, disruption of pro-tumorigenic CSC-microenvironment interactions, anti-angiogenic therapy, etc.

References

Bracken AP, Helin K (2009) Polycomb group proteins: navigators of lineage pathways led astray in cancer. Nat Rev Cancer 9:773–784.
Budhu A, Jia HL, Forgues M et al (2008) Identification of metastasis-related microRNAs in hepatocellular carcinoma. Hepatology 47:897–907.
Challen GA, Little MH (2006) A side order of stem cells: the SP phenotype. Stem Cells 24:3–12.
Chiba T, Kita K, Zheng YW, et al (2006) Side population purified from hepatocellular carcinoma cells harbors cancer stem cell-like properties. Hepatology 44:240–251.
Chiba T, Miyagi S, Saraya A, et al (2008) The polycomb gene product BMI1 contributes to the maintenance of tumor-initiating side population cells in hepatocellular carcinoma. Cancer Res 68: 7742–7749.
de Boer CJ, van Kricken JH, Janssen van Rhijn CM, et al (1999) Expression of Ep-CAM in normal, regenerating, metaplastic, and neoplastic liver. J Pathol 188:201–206.
deSano JT, Xu L (2009) microRNA regulation of cancer stem cells and therapeutic implications. The AAPS Journal 11:682–692.
Esquela-Kerscher A, Slack FJ (2006) Oncomirs – microRNAs with a role in cancer. Nat Rev Cancer 6:259–269.
Frank NY, Schatton T, Frank MH (2010) The therapeutic promise of the cancer stem cell concept. J Clin Invest 120:41–50.
Goodell MA, Brose K, Paradis G, et al (1996) Isolation and functional properties of murine hematopoietic stem cells that are replicating *in vivo*. J Exp Med 183:1797–1806.
Haraguchi N, Utsunomiya T, Inoue H, et al (2006) Characterization of a side population of cancer cells from human gastrointestinal system. Stem Cells 24:506–513.

Hess DA, Wirthlin L, Craft TP, et al (2006) Selection based on CD133 and high aldehyde dehydrogenase activity isolates long-term reconstituting human hematopoietic stem cells. Blood 107: 2162–2169.

Iwama A, Oguro H, Negishi M, et al (2004) Enhanced self-renewal of hematopoietic stem cells mediated by the polycomb gene product Bmi-1. Immunity 21:843–851.

Ji J, Yamashita T, Budhu A, et al (2009) Identification of microRNA-181 by genome-wide screening as a critical player in EpCAM-positive hepatic cancer stem cells. Hepatology 50:472–480.

Kim JW, Ye Q, Forgues M, et al (2004) Cancer-associated molecular signature in the tissue samples of patients with cirrhosis. Hepatology 39:518–527.

Ma S, Chan KW, Hu L, et al (2007) Identification and characterization of tumorigenic liver cancer stem/progenitor cells. Gastroenterology 132:2542–2556.

Ma S, Lee TK, Zheng BJ, et al (2008a) CD133+ HCC cancer stem cells confer chemoresistance by preferential expression of the Akt/PKB survival pathway. Oncogene 27:1749–1758.

Ma S, Chan KW, Lee TK, et al (2008b) Aldehyde dehydrogenase discriminates the CD133 liver cancer stem cell populations. Mol Cancer Res 6:1146–1153.

Ma S, Tang KH, Chan YP, et al (2010) miR-130b promotes CD133$^+$ liver tumor-initiating cell growth and self-renewal via tumor protein 53-induced nuclear protein 1. Cell Stem Cell 7:694–707.

Molofsky AV, Pardal R, Iwashita T, et al (2003) Bmi-1 dependence distinguishes neural stem cell self-renewal from progenitor proliferation. Nature 425:962–967.

Moserle L, Ghisi M, Amadori A, et al (2010) Side population and cancer stem cells: therapeutic implications. Cancer Lett 288:1–9.

Park IK, Qian D, Kiel M, et al (2003) Bmi-1 is required for maintenance of adult self-renewing haematopoietic stem cells. Nature 423:302–305.

Pearce DJ, Taussig D, Simpson C, et al (2005) Characterization of cells with a high aldehyde dehydrogenase activity from cord blood and acute myeloid leukemia samples. Stem Cells 23:752–60.

Song W, Li H, Tao K, et al (2008) Expression and clinical significance of the stem cell marker CD133 in hepatocellular carcinoma. Int J Clin Pract 62:1212–1218.

Suetsugu A, Nagaki M, Aoki H, et al (2006) Characterization of CD133$^+$ hepatocellular carcinoma cells as cancer stem/progenitor cells. Biochem Biophys Res Commun 351:820–824.

Tang Y, Kitisin K, Jogunoori W, et al (2008) Progenitor/stem cells give rise to liver cancer due to aberrant TGF-beta and IL-6 signaling. Proc Natl Acad Sci USA 105:2445–2450.

Yamashita T, Forgues M, Wang W, et al (2008) EpCAM and alpha-fetoprotein expression defines novel prognostic subtypes of hepatocellular carcinoma. Cancer Res 68:1451–1461.

Yamashita T, Ji J, Budhu A, et al (2009) EpCAM-positive hepatocellular carcinoma cells are tumor-initiating cells with stem/progenitor cell features. Gastroenterology 136:1012–1024.

Yang W, Yan HX, Chen L, et al (2008a) Wnt/beta-catenin signaling contributes to activation of normal and tumorigenic liver progenitor cells. Cancer Res 68:4287–4295.

Yang ZF, Ngai P, Ho DW, et al (2008b) Identification of local and circulating cancer stem cells in human liver cancer. Hepatology 47:919–928.

Yang ZF, Ho DW, Ng MN, et al (2008c) Significance of CD90$^+$ cancer stem cells in human liver cancer. Cancer Cell 13:153–166.

Yin S, Li J, Hu C, et al (2007) CD133 positive hepatocellular carcinoma cells possess high capacity for tumorigenicity. Int J Cancer 120:1444–1450.

You H, Ding W, Rountree CB (2010) Epigenetic regulation of cancer stem cell marker CD133 by transforming growth factor-beta. Hepatology 51:1635–1644.

Zhou BB, Zhang H, Damelin M, et al (2009) Tumor-initiating cells: challenges and opportunities for anticancer drug discovery. Nat Rev Drug Discov 8:806–823.

Zhu Z, Hao X, Yan M, et al (2010) Cancer stem/progenitor cells are highly enriched in CD133(+) CD44(+) population in hepatocellular carcinoma. Int J Cancer 126:2067–2078.

Chapter 12
Pancreatic Cancer Stem Cells

Erica N. Proctor and Diane M. Simeone

Introduction

Pancreatic adenocarcinoma (PDAC) is a highly lethal malignancy with no known cure and limited effective therapies. Despite substantial research efforts and significant improvement in diagnostic modalities and complex pancreatic surgery, the prognosis for patients diagnosed with pancreatic cancer remains dismal with a 5-year survival of less than 5% and median survival of only 4–6 months in patients with metastatic disease (Jemal et al. 2007). The median survival of patients with localized and unresectable lesions is 8–10 months (Philip et al. 2009). The high mortality and poor clinical outcomes associated with the diagnosis of pancreatic cancer are due to the characteristically advanced stage of disease at presentation, extensive local tumor invasion, early systemic dissemination, and frequent resistance to conventional chemotherapeutic agents and radiation. In the USA alone, an estimated 43,140 new cases of PDAC will be diagnosed in 2010. The annual death rate will approach the annual incidence rate with 36,880 patients estimated to succumb to pancreatic cancer in 2010. The lack of substantial progress in improving mortality associated with PDAC portends the need for novel treatment strategies and research efforts aimed at elucidating the underlying mechanisms for pancreatic tumorigenesis, metastasis, and chemoresistance.

E.N. Proctor • D.M. Simeone (✉)
Departments of Surgery and Molecular and Integrative Physiology,
University of Michigan Medical Center, 1500 E Medical Center Drive,
TC 2210B Box 5343, Ann Arbor, MI 48109, USA
e-mail: simeone@med.umich.edu

Cancer Stem Cell Theory

Emerging research has demonstrated marked heterogeneity in malignant pancreatic tumors and suggests that PDAC tumors are composed of a large population of differentiated cells with limited proliferative capacity and a much smaller subpopulation of stem-like cells, termed cancer stem cells (CSCs), that are responsible for tumorigenesis, maintenance of tumor growth, and metastasis (Visvader and Lindeman 2008). The CSC theory posits that a small, variable population of tumor-initiating cells exists with the defining features of self-renewal, the ability to differentiate, and the ability to migrate giving rise to secondary tumors (Wicha et al. 2006; Reya et al. 2001). The early work on putative CSCs was performed in hematologic malignancies by Dick et al. who first isolated CSCs in myeloid leukemia using cell surface marker expression and the ability of human leukemia cells to engraft in nonobese diabetic severe combined deficiency (NOD-SCID) mice and be serially passaged (Bonnet and Dick 1997). These findings were the impetus for investigation of putative CSCs in solid organ malignancies, and in 2003 Al-Hajj et al. reported the first identified epithelial solid organ CSCs in breast cancer. This study reported a phenotypically distinct and relatively rare population of tumor cells with the cell surface marker expression of $CD44^+/CD24^{-/low}/ESA^+$ (epithelial-specific antigen) that were highly tumorigenic and possessed the ability to recapitulate tumors cognate to the primary tumor in immunocompromised mice (Al-Hajj et al. 2003). Additionally, these $CD44^+/CD24^{-/low}/ESA^+$ cells could be serially transplanted without loss of tumorigenicity. The existence of CSCs has now been validated in several solid tumors, including glioblastoma (Singh et al. 2004), colon (Ricci-Vitiani et al. 2007), and liver (Ma et al. 2007). Studies demonstrating the ability to identify CSCs in solid tumors lead to work by Li et al. to prospectively identify pancreatic CSCs (Li et al. 2007).

Identification of Pancreatic Cancer Stem Cells

To investigate the presence of a putative CSC population in primary human PDAC, Li et al. adapted the techniques employed by Al-Hajj and colleagues in malignant breast tumors. Several primary human PDAC samples were obtained and xenografts were established by inserting minced pieces of patient tumor in a subcutaneous pocket in the abdomen of immunocompromised mice. After xenograft expansion of the tumor samples, tumors were procured and mechanically and enzymatically dissociated with collagenase to produce a single cell suspension. To identify prospective cell surface markers, cells were stained with fluorescently conjugated antibodies to CD44, CD24, and ESA, which had been previously studied in analyses of CSC populations in both solid and hematopoietic malignancies. Fluorescence-activated cell sorting (FACS) was then used to separate the heterogeneous cell populations into up to four separate populations at a time, based upon light scattering and fluorescent characteristics of each cell (Li et al. 2007).

12 Pancreatic Cancer Stem Cells

Table 12.1 Tumor formation ability of sorted pancreatic cancer cells using cell surface markers

Number of cells injected	10^4	10^3	500	100
Unsorted	4/6	0/6	0/3	0/3
CD44+	8/16	7/16	5/16	4/16
CD44-	2/16	1/16	1/16	0/16
P	0.022*	0.014*	0.07	0.03*
ESA+	12/18	13/18	8/18	0/18
ESA-	3/18	1/18	1/18	0/18
P	0.002*	0.0001*	0.007*	N/A
CD24+	11/16	10/16	7/16	1/16
CD24-	2/16	1/16	0/16	0/16
P	0.001*	0.001*	0.003*	0.31
CD44+ESA+	9/16	10/16	7/16	4/16
CD44-ESA-	3/16	2/16	0/16	0/16
P	0.03*	0.004*	0.003*	0.033*
CD24+ESA+	6/8	5/8	5/8	2/8
CD24-ESA-	2/8	1/8	0/8	0/8
P	0.05*	0.04*	0.007*	0.13
CD44+CD24+	6/8	5/8	4/8*	2/8
CD44-CD24-	1/8	1/8	0/8	0/8
P	0.01*	0.04*	0.02*	0.13
CD44+CD24+ESA+	10/12	10/12	7/12	6/12
CD44-CD24-ESA-	1/12	0/12	0/12	0/12
P	0.0002*	0.0001*	0.001*	0.004*

Note: Cells were isolated by flow cytometry as described in Fig. 12.1 based on expression of the combinations of the indicated markers and assayed for the ability to form tumors after injection into the subcutaneum of the flank of NOD/SCID mice at 100, 500, 103, and 104 cells per injection. Mice were examined for tumor formation by palpation and subsequent autopsy. The analysis was completed 16 weeks following injection. Data are expressed as number of tumors formed/number of injections. P values are listed comparing tumor formation for each marker at different cell dilutions

*P values <0.05 compared with results with marker-negative cells (reproduced from Li et al. 2007)

FACS analysis of primary or low passage (1–2) xenograft primary human PDAC tumors using the CD44, CD24, and ESA markers alone or in combination facilitated the development of a staining profile that identified multiple subpopulations of tumor cells. To delineate which populations were responsible for tumor initiation in pancreatic cancer, each population alone or in combination with other markers was sorted and subcutaneously implanted into the abdomen of NOD-SCID mice to assess their tumor-initiating potential (Table 12.1). Initial observations using ESA+ cells individually and either CD44+ or CD24+ in combination with ESA+ revealed populations of cells that had a tumor initiation rate of one in four animals with as few as 100 viable human cells injected. To identify a more enriched CSC population all three markers were used in combination and identified a population of CD44+CD24+ESA+ cells comprising only 0.2–0.8% of all human pancreatic cancer cells in the pancreatic tumors examined. As few as 100 CD44+CD24+ESA+ cells injected in NOD-SCID mice were able to generate tumors in 50% of the animals (6 of 12), while CD44⁻CD24⁻ESA⁻ cells did not form tumors until at least 10,000 cells were injected. Of note, only 1 of 12 animals formed a tumor from these triple marker-negative cells, reflecting a 100-fold greater tumor-initiating potential in the CD44⁺CD24⁺ESA⁺ population. Additionally, FACS analysis of CD44⁺CD24⁺ESA⁺ derived xenograft tumors displayed a staining profile with CSC and nontumorigenic cells represented in populations equivalent to the staining levels in the primary tumor. These populations remained stable in subsequent passages in NOD-SCID animals with up to four passages tested. These data provided strong evidence for a self-renewing, multipotent population of pancreatic tumor initiating cells in human PDAC.

Studies in brain and colon cancer have demonstrated that cancer cells expressing the surface marker CD133 also have properties of CSCs (O'Brien et al. 2007; Singh et al. 2004). Similarly, Hermann et al. (2007) found that CD133⁺ cells in primary pancreatic cancers and pancreatic cancer cell lines also identified cells with enhanced proliferative capacity and CSC traits. They demonstrated that CD133⁺ cells comprised approximately 1–3% of PDAC cells analyzed in the study, and injection of 500 cells into immunocompromised mice generated tumors that recapitulated the primary PDAC tumor. Additional findings included an observed overlap between CD44⁺/CD24⁺/ESA⁺ subpopulation and the CD133⁺ population (Hermann et al. 2007). More recently, Mueller et al. used CD133 to investigate a novel therapeutic strategy targeting this subpopulation of human pancreatic cancer cells that is highly enriched for tumor-promoting CSCs both in primary pancreatic cancer cells and the xenografted, highly aggressive pancreatic cancer cell line L3.6pl (Mueller et al. 2009). These findings call into question the existence of more than one population of putative CSCs. In the breast cancer literature, Wright et al. suggests that there are two distinct phenotypes of stem cells in breast cancer denoted by CD44⁺/CD24⁺ and CD133⁺ with no overlap of marker expression depending on the tumor used to isolate the CSC populations. Each stem-cell population behaved similarly with equal potency for tumor formation despite distinct surface marker expression without overlap (Wright et al. 2008). In contrast, Hermann et al. reported an overlap of 14% between CD44⁺/CD24⁺/ESA⁺ and CD133⁺ pancreatic cancer cells (Hermann et al. 2007). Further in vivo tumorigenicity experiments are needed to determine if CD44⁺/CD24⁺/ESA⁺ and CD133⁺ pancreatic cancer cells represent distinct CSC populations, or if a pancreatic CSC population expressing all four markers is the most highly enriched subset for tumor initiation and CSC functions.

In addition to the gold standard in vivo dilutional tumor propagation assays used to identify CSCs, cancer stem cells have also been studied using in vitro sphere-forming assays. It has been demonstrated in both normal and cancerous neural tissue that the ability of cells to form floating colonies in spherical aggregates in nonadherent culture conditions is reflective of self-renewal capacity (Singh et al. 2004; Ishibashi et al. 2004). Using a version of this assay and conditions with minimally modified culture media, the Simeone lab has found that visually inspected and plated, single CD44⁺/CD24⁺/ESA⁺ pancreatic cancer cells form spheres, coined

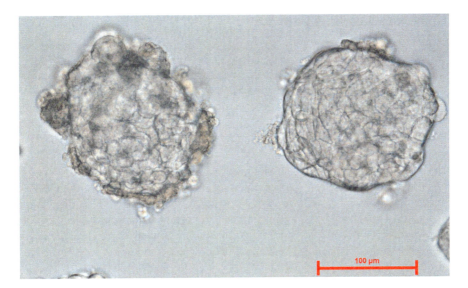

Fig. 12.1 Pancreatic cancer tumorspheres

pancreatic tumorspheres, while the differentiated CD44$^-$/CD24$^-$/ESA$^-$ cells do not form such spheres (Fig. 12.1). These CD44$^+$/CD24$^+$/ESA$^+$ tumorspheres can be passaged serially without loss of tumorsphere forming capability thus demonstrating self-renewal capacity in vitro. Furthermore, analysis of the tumorspheres by FACS analysis following 7–10 days in culture revealed that the spheres contain both CSC and marker-negative cell populations, demonstrating that CSCs give rise to differentiated progeny in addition to their self-renewal capacity.

Critical Stem Cell Signaling Pathways

While distinct populations of highly tumorigenic cancer cell populations have now been isolated from several solid organ malignancies, the cellular pathways underlying their unique stem-like properties and tumor-initiating capacity are the subject of ongoing research. One hypothesis is that embryonic gene pathways as well as pathways that affect normal stem cell function are aberrantly regulated in CSCs. Recent studies have suggested that cancer is triggered by the reactivation of developmental signaling pathways that are typically downregulated following the completion of embryonic development (Hruban et al. 2006; Bailey et al. 2007; Wilson and Radtke 2006). Specifically, developmental signaling pathways such as the Notch and Hedgehog pathways have been implicated in pancreatic carcinogenesis while canonical signaling pathways such as Bmi-1 and Wnt have also been linked to oncogenesis.

Hedgehog Signaling Pathway

While normally suppressed in the adult pancreas, the Hedgehog signaling pathway is frequently found to be upregulated in pancreatic cancer. The hedgehog pathway (Hh) plays a critical role during the development of the gastrointestinal system and in specification of embryonic tissues. Active Hh signaling is stimulated by three ligands: Sonic hedgehog (SHh), Indian hedgehog, and Desert hedgehog. In the absence of a ligand, the Hh plasma membrane ligand receptor Patched1 (PTCH1), represses the activity of Smoothened (SMO). In this state, the GLI transcription factors are phosphorylated and repressed. Hedgehog ligand binding releases PTCH1 inhibition of SMO via the internalization of the receptor and activation of SMO. A signaling cascade downstream of SMO leads to activation of GLI transcription factors, thus activating transcription of downstream target genes, including pathway components PTCH1, GLI1, and HIP (Rubin and de Sauvage 2006). Regulation of pathway components facilitates tight molecular regulation of the Hh pathway activity through complex feedback mechanisms. Furthermore, other observed downstream targets include known cell proliferation and differentiation factors Wnt, TGF_3, and FGF pathway components in addition to cell cycle regulators p21 and cyclin D1 (Pasca di Magliano and Hebrok 2003).

Evidence for a role of Hh signaling in CSCs has emerged from solid tumor models of cancer. In breast CSC populations, CSCs were observed to have a 30-fold higher level of expression of GLI1 and upregulation of PTCH1 and GLI2 compared to nontumorigenic cells (Liu et al. 2006). Liu et al. also observed that adding SHH to cultures of normal stem cell mammosphere colonies is a potent mitogen and upregulates self-renewal pathways including expression of the polycomb gene Bmi-1. Of note, treated mammospheres show increased secondary sphere formation, an indicator of self-renewal, and an increase in the amount of multipotent cells following differentiation. These findings were reversed by the addition of the Hedgehog pathway inhibitor, cyclopamine (Liu et al. 2006).

In our own studies, we have identified that direct isolation and qRT-PCR of pancreatic cancer stems cells revealed higher levels of SHh expression compared to the nontumorigenic population (Li et al. 2007). We found that the expression of SHh transcript was upregulated over 40-fold compared to nontumorigenic cells and normal pancreatic epithelial cells. Our lab is currently engaged in ongoing research to better characterize the role of the hedgehog signaling pathway in pancreatic CSC function using primary human pancreatic cancer samples. Feldmann et al. have indirectly tested the role of Hh signaling in pancreatic CSCs by treatment of a metastatic cell line of pancreatic cancer with the Hedgehog pathway inhibitor, cyclopamine (Feldmann et al. 2007). These treatments exhibited a significant effect on preventing tumor metastasis and a decrease of the CSC population as assessed by a reduction in aldehyde dehydrogenase activity. Given the recent study describing a paracrine requirement for Hedgehog signaling in pancreatic cancer (Yauch et al. 2008), the prevention of metastasis observed by Feldmann et al. may be mediated by inhibition of both Hh signaling and cross-talk in the tumor stroma that is critical to pancreatic CSC maintenance. As we develop in vitro and in vivo models that allow us to better evaluate the tumor microenvironment, looming questions about the nature of Hedgehog signaling in CSC function and maintenance may be answered.

Bmi-1

Bmi-1 is a polycomb gene family member that regulates self-renewal in normal and CSC systems. It was initially characterized as a c-myc cooperative oncogene that induced murine lymphoma formation when overexpressed (van Lohuizen et al. 1991; Haupt et al. 1993). Bmi-1 acts a transcriptional repressor of the INK4a/ARF locus, and premature cellular senescence is observed when Bmi-1 is deleted and p16 and p19 cyclin dependent kinase inhibitor expression is upregulated (Jacobs et al. 1999). Bmi-1 is also functionally important in stem cell biology by promoting stem cell self-renewal, as demonstrated in the studies of the adult hematopoietic system (Lessard and Sauvageau 2003; Park et al. 2003). Studies performed with leukemic stem cells also demonstrated a requirement for Bmi-1 in maintaining the leukemic stem cell proliferation and self-renewal (Lessard and Sauvageau 2003). In solid neoplasms, overexpression of Bmi-1 has been shown to play a role in the invasive potential of colon, brain, oral, and breast cancers (Kim et al. 2004a, b; Cui et al. 2007; Kang et al. 2007).

To investigate differential expression of Bmi-1 in pancreatic CSC populations, our lab has performed qRT-PCR on tumorigenic and nontumorigenic pancreatic tumor cell populations. We identified a fivefold increase in BMI-1 expression in CD44$^+$CD24$^+$ESA$^+$ cells compared to the nontumorigenic population. To determine the role of Bmi-1 in PDAC cell proliferation and invasion, shRNA targeting Bmi-1 was used to alter Bmi-1 levels in MiaPaCa2 and Panc1 cell lines, by silencing and overexpression, respectively. We observed that increased expression of Bmi-1 in MiaPaCa2 cells enhanced cellular proliferation. Conversely, silencing of Bmi1 in Panc1 cells dramatically reduced cellular proliferation and invasion via changes in the cell cycle distribution of cells (unpublished observations). Interestingly, Bmi-1 was also observed to be activated in the early stages of pancreatic cancer progression, as a significant proportion of pancreatic cancer precursor PanIN lesions were found to express BMI-1 (unpublished observations). Ongoing studies utilizing the in vitro tumorsphere model and in vivo orthotopic implantation are allowing us to further elucidate the role of Bmi-1 in pancreatic cancer tumorigenesis and the maintenance and function of the pancreatic CSC population.

Pancreatic Cancer Stem Cells and Metastasis

Metastatic pancreatic cancer is incurable and a better understanding of the molecular mechanisms driving the migration of pancreatic cancer cells to distant sites may have significant implications for the development of effective targeted therapeutics to prevent systemic dissemination. The role of CSCs in pancreatic cancer progression and metastasis has emerged in recent studies. Notably, Hermann et al. characterized CD133+ pancreatic CSCs and their involvement in tumor metastasis. They identified a subpopulation of CD133+/CXCR4+ cells that were observed to display high migratory activity toward gradients of the CXCR4 ligand stromal derived factor-1 (SDF-1). Inhibition of CD133+/CXCR4+ cell migration in vitro was accomplished using anti-CXCR4 neutralizing antibodies and the small molecule inhibitor AMD3100. Upon orthotopic implantation of separate populations of CD133+/CXCR4+ and CD133+/CXCR4− cells in immunocompromised mice, they found that while both populations formed tumors, only the CD133+/CXCR4+ cells population gave rise to liver and splenic metastases and tumor cells in the circulating blood. As in the in vitro experiments, blockade of CXCR4 significantly reduced the ability of these cells to become metastatic in vivo, suggesting that coexpression of CD133 and CXCR4 play a role in the generation of metastasis (Hermann et al. 2007).

Further evidence supporting the role of a putative CSC population in pancreatic cancer comes from work performed by Feldmann and colleagues who examined the invasion potential of the aggressive and metastatic PDAC cell line, E3LZ10.7, in an orthotopic xenograft tumor model. Using cyclopamine, a specific Hedgehog pathway inhibitor, they were able to demonstrate that following 30 days of cyclopamine treatment, only 14% of animals were found to have metastatic lesions compared to 100% of the animals in the control group. Interestingly, there was no significant difference in tumor size between the control and treated groups, and the reduction in metastatic potential corresponded with a threefold decrease in ALDH+ cells, which are thought to be a prospective pancreatic CSC marker (Feldmann et al. 2007).

Another theory regarding CSC involvement in metastasis is that tumorigenic CSCs acquire a migrating phenotype during an epithelial–mesenchymal-transition (EMT) process, enabling them to disseminate systemically. EMT is characterized by downregulation of cell adhesion proteins, loss of cell–cell junction connections, and an increase in cell mobility. Recent work in the study of EMT, a key step in the formation of metastasis, has provided clues as to how CSCs may be involved. EMT-related transcription factors, including Twist, Snail, and Slug, are found to be overexpressed in many cancer subtypes (Yang et al. 2004; Barbera et al. 2004; Hajra et al. 2002). Moreover, these transcription factors are implicated in suppression of E-cadherin and the transition to motile and highly proliferative cells. Evidence for the role of EMT in metastasis was provided by Wellner et al. who reported that the EMT-inducer ZEB1 supports metastasis not only by promoting tumor cell mobility and dissemination, but also by maintaining a stem cell phenotype through inhibition of miR200 family members (Wellner et al. 2009). Further investigation of the role of EMT in the acquisition and maintenance of stem-like characteristics was performed by Mani et al. in immortalized human mammary epithelial cells (Mani et al. 2008). Normal immortalized human mammary epithelial cells were induced to EMT by the ectopic expression of either Twist or Snail. FACS analysis of these induced cells for CD44 and CD24 showed that the majority of cells displayed a CD44^{high}/CD24^{low} expression pattern that mimicked the marker pattern observed in breast CSCs. In vitro, the EMT-induced cells had a 30-fold higher rate of mammosphere formation, an indicator of self-renewal, compared to normal mammary epithelial cells. Additionally, overexpressing Twist or Snail in transformed mammary epithelial cells resulted in greater tumor initiation in xenograft models (Mani et al. 2008). These data support the possibility that the migratory and metastatic potential of CSCs may indeed be conferred during the EMT process. Given the certain 100% mortality of metastatic pancreatic cancer, further elucidating the role of CSCs in pancreatic cancer metastasis may have a significant impact on the development of treatments to prevent relapse and the devastating prognosis of systemic dissemination.

Pancreatic Cancer Stem Cells and Resistance to Therapy

Resistance to chemotherapy and radiotherapy has been reported in several solid tumor CSC populations and is best characterized in brain, colon, and breast tumors. $CD133^+$ CSCs have been found to mediate tumor radiotherapy resistance both in vivo and in vitro in primary human gliomas (Bao et al. 2006). Bao and colleagues reported that exposure of glioma xenografts to radiation led to enrichment of $CD133^+$ CSCs. In vitro resistance of the $CD133^+$ subpopulation was mediated by the Chk1/Chk2 pathway, and $CD133^+$ cells were observed to preferentially activate the DNA-damage apparatus. Through upregulation of DNA damage checkpoint response activation, $CD133^+$ cells were able to more efficiently repair radiation-induced DNA damage than $CD133^-$ cells. Conversely, use of inhibitors against the DNA damage checkpoint protein Chk1 in synergy with ionizing radiation proved effective in preventing the radioresistance of $CD133^+$ brain CSCs (Bao et al. 2006). The ability of $CD133^+$ stem cells to evade standard cytotoxic therapy was also demonstrated by Dylla et al. who reported resistance of $CD133^+$ colon CSCs to cyclophosphamide and irinotecan (Dylla et al. 2008). In the pancreatic cancer literature, Hermann et al. described enrichment of the $CD133^+$ subpopulation following treatment of the L3.6pl pancreatic cancer cell line with gemcitabine (Hermann et al. 2007). Additionally, L3.6pl and AsPC-1 cell line treatment with gemcitabine also led to the relative enrichment of the $CD44^+/CD24^+/ESA^+$ CSC subpopulation. In experiments that parallel the previous work on pancreatic CSC resistance, we also have found that treatment with the standard pancreatic cancer chemotherapeutic agent gemcitabine and ionizing radiation results in enrichment of the $CD44^+/CD24^+/ESA^+$ population in human primary PDAC xenografts (unpublished observations). Interestingly, Shah et al. showed that pancreatic cancer cell lines selectively grown in culture media containing therapeutic doses of gemcitabine demonstrated properties of EMT. In addition, relative to the parental cells from which they were derived, these gemcitabine-resistant cells expressed an increased level of CD44, CD24, and ESA cell surface markers (Shah et al. 2007). These data provide strong evidence for the critical involvement of pancreatic CSCs in the failure of standard radiation and chemotherapy. Further investigation to determine the mechanisms by which putative CSCs evade standard therapies in PDAC are ongoing and will be critical to our ability to therapeutically address the burden of relapsed disease.

Cancer Stem Cell-Based Therapeutics

The dire need to identify new agents against pancreatic cancer is underscored by the less than 5% survival rate for PDAC which has been unchanged over the past 40 years. The only cytotoxic drug approved by the Food and Drug Administration for PDAC is gemcitabine, which is not curative and only marginally prolongs life. Moreover, it is clear that the standard therapy does not address the heterogeneous populations of cells that comprise PDAC lesions such as CSCs that employ unique survival mechanisms. Emerging and strong evidence for resistance of pancreatic CSCs to ionizing radiation and chemotherapy reinforces the need for therapies that specifically target CSCs to increase the probability of tumor eradication and improved clinical outcomes. However, several barriers to targeting CSCs remain. Selective targeting of CSCs will require better characterization of optimal markers to identify this cell subpopulation. Additionally, while CSCs signaling pathways provide a rich target, we must address the likelihood of overlap between critical pathways that exist in normal stem cells and those in CSCs. Perhaps driving CSC to differentiate, thereby making them vulnerable to standard cytotoxic agents, will prove to be a promising therapeutic strategy. Another important aspect of testing novel CSC therapeutics will be the utilization of an optimal preclinical model system. Our research group considers the primary pancreatic cancer orthotopic xenograft model system as optimal for testing potential therapeutics, as this model system best reflects the tumor heterogeneity that is observed in actual patients and reproduces the challenges of drug delivery to the tumor site. The orthotopic xenograft model system may be strengthened by simultaneous engraftment of human pancreatic stromal cells to recreate human tumor conditions, as cellular signaling cross-talk in the local microenvironment may affect the biology of the tumor. Therapeutics targeted to the CSC population are currently under development and in the early testing phases (Garber 2007). Clinical trials of a Hedgehog antagonist and a gamma-secretase inhibitor to block the Hedgehog and Notch developmental signal pathways, respectively, in pancreatic cancer are underway.

For clinical trials testing targeted pancreatic CSC therapeutics, new measures of efficacy will likely be needed as reduction in bulk tumor volume does not correlate with significant or lasting effects on the CSC population. Measuring the effects of new drugs on the pancreatic CSC population in patients may prove to be an obstacle given the less than ideal anatomic location of the pancreas for biopsy. Additionally, tumor shrinkage is essential to stemming the burden of disease, and it is likely that the most effective novel therapeutics will be multimodal, addressing both the highly tumorigenic and migratory CSC subpopulation and the much larger population of differentiated tumor cells. The data obtained in clinical trials will be invaluable in determining if targeting CSCs will decrease mortality and result in long-term disease-free survival or cure.

Conclusion

The identification of CSCs in solid tumors has engendered a new paradigm in our understanding of tumorigenesis, metastasis, and resistance to therapy. CSCs also provide a novel target for therapeutics that may effectively quell tumorigenesis, capacity for self-renewal, and multipotent differentiation. In pancreatic cancer, the discovery of CSCs and their characteristic resistance to standard chemotherapy and ionizing radiation has provided renewed hope for a cure for one of the most devastating solid organ malignancies. More research is needed in several areas of CSC biology. Further elucidating the molecular machinery that drive the stem-like activity of CSCs, confer their resistance to standard therapy, allow migration throughout the host and differentiate them from normal stem cells will provide important insights to improve therapeutic strategies in PDAC. While effectively targeting CSCs poses a great challenge, our success may provide an even greater reward for patients suffering from PDAC.

References

Al-Hajj M, Wicha MS, Benito-Hernandez A, Morrison SJ, Clarke MF (2003) Prospective identification of tumorigenic breast cancer cells. Proc Natl Acad Sci USA 100 (7):3983–3988. doi:10.1073/pnas.0530291100 0530291100 [pii]

Bailey JM, Singh PK, Hollingsworth MA (2007) Cancer metastasis facilitated by developmental pathways: Sonic hedgehog, Notch, and bone morphogenic proteins. J Cell Biochem 102 (4):829–839. doi:10.1002/jcb.21509

Bao S, Wu Q, McLendon RE, Hao Y, Shi Q, Hjelmeland AB, Dewhirst MW, Bigner DD, Rich JN (2006) Glioma stem cells promote radioresistance by preferential activation of the DNA damage response. Nature 444 (7120):756–760. doi:nature05236 [pii] 10.1038/nature05236

Barbera MJ, Puig I, Dominguez D, Julien-Grille S, Guaita-Esteruelas S, Peiro S, Baulida J, Franci C, Dedhar S, Larue L, Garcia de Herreros A (2004) Regulation of Snail transcription during epithelial to mesenchymal transition of tumor cells. Oncogene 23 (44):7345–7354. doi:10.1038/sj.onc.1207990 1207990 [pii]

Bonnet D, Dick JE (1997) Human acute myeloid leukemia is organized as a hierarchy that originates from a primitive hematopoietic cell. Nat Med 3 (7):730–737

Cui H, Hu B, Li T, Ma J, Alam G, Gunning WT, Ding HF (2007) Bmi-1 is essential for the tumorigenicity of neuroblastoma cells. Am J Pathol 170 (4):1370–1378. doi:170/4/1370 [pii] 10.2353/ajpath.2007.060754

Dylla SJ, Beviglia L, Park IK, Chartier C, Raval J, Ngan L, Pickell K, Aguilar J, Lazetic S, Smith-Berdan S, Clarke MF, Hoey T, Lewicki J, Gurney AL (2008) Colorectal cancer stem cells are enriched in xenogeneic tumors following chemotherapy. PLoS One 3 (6):e2428. doi:10.1371/journal.pone.0002428

Feldmann G, Dhara S, Fendrich V, Bedja D, Beaty R, Mullendore M, Karikari C, Alvarez H, Iacobuzio-Donahue C, Jimeno A, Gabrielson KL, Matsui W, Maitra A (2007) Blockade of hedgehog signaling inhibits pancreatic cancer invasion and metastases: a new paradigm for combination therapy in solid cancers. Cancer Res 67 (5):2187–2196. doi:67/5/2187 [pii] 10.1158/0008-5472.CAN-06-3281

Garber K (2007) Notch emerges as new cancer drug target. J Natl Cancer Inst 99 (17):1284–1285. doi:djm148 [pii] 10.1093/jnci/djm148

Hajra KM, Chen DY, Fearon ER (2002) The SLUG zinc-finger protein represses E-cadherin in breast cancer. Cancer Res 62 (6):1613–1618

Haupt Y, Bath ML, Harris AW, Adams JM (1993) bmi-1 transgene induces lymphomas and collaborates with myc in tumorigenesis. Oncogene 8 (11):3161–3164

Hermann PC, Huber SL, Herrler T, Aicher A, Ellwart JW, Guba M, Bruns CJ, Heeschen C (2007) Distinct populations of cancer stem cells determine tumor growth and metastatic activity in human pancreatic cancer. Cell Stem Cell 1 (3):313–323. doi:S1934-5909(07)00066-5 [pii] 10.1016/j.stem.2007.06.002

Hruban RH, Rustgi AK, Brentnall TA, Tempero MA, Wright CV, Tuveson DA (2006) Pancreatic cancer in mice and man: the Penn Workshop 2004. Cancer Res 66 (1):14–17. doi:66/1/14 [pii] 10.1158/0008-5472.CAN-05-3914

Ishibashi S, Sakaguchi M, Kuroiwa T, Yamasaki M, Kanemura Y, Shizuko I, Shimazaki T, Onodera M, Okano H, Mizusawa H (2004) Human neural stem/progenitor cells, expanded in long-term neurosphere culture, promote functional recovery after focal ischemia in Mongolian gerbils. J Neurosci Res 78 (2):215–223. doi:10.1002/jnr.20246

Jacobs JJ, Kieboom K, Marino S, DePinho RA, van Lohuizen M (1999) The oncogene and Polycomb-group gene bmi-1 regulates cell proliferation and senescence through the ink4a locus. Nature 397 (6715):164–168. doi:10.1038/16476

Jemal A, Siegel R, Ward E, Murray T, Xu J, Thun MJ (2007) Cancer statistics, 2007. CA Cancer J Clin 57 (1):43–66. doi:57/1/43 [pii]

Kang MK, Kim RH, Kim SJ, Yip FK, Shin KH, Dimri GP, Christensen R, Han T, Park NH (2007) Elevated Bmi-1 expression is associated with dysplastic cell transformation during oral carcinogenesis and is required for cancer cell replication and survival. Br J Cancer 96 (1):126–133. doi:6603529 [pii] 10.1038/sj.bjc.6603529

Kim JH, Yoon SY, Jeong SH, Kim SY, Moon SK, Joo JH, Lee Y, Choe IS, Kim JW (2004a) Overexpression of Bmi-1 oncoprotein correlates with axillary lymph node metastases in invasive ductal breast cancer. Breast 13 (5):383–388. doi:10.1016/j.breast.2004.02.010 S09609776 04000372 [pii]

Kim JH, Yoon SY, Kim CN, Joo JH, Moon SK, Choe IS, Choe YK, Kim JW (2004b) The Bmi-1 oncoprotein is overexpressed in human colorectal cancer and correlates with the reduced p16INK4a/p14ARF proteins. Cancer Lett 203 (2):217–224. doi:S030438350300692X [pii]

Lessard J, Sauvageau G (2003) Bmi-1 determines the proliferative capacity of normal and leukaemic stem cells. Nature 423 (6937):255–260. doi:10.1038/nature01572 nature01572 [pii]

Li C, Heidt DG, Dalerba P, Burant CF, Zhang L, Adsay V, Wicha M, Clarke MF, Simeone DM (2007) Identification of pancreatic cancer stem cells. Cancer Res 67 (3):1030–1037. doi:67/3/1030 [pii] 10.1158/0008-5472.CAN-06-2030

Liu S, Dontu G, Mantle ID, Patel S, Ahn NS, Jackson KW, Suri P, Wicha MS (2006) Hedgehog signaling and Bmi-1 regulate self-renewal of normal and malignant human mammary stem cells. Cancer Res 66 (12):6063–6071. doi:66/12/6063 [pii] 10.1158/0008-5472.CAN-06-0054

Ma S, Chan KW, Hu L, Lee TK, Wo JY, Ng IO, Zheng BJ, Guan XY (2007) Identification and characterization of tumorigenic liver cancer stem/progenitor cells. Gastroenterology 132 (7):2542–2556. doi:S0016-5085(07)00786-X [pii] 10.1053/j.gastro.2007.04.025

Mani SA, Guo W, Liao MJ, Eaton EN, Ayyanan A, Zhou AY, Brooks M, Reinhard F, Zhang CC, Shipitsin M, Campbell LL, Polyak K, Brisken C, Yang J, Weinberg RA (2008) The epithelial-mesenchymal transition generates cells with properties of stem cells. Cell 133 (4):704–715. doi:S0092-8674(08)00444-3 [pii] 10.1016/j.cell.2008.03.027

Mueller MT, Hermann PC, Witthauer J, Rubio-Viqueira B, Leicht SF, Huber S, Ellwart JW, Mustafa M, Bartenstein P, D'Haese JG, Schoenberg MH, Berger F, Jauch KW, Hidalgo M, Heeschen C (2009) Combined targeted treatment to eliminate tumorigenic cancer stem cells in human pancreatic cancer. Gastroenterology 137 (3):1102–1113. doi:S0016-5085(09)00901-9 [pii] 10.1053/j.gastro.2009.05.053

O'Brien CA, Pollett A, Gallinger S, Dick JE (2007) A human colon cancer cell capable of initiating tumour growth in immunodeficient mice. Nature 445 (7123):106–110. doi:nature05372 [pii] 10.1038/nature05372

Park IK, Qian D, Kiel M, Becker MW, Pihalja M, Weissman IL, Morrison SJ, Clarke MF (2003) Bmi-1 is required for maintenance of adult self-renewing haematopoietic stem cells. Nature 423 (6937):302–305. doi:10.1038/nature01587 nature01587 [pii]

Pasca di Magliano M, Hebrok M (2003) Hedgehog signalling in cancer formation and maintenance. Nat Rev Cancer 3 (12):903–911. doi:10.1038/nrc1229 nrc1229 [pii]

Philip PA, Mooney M, Jaffe D, Eckhardt G, Moore M, Meropol N, Emens L, O'Reilly E, Korc M, Ellis L, Benedetti J, Rothenberg M, Willett C, Tempero M, Lowy A, Abbruzzese J, Simeone D, Hingorani S, Berlin J, Tepper J (2009) Consensus report of the national cancer institute clinical trials planning meeting on pancreas cancer treatment. J Clin Oncol 27 (33):5660–5669. doi:JCO.2009.21.9022 [pii] 10.1200/JCO.2009.21.9022

Reya T, Morrison SJ, Clarke MF, Weissman IL (2001) Stem cells, cancer, and cancer stem cells. Nature 414 (6859):105–111. doi:10.1038/35102167 35102167 [pii]

Ricci-Vitiani L, Lombardi DG, Pilozzi E, Biffoni M, Todaro M, Peschle C, De Maria R (2007) Identification and expansion of human colon-cancer-initiating cells. Nature 445 (7123):111–115. doi:nature05384 [pii] 10.1038/nature05384

Rubin LL, de Sauvage FJ (2006) Targeting the Hedgehog pathway in cancer. Nat Rev Drug Discov 5 (12):1026–1033. doi:nrd2086 [pii] 10.1038/nrd2086

Shah AN, Summy JM, Zhang J, Park SI, Parikh NU, Gallick GE (2007) Development and characterization of gemcitabine-resistant pancreatic tumor cells. Ann Surg Oncol 14 (12):3629–3637. doi:10.1245/s10434-007-9583-5

Singh SK, Hawkins C, Clarke ID, Squire JA, Bayani J, Hide T, Henkelman RM, Cusimano MD, Dirks PB (2004) Identification of human brain tumour initiating cells. Nature 432 (7015):396–401. doi:nature03128 [pii] 10.1038/nature03128

van Lohuizen M, Verbeek S, Scheijen B, Wientjens E, van der Gulden H, Berns A (1991) Identification of cooperating oncogenes in E mu-myc transgenic mice by provirus tagging. Cell 65 (5):737–752. doi:0092-8674(91)90382-9 [pii]

Visvader JE, Lindeman GJ (2008) Cancer stem cells in solid tumours: accumulating evidence and unresolved questions. Nat Rev Cancer 8 (10):755–768. doi:nrc2499 [pii] 10.1038/nrc2499

Wellner U, Schubert J, Burk UC, Schmalhofer O, Zhu F, Sonntag A, Waldvogel B, Vannier C, Darling D, zur Hausen A, Brunton VG, Morton J, Sansom O, Schuler J, Stemmler MP, Herzberger C, Hopt U, Keck T, Brabletz S, Brabletz T (2009) The EMT-activator ZEB1 promotes tumorigenicity by repressing stemness-inhibiting microRNAs. Nat Cell Biol 11 (12):1487–1495. doi:ncb1998 [pii] 10.1038/ncb1998

Wicha MS, Liu S, Dontu G (2006) Cancer stem cells: an old idea--a paradigm shift. Cancer Res 66 (4):1883–1890; discussion 1895–1886. doi:66/4/1883 [pii] 10.1158/0008-5472.CAN-05-3153

Wilson A, Radtke F (2006) Multiple functions of Notch signaling in self-renewing organs and cancer. FEBS Lett 580 (12):2860–2868. doi:S0014-5793(06)00326-7 [pii] 10.1016/j.febslet.2006.03.024

Wright MH, Calcagno AM, Salcido CD, Carlson MD, Ambudkar SV, Varticovski L (2008) Brca1 breast tumors contain distinct CD44+/CD24- and CD133+ cells with cancer stem cell characteristics. Breast Cancer Res 10 (1):R10. doi:bcr1855 [pii] 10.1186/bcr1855

Yang J, Mani SA, Donaher JL, Ramaswamy S, Itzykson RA, Come C, Savagner P, Gitelman I, Richardson A, Weinberg RA (2004) Twist, a master regulator of morphogenesis, plays an essential role in tumor metastasis. Cell 117 (7):927–939. doi:10.1016/j.cell.2004.06.006 S0092867404005768 [pii]

Yauch RL, Gould SE, Scales SJ, Tang T, Tian H, Ahn CP, Marshall D, Fu L, Januario T, Kallop D, Nannini-Pepe M, Kotkow K, Marsters JC, Rubin LL, de Sauvage FJ (2008) A paracrine requirement for hedgehog signalling in cancer. Nature 455 (7211):406–410. doi:nature07275 [pii] 10.1038/nature07275

Chapter 13
Cancer Stem Cells and Renal Carcinoma

Benedetta Bussolati and Giovanni Camussi

Renal Carcinoma

Renal carcinoma is a common urological tumor and accounts for ≈3% of all human malignancies. The renal carcinoma is not a single entity, but comprises a group of tumors that arise from the epithelium of renal tubules: clear cell carcinoma, the most common histological subtype, papillary carcinoma, and chromophobe carcinoma. Genetic or epigenetic inactivation of the von Hippel–Lindau tumor suppressor gene and subsequent activation of the hypoxia response pathway is recognized as the tumorigenic event in clear cell carcinomas (Arai and Kanai 2010). Among urologic tumors, it is the worst in cancer-specific mortality, since more than 40% of the patients with RCC die of the disease, opposite to the 20% mortality observed in prostate cancer or bladder carcinoma (Pascual and Borque 2008; Chow et al. 2010). The annual mortality-to-incidence ratio for renal carcinoma is significantly higher than for other urological malignancies since renal carcinoma is insensitive to traditional cytotoxic drugs as well as radiotherapy. During the past decades, immunotherapy with cytokines based on interferon-alpha and interleukin-2 have been the standard therapies for metastatic renal carcinoma, even if results have been poor (Di Lorenzo et al. 2010). New therapies, directed at specific molecular targets implicated in angiogenesis and tumor proliferation has been investigated, leading to encouraging results. Among them, inhibitors of the vascular endothelial growth factor (VEGF), tyrosine-kinase inhibitors, epithelial growth factor (EGF) inhibitors, and m-TOR inhibitors (Heldevein et al. 2009).

If tumors are derived from cancer stem cells (CSCs), then drugs that kill these cells could prove highly effective treatments of cancer (Sehl et al. 2009). Recent

---

B. Bussolati (✉) • G. Camussi
Renal and Vascular Physiopathology Laboratory, Department of Internal Medicine,
Molecular Biotechnology Centre and Research Centre for Molecular Medicine,
University of Torino, Cso Dogliotti 14, 10126 Torino, Italy
e-mail: benedetta.bussolati@unito.it

encouraging data have provided proof of principle that selective targeting of CSCs is possible (Yilmaz et al. 2006; Smith et al. 2010). Strategies of targeting CSCs should, therefore, be taken into account also in renal carcinomas.

Embryonic Renal Stem Cells and Wilm's Tumor

According to the hierarchical lineage view of tumors (Sell 2010), renal tumors may arise from the embryonic stem cell compartment, as well as from the stem cell pool of the adult kidney or from the deriving progenitors. Tumors due to mutations of embryonic stem cells might give rise to the Wilm's tumor, whereas mutations occurring in the adult stem cell compartment could give rise to the different histologic types of carcinomas. Embryonic stem cells have been described in the embryonic kidney until relatively late in gestation in the nephrogenic zone, from which they have been isolated and characterized (Pleniceanu et al. 2010). Comparative analysis of embryonic stem cells and of the pediatric renal malignancy Wilms' tumor showed that Wilm's tumor resulted from a differentiation arrest of embryonic progenitors committed to the nephrogenic lineage (Dekel et al. 2006). Wilms' tumor, a common pediatric kidney cancer, can be considered a primitive malignancy of embryonic renal precursors, which fail to terminally differentiate into epithelium and continue to proliferate. The multipotency of these cells is supported by a characteristic histology of the tumor, which includes, apart from blastemal components, more mature epithelial and stromal cells and suggests that blastemal cells have differentiated at least in part in renal-differentiated elements. In addition, it was shown by Metsuyanim et al. (2008) that stem-like cells of the Wilm's tumor present epigenetic alterations involving polycomb activation and epigenetic modifications of nephric-progenitor genes, suggesting a role for epigenetic modification of normal renal stem cells in the initiation and progression of renal cancer.

Renal Adult Stem Cells

In the human adult kidney, CD133$^+$ renal progenitor cells have been characterized by our group in the renal cortex from the tubule/interstitium (Bussolati et al. 2005). Once isolated, these cells lacked the expression of hematopoietic markers (CD34 and CD45), whereas they expressed some mesenchymal stem cell markers, such as CD29, CD90, CD44, and CD73. Moreover, they expressed Pax-2, an embryonic renal marker (Dressler and Douglass 1992; Bruno et al. 2009), suggesting their renal origin. These cells were shown to undergo epithelial and endothelial differentiation both in vitro and in vivo (Bussolati et al. 2005). When injected in vivo subcutaneously in Matrigel, CD133$^+$ cells spontaneously differentiated in tubular structures expressing proximal and distal tubular epithelial markers. In vivo, when injected subcutaneously in Matrigel, endothelial-differentiated CD133⁺ cells formed vessels connected with the mouse vasculature. Moreover, when injected into mice with glycerol-induced acute renal injury, CD133⁺ renal progenitors homed to the kidney and integrated into proximal and distal tubules during the repair (Bussolati et al. 2005).

In addition, multipotent CD133⁺/CD24⁺ stem cells were isolated from the Bowman's capsule (Sagrinati et al. 2006). A genomic characterization of multipotent CD133⁺/CD24⁺ renal progenitor cells from glomeruli and tubules of adult human kidney revealed no significant differences in the gene expression patterns, suggesting that tubular and glomerular renal progenitor cells represent a genetically homogeneous population (Sallustio et al. 2010). Indeed, the presence of cytokeratin expression by the CD133⁺/CD24⁺ cells suggests an epithelial commitment that characterizes these cells as epithelial progenitors.

CD133⁺/CD34⁻ Cells and Renal Carcinomas

Following the stem cell view of tumor generation (Clarke and Fuller 2006; Alison et al. 2010), CD133 has been investigated as a marker for the identification of CSCs in renal carcinomas. A small population of CD133⁺/CD34⁻ cells (less than 1% of the total cells) was found in human renal carcinomas (Bruno et al. 2006). The lack of CD34 expression indicated that they were not endothelial progenitor cells derived from circulating elements. Indeed, these cells, that represented a progenitor cell population in the normal kidney, showed the same mesenchymal phenotype and differentiative ability of their normal counterpart (Bussolati et al. 2005). They expressed CD73, CD44, CD29, the developmental renal marker PAX-2, and the mesenchymal marker vimentin and were able to differentiate both in endothelial and epithelial cells in vitro and in vivo. When injected subcutaneously within Matrigel in immunodeficient mice, CD133⁺/CD34⁻ stem cells were not able to form tumors. These data indicate that CD133⁺/CD34⁻ cells are not a population of tumor-initiating cells, at variance of CD133⁺ cells derived from brain, prostate, colon, and pulmonary tumors (Singh et al. 2003; Collins et al. 2005; O'Brien et al. 2007; Eramo et al. 2008). As culture of CD133⁺/CD34⁻ cells in the presence of the tumor supernatant induced their differentiation into endothelial cells, it could be speculated that the tumor microenvironment could be involved in the endothelial commitment of these renal progenitors. Indeed, when co-transplanted with renal tumor cells, at a 1:100 ratio (the same ratio present in renal carcinomas), CD133⁺/CD34⁻ cells significantly enhanced tumor engraftment, growth, and vascularization, suggesting that these progenitors may produce a growth factor environment favoring tumor growth (Bruno et al. 2006) and vascularization. Recently, D'Alterio et al. (2010) evaluated the expression of CD133 on samples of human renal clear cell carcinoma, showing that CD133 expression did not correlate to clinical pathological features or affected patients prognosis.

CD105⁺ Renal Cancer Stem Cells

Based on the mesenchymal origin of the kidney and on the mesenchymal phenotype of stem cells found in normal rodent kidney (Gupta et al. 2006; Da Silva et al. 2006; Plotkin and Goligorsky 2006) as well as in the human embryo (Metsuyanim et al. 2009), mesenchymal markers were successfully used to identify a population of tumor-initiating cells in renal carcinomas. In particular, a population of CD105⁺ tumor-initiating cells was found in renal human carcinomas independently from the histologic type of origin (Bussolati et al. 2008). The lack of CD133 and CD24 expression, which are present in adult and embryonic renal progenitors (Bussolati et al. 2005; Lazzeri et al. 2007), by tumor-initiating CD105⁺ cells suggests that they are not derived from this population. Moreover, CD133⁺ previously isolated from renal tumors did not express CD105 and were not tumorigenic (see above).

By magnetic cell sorting of specimens of human renal carcinomas, we isolated (Bussolati et al. 2008) a subpopulation of cell expressing the mesenchymal marker CD105, representing around 8% of the tumor mass. The CD105⁺ population induced tumors in SCID mice with 100% incidence, whereas the CD105⁻ population induced tumors with only 10% incidence. CD105⁺ cells were cloned to avoid contamination of non-tumor cell types expressing the CD105 marker (Bussolati et al. 2008). Characterization of the phenotype of CD105⁺ clones revealed the expression of markers characteristic of mesenchymal stem cells (CD44, CD90, CD146, CD73, CD29, and vimentin) and of embryonic stem cells markers (Nanog, Oct4, Musashi, Nestin, and the embryonic marker Pax2) and lack of differentiative epithelial markers. Moreover, they presented several stem cells properties, such as clonogenic ability, sphere-formation in the presence of non-adhesive cell culture medium and in vitro differentiation on both endothelial and epithelial cell types. In addition, in vivo they generated serially transplantable carcinomas containing a small population of undifferentiated CD105⁺ tumorigenic cells and differentiated CD105⁻ tumor epithelial cells. At variance of CD105⁺ cells derived from the stroma that forms mesenchymal tumors, tumor initiating cells were able to generate carcinomas expressing an epithelial phenotype. In vivo, CD105⁺ cells were able to maintain the tumor-initiating CD105⁺ population expressing stem cell properties and lacking differentiative markers. Moreover, CD105⁺ clones were able to generate a progeny of differentiated CD105⁻ cells unable to generate the tumor and expressing cytokeratin.

These data suggest that the CD105⁺ cells represent a tumor-initiating cell population that may originate from resident renal stem cells with mesenchymal characteristics. However, it cannot be excluded that the CD105⁺ stem cell population identified in renal carcinomas may derive from mutated stromal/mesenchymal cells of the tumor or from bone marrow-derived stem cells. Indeed, stem cells derived from the bone marrow cells have been suggested to contribute to tumor development (Houghton et al. 2004; Aractingi et al. 2005). In particular, generation of a renal carcinoma of recipient cell origin arising in a grafted kidney was recently reported, suggesting the integration in the grafted kidney of circulating cells originating in the recipient and their subsequent malignant transformation in the graft (Boix et al. 2009).

Moreover, mesenchymal cells present in tumor stroma were shown to be able to follow an autonomous fate, developing into rapidly growing, highly vascularized and invasive mesenchymal tumors (Galiè et al. 2008). There are reports suggesting the possibility that these tumor mesenchymal cells may undergo tumorigenic phenotypic changes induced by the neoplastic microenvironment (Kurose et al. 2002). Indeed, various studies showed chromosomal alterations in tumor stroma (Hu et al. 2005).

Side Population in Renal Carcinomas

A useful tool to isolate stem cell-like populations by cytofluorimetric analysis is the Hoechst 33342 dye efflux model, which has been shown to isolate populations of hemopoietic stem cells, so-called side population (SP) cells, from blood, bone marrow as well as from various organs (Goodell et al. 1996). To bypass the need of specific cell markers for CSCs, SP cells were identified and characterized in both normal and malignant renal epithelial cells (Addla et al. 2008). The SP of normal kidney expressed the same markers identified by Bussolati et al. (2005) in renal progenitors. In addition, the authors found a differential expression of CD133 marker between the side population of normal and malignant kidney, being CD133 only expressed by the normal SP. These data, in agreement with the lack of CD133 by CSCs (Bussolati et al. 2008), may suggest that the loss of CD133 might be a very early event in stem cell differentiation and possibly in malignant transformation (Addla et al. 2008). Cells gated as SP fraction were reported to be around 6% of the total epithelial population (Addla et al. 2008; Oates et al. 2009), a high percentage in respect to other malignancies (Oates et al. 2009) and similar to that estimated by Bussolati et al. (2008). The SP fraction showed increased proliferation, expression of proliferative and putative stem markers, clonogenicity and sphere forming ability in respect to the non-SP fraction (Addla et al. 2008; Oates et al. 2009). The subsequent characterization of SP cells using high brilliance synchrotron-FITR spectroscopy revealed the presence of different subpopulations of cells with the SP renal cancer population, with different cellular biochemistry (Hughes et al. 2010). The differential role of these subpopulations in carcinogenesis, and the presence of specific markers is still undetermined.

Sphere-Derived CSCs

The presence of CSCs with tumor-initiating ability has also been confirmed in a renal tumor cell line. Generation of spheres is considered a useful culture system to select for CSCs, relaying on the ability of CSCs to growth in non-adhesive spheres in serum-free medium supplemented with EGF and bFGF (Ponti et al. 2005). Using this selection system, cells growing as tumor spheres were isolated from the renal carcinoma cell line SK-RC-42 (Zhong et al. 2010). This sphere-forming population showed the ability of self-renewing in vitro and in vivo, higher mRNA expression levels of several stemness genes, including Oct-3/4, Bmi, β-catenin, and Nanog compared with the monolayer adherent cells and stronger tumorigenicity and resistance to chemotherapeutic agents and irradiation. Furthermore, a detailed characterization of surface molecules involved in the immunophenotype of the sphere forming cells showed that they displayed several molecules involved in the evasion from immune surveillance and from complement-mediated cell killing (Zhong et al. 2010).

Renal CSCs and Endothelial Differentiation

The stemness and the origin of CSCs from tissue stem/progenitor cells may support the capacity of CSCs to differentiate in cell types present in the tumor other than the epithelial tumor cells. In renal carcinomas, CD105$^+$ CSCs were shown to be bipotent, as they were able to differentiate into tumor epithelial and endothelial cells both in vitro and in vivo (Bussolati et al. 2008). The evidence of an in vivo differentiation of stem cells into endothelial cells was provided by the observation that at least a fraction of the vessels present in the transplanted tumors originated from tumor stem cells were of human origin. Clonal studies showing endothelial differentiation of single cell-derived spheres or clonal cell lines derived from renal CSCs confirmed the multipotency of renal CSCs. This endothelial differentiation has also been shown for CSCs derived from glioblastomas (Wang et al. 2010; Dong et al. 2010; Ricci-Vitiani et al. 2010; Zhao et al. 2010), ovarian (Alvero et al. 2009), and breast cancer (Bussolati et al. 2009), suggesting that this is rather a general phenomenon applicable to stem cells in different tumors, possibly due to the maintenance of stem properties in CSCs. Of interest, hypoxia was reported as a mechanism involved in the endothelial differentiation of tumor stem cells (Bussolati et al. 2009). This concept is of particular relevance in tumor anti-angiogenic therapy, as therapy-induced hypoxia may promote alternative strategies to support tumor vascularization and induce a switch from normal to cancer stem-dependent vascularization (Fig. 13.1). Anti-angiogenic therapies currently implied in the treatment of renal carcinoma should, therefore, be aimed to target not only normal but also tumor-derived endothelial cells.

Conclusion

In renal tumors, the data of the literature demonstrate the presence of cells showing the properties of CSCs in vitro and in vivo. In vitro, renal CSCs showed the expression of stem markers, clonogenicity, ability to growth in spheres, and chemoresistance. In vivo, they showed ability to initiate tumors that recapitulated the tumor

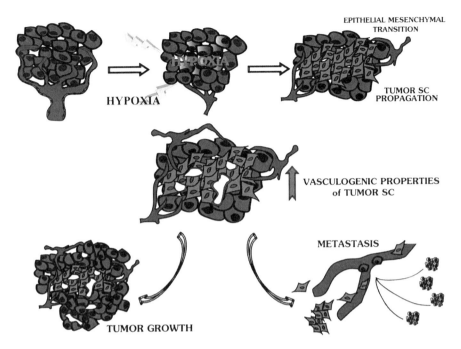

Fig. 13.1 Vasculogenic properties of renal CSCs. Renal tumor vessels may in part derive from CSCs undergoing a vasculogenic differentiation. Hypoxia and epithelial-to-mesenchymal transition occurring after anti-angiogenic therapy and the subsequent hypoxia may increase the vasculogenic property of CSCs and favor the switch from a normal to a cancer-dependent tumor vascularization

of origin and to generate serially transplantable tumors maintaining a CSC undifferentiated tumorigenic population and a non-tumorigenic-differentiated population (Table 13.1).

Concerning the stem cell origin of renal CSCs, the data are still discordant. The lack of tumorigenicity of CD133+ cells (Bruno et al. 2006) is in contrast with the idea that, also in the kidney, carcinomas originate from renal progenitors expressing CD133. A possible explanation is the origin of renal carcinomas from of a more undifferentiated stem cell compartment. Alternatively, it could be postulated that a true stem cell compartment is lacking in the renal tubuli. In particular, the dynamic phenotype of tubular cells, evidenced by the finding that they are in the G1 phase of the cell cycle (Vogetseder et al. 2008), can suggested that tubular cells may modulate their phenotype towards stemness in response to environmental stimuli. Recent data have proposed that CSCs may not be static and well-defined entities, but rather tumor cells that transiently acquire stemness properties depending on the tumor microenvironment. Accordingly, it has been shown that the epithelial mesenchymal transition of tumor cells may induce markers and phenotypic properties of CSCs (Mani et al. 2008). Knowledge on identity and mechanisms of generation of renal CSCs could be of great value in the management of this aggressive and angiogenic cancer.

Table 13.1 In vitro and in vivo properties of the different CSC populations identified in human renal carcinomas

Identification method	CD105	SP	Spheres
Mesenchymal markers	+	+	+
Embryonic markers	+	+	+
SP	ND	+	+
Sphere formation	+	+	+
Clonogenicity	+	+	+
Endothelial differentiation	+	ND	ND
Chemoresistance	ND	+[a]	+
Tumor initiation	+	ND	+
Recapitulation of the tumor of origin	+	ND	+
Serially transplantable tumor generation	+	ND	ND
References	Bussolati et al. (2008)	Addla et al. (2008)	Zhong et al. (2010)

ND not done
[a]Indirect evidence as expression of the multidrug resistance protein

References

Addla S, Brown M, Hart C et al (2008) Characterization of the Hoechst 33342 side population from normal and malignant human renal epithelial cells. Am J Physiol Renal Physiol 295:F680–F687

Alison MR, Islam S, Wright NA (2010) Stem cells in cancer: instigators and propagators? J Cell Sc 123:2357–68

Alvero AB, Fu HH, Holmberg J et al (2009) Stem-like ovarian cancer cells can serve as tumor vascular progenitors. Stem Cells 27:2405–13

Aractingi S, Kanitakis J, Euvaard S et al (2005) Skin carcinoma arising from donor cells in a kidney transplant recipient. Cancer Res 65:1755–60

Arai E, Kanai Y (2010) Genetic and epigenetic alterations during renal carcinogenesis. Int J Clin Exp Pathol 4:58–73

Boix R, Sanz C, Mora M et al (2009) Primary renal cell carcinoma in a transplanted kidney: genetic evidence of recipient origin. Transplantation 87:1057–61

Bruno S, Bussolati B, Grange C et al (2006) CD133+ renal progenitor cells contribute to tumor angiogenesis. Am J Pathol 169:2223–35

Bruno S, Bussolati B, Grange C et al (2009) Isolation and characterization of resident mesenchymal stem cells in human glomeruli. Stem Cells Dev 18(6):867–80

Bussolati B, Bruno S, Grange C et al (2005) Isolation of renal progenitor cells from adult human kidney. Am J Pathol 166:545–55

Bussolati B, Bruno S, Grange C et al (2008) Identification of a tumor-initiating stem cell population in human renal carcinomas. Faseb J 22:3696–705

Bussolati B, Grange C, Sapino A et al (2009) Endothelial cell differentiation of human breast tumour stem/progenitor cells. J Cell Mol Med 13:309–19

Chow WH, Dong LM, Devesa SS (2010) Epidemiology and risk factors for kidney cancer. Nat Rev Urol 7:245–57

Clarke MF, Fuller M (2006) Stem cells and cancer: two faces of eve. Cell 124:1111–5

Collins AT, Berry PA, Hyde C et al (2005) Prospective identification of tumorigenic prostate cancer stem cells. Cancer Res 65:10946–51

D'Alterio C, Cindolo L, Polimeno M et al (2010) Differential role of CD133 and CXCR4 in renal cell carcinoma. Cell Cycle 9:4492–500

Da Silva Meirelles L, Chagastelles PC, Nardi NB (2006) Mesenchymal stem cells reside in virtually all post-natal organs and tissues. J Cell Science 119:2204–13

Dekel B, Metsuyanim S, Schmidt-Ott KM et al (2006) Multiple imprinted and stemness genes provide a link between normal and tumor progenitor cells of the developing human kidney. Cancer Res 66:6040–9

Di Lorenzo G, Buonerba C, Biglietto M et al (2010) The therapy of kidney cancer with biomolecular drugs. Cancer Treat Rev 3:S16–20

Dong J, Zhao Y, Huang Q et al (2010) Glioma stem/progenitor cells contribute to neovascularization via transdifferentiation. Stem cell rev [Epub ahead of print]

Dressler GR, Douglass EC (1992) Pax-2 is a DNA-binding protein expressed in embryonic kidney and Wilms tumor. Proc Natl Acad Sci USA 89:1179–83

Eramo A, Lotti F, Sette G et al (2008) Identification and expansion of the tumorigenic lung cancer stem cell population. Cell Death Differ 15:504–14

Galiè M, Konstantinidou G, Peroni D et al (2008) Mesenchymal stem cells share molecular signature with mesenchymal tumor cells and favor early tumor growth in syngeneic mice. Oncogene 27:2542–51

Goodell MA, Brose K, Paradis G et al (1996) Isolation and functional properties of murine hematopoietic stem cells that are replicating in vivo. J Exp Med 183:1797–806

Gupta S, Verfaillie C, Chmielewski D et al (2006) Isolation and characterization of kidney-derived stem cells. J Am Soc Nephrol 17:3028–40

Heldevein F, Escudier B, Smyth G et al (2009) Metastatic renal cell carcinoma management. Int Braz J Urol 35:256–70

Houghton J, Stoicov C, Nomura S et al (2004) Gastric cancer originating from bone marrow-derived cells. Science 306:1568–71

Hu M, Yao J, Cai L et al (2005) Distinct epigenetic changes in the stromal cells of breast cancers. Nat Genet 37:899–905

Hughes C, Liew M, Sachdeva A et al (2010) SR-FTIR spectroscopy of renal epithelial carcinoma side population cells displaying stem cell-like characteristics. Analyst 135:3133–41

Kurose K, Gilley K, Matsumoto S et al (2002) Frequent somatic mutations in PTEN and TP53 are mutually exclusive in the stroma of breast carcinomas. Nat Genet 32:355–7

Lazzeri E, Crescioli C, Ronconi E et al (2007) Regenerative potential of embryonic renal multipotent progenitors in acute renal failure. J Am Soc Nephrol 18.3128–38

Mani SA, Guo W, Liao MJ et al (2008) The epithelial-mesenchymal transition generates cells with properties of stem cells. Cell 133:704–15

Metsuyanim S, Harari-Steinberg O, Buzhor E et al (2009) Expression of stem cell markers in the human fetal kidney. PLoS One 4:e6709

Metsuyanim S, Pode-Shakked N, Schmidt-Ott KM et al (2008) Accumulation of malignant renal stem cells is associated with epigenetic changes in normal renal progenitor genes. Stem Cells 26:1808–17

Oates JE, Grey BR, Addla SK, et al (2009) Hoechst 33342 side population identification is a conserved and unified mechanism in urological cancers. Stem Cells Dev 18:1515–22

O'Brien CA, Pollett A, Gallinger S et al (2007) A human colon cancer cell capable of initiating tumour growth in immunodeficient mice. Nature 445:106–10

Pascual D, Borque A (2008) Epidemiology of kidney cancer. Adv Urol. 782381

Pleniceanu O, Harari-Steinberg O, Dekel B (2010) Concise review: Kidney stem/progenitor cells: differentiate, sort out, or reprogram? Stem Cells 28:1649–60

Plotkin MD, Goligorsky MS (2006) Mesenchymal cells from adult kidney support angiogenesis and differentiate into multiple interstitial cell types including erythropoietin-producing Fibroblasts. Am J Physiol Renal Physiol 291: F902–F912

Ponti D, Costa A, Zaffaroni N et al (2005) Isolation and in vitro propagation of tumorigenic breast cancer cells with stem/progenitor cell properties. Cancer Res 65:5506–11

Ricci-Vitiani L, Pallini R, Biffoni M et al (2010) Tumor vascularization via endothelial differentiation of glioblastoma stem-like cells. Nature 468:824–8

Sagrinati C, Netti GS, Mazzinghi B et al (2006) Isolation and characterization of multipotent progenitor cells from the Bowman's capsule of adult human kidneys. J Am Soc Nephrol 17: 2443–5

Sallustio F, De Benedictis L, Castellano G et al (2010) TLR2 plays a role in the activation of human resident renal stem/progenitor cells. Faseb J 24: 514–25

Sehl ME, Sinsheimer JS, Zhou H et al (2009) Differential destruction of stem cells: implications for targeted cancer stem cell therapy. Cancer Res 69:9481–9

Sell S (2010) On the stem cell origin of cancer. Am J Pathol 176:2584–94

Singh SK, Clarke ID, Terasaki M et al (2003) Identification of a cancer stem cell in human brain tumors. Cancer Res 63: 5821–28

Smith KM, Datti A, Fujitani M et al (2010) Selective targeting of neuroblastoma tumour-initiating cells by compounds identified in stem cell-based small molecule screens. EMBO Mol Med 2:371–84

Vogetseder A, Picard N, Gaspert A et al (2008) Proliferation capacity of the renal proximal tubule involves the bulk of differentiated epithelial cells. Am J Physiol Cell Physiol 294:C22–28

Wang R, Chadalavada K, Wilshire J et al (2010) Glioblastoma stem-like cells give rise to tumour endothelium Nature 468:829–33

Yilmaz OH, Valdez R, Theisen BK et al (2006) Pten dependence distinguishes haematopoietic stem cells from leukaemia-initiating cells. Nature. 441:475–82

Zhao Y, Dong J, Huang Q et al (2010) Endothelial cell transdifferentiation of human glioma stem progenitor cells in vitro Brain Res Bull 82:308–12

Zhong Y, Guan K, Guo S et al (2010) Spheres derived from the human SK-RC-42 renal cell carcinoma cell line are enriched in cancer stem cells. Cancer Lett 299:150–60

Chapter 14
Cancer Stem Cells: Proteomic Approaches for New Potential Diagnostic and Prognostic Biomarkers

Patrizia Bottoni, Bruno Giardina, and Roberto Scatena

Introduction

After the first hypothesis, suggested by Virchow back in 1855, that some tumours could arise from misplaced embryonic cells, and the first identification, by Bonnet and Dick in 1997, of an acute myeloid leukaemia-initiating cell that was capable of initiating the systemic disease when transplanted into severe combined immune-deficient (SCID) mice, several different approaches have been applied leading to the isolation and characterization of CSCs from all of the major types of human solid tumours, including breast (Al-Hajj et al. 2003), colon (O'Brien et al. 2007; Dalerba et al. 2007), prostate (Patrawala et al. 2006), liver (Yang et al. 2008), pancreas (Li et al. 2007), and brain tumours (Singh et al. 2004). A great many data that have supplied information about specific cell surface antigens and gene expression in pluripotent hESCs were obtained by fluorescence-activated cell sorting (FACS) and by RT-PCR or microarrays (Sperger et al. 2003; Brimble et al. 2004).

In recent years, the proteomic field has rapidly evolved with the aim at systematically studying protein structure, function, expression levels and interaction network. By providing a snapshot of the proteins expressed at the given time and conditions from a biological system, proteomic analyses could facilitate the identification of proteins or protein expression patterns that have important pathogenetic, diagnostic, and prognostic value, with numerous potential applications in clinical research in general and in oncology in particular (Scatena et al. 2008). A classical proteomic approach is conducted by using two-dimensional electrophoresis (2-DE) as powerful separation method and mass spectrometry (MS spectrometry) as efficacious identification method. The recent introduction (Unlu et al. 1997) of labelling methodologies like DIGE has enhanced notably the versatility of 2-DE, allowing

P. Bottoni (✉) • B. Giardina • R. Scatena
Department of Laboratory Medicine, Catholic University,
Largo A. Gemelli 8, 00168 Rome, Italy
e-mail: patrizia.bottoni@rm.unicatt.it

not only the identification of low abundant proteins but also considerably improving the reproducibility of the quantitative proteomic analysis. Other methods frequently used in proteomics for relative quantification of proteins and peptides are isotope-coded affinity tag (ICAT) and isobaric tag for relative and absolute quantitation (iTRAQ). Additionally, proteomic technologies, employing mass spectrometry instruments associated with biostatistic/bioinformatic tools, permit to carry out different strategies of study, including various gel-free MS-based approaches. In Table 14.1 we summarized various proteomic methodologies currently utilized for studying cell proteome. The delineation of the CSC proteome could significantly contribute not only to identify cell-specific surface markers but also to elucidate the complex cellular mechanisms leading carcinogenesis and potentially discriminate every protein that plays a significant pathogenetic role in cancer with important clinical consequences in terms of prevention, diagnosis, and above all therapy. In addition, studies of protein expression profiles may also support and implement microarray-based transcriptome analyses (Lottaz et al. 2010), by providing further information on potential posttranslational modifications (PTMs) (e.g. methylation, acetylation, ubiquitination, and phosphorylation) and protein interactions. Moreover, it could be useful to stress that the expression levels of proteins involved in various processes do not always correlate with the changes of corresponding mRNA levels (Foss et al. 2007). A number of studies showed differences in the transcriptomic and proteomic expression levels during ESC differentiation process (Unwin et al. 2006; Spooncer et al. 2008; Fathi et al. 2009) and stressed the need to perform proteomic analysis in an attempt to clarify some aspects in the SC development and maintenance of pluripotency. It is evident that an accurate integration of proteomic and genomic data and their functional interpretation together with clinical evaluations could permit a more thorough understanding of complex biological processes, emphasizing different aspects to provide a complete picture of CSCs behaviour.

As a relatively recent topic, it is not surprising that the proteomics of CSCs are still developing, and to date a limited, but promising, number of studies have been published on the proteomic profiles of CSCs. SC proteome analyses have been, on the contrary, the object of a larger number of studies.

Notwithstanding the variability related to the use of various experimental protocols, which renders often difficult to directly compare results obtained from different studies and different laboratories, the proteomic research has recently generated a list of ESC-specific proteins and the ESC-derived proteome profile is now beginning to emerge. Such data could be interesting for an inside approach to CSC morphofunctional definition.

The Stem Cell Proteome

For their unique ability to self-renew and differentiate into specialized cell types under the appropriate physiological or experimental conditions, there is great interest in using SCs in the promising area of regenerative medicine, that aims to replace damaged tissue, especially in organs whose repairing capacity is particularly low

Table 14.1 Overview on proteomic technologies for studying CSCs proteome

Technology	Principle
2-DE (Two-dimensional electrophoresis)	The proteins are separated in the first dimension according to their isoelectric point and in the second dimension during SDS-PAGE by their molecular mass. The stained gels are visualized and subjected to an image analysis to highlight the differences in spot intensities among different gels. Protein spots of interest can undergo a tryptic digestion for identification by mass spectrometry
2D-DIGE (Difference in gel electrophoresis)	Modification of 2-DE in which protein samples can be labelled with different fluorescent dyes and then mixed and analyzed on a single 2-DE gel, that is scanned with excitation wavelength of each dye and detected using a fluorescence imaging scanner. This method assures an accurate analysis of differences in protein abundance between samples, by reducing inter-gel variations
LC-MS MS (Liquid chromatography-mass spectrometry)	High sensitivity technique that permits the physical separation of a mixture of peptides by liquid chromatography and the identification of their masses by MS spectrometry
MALDI-TOF MS (Matrix-assisted laser desorption/ionization)	Soft ionization technique that allows the desorption of proteins (or tryptic digest) previously mixed with a chemical matrix, aimed to obtain the accurate measurement of their masses and primary sequence information by time of flight
SELDI-TOF MS (Surface-enhanced laser desorption/ionization)	Variation of MALDI-TOF MS in which protein samples are spotted on a specific chromatographic surface to achieve a separation step based on the biochemical affinity and to render easier the protein mass analysis
ICAT (Isotope-coded affinity tags)	Non-gel based technique for quantitative proteomics. Proteins or peptides derived from two different samples are derivatized with heavy and light stable isotopic labels on cysteine residues. The labelled samples are then mixed and analyzed by LC-MS to calculate the relative abundance levels by comparing signal intensities of the heavy and light labelled peptides
iTRAQ (Isobaric tag for relative and absolute quantitation)	A gel-free method that is based on chemically labelling the N-terminus of proteins or peptides to enable relative quantification comparisons (up to eight different proteomic samples can be used to label peptides from different samples or treatments). The labelled samples are then mixed and analysed by LC-MS MS
Protein microarrays	Technology that makes use of various different capture molecules, frequently monoclonal antibodies, that are deposited on a chip surface for binding specific proteins from a sample. Bound proteins are detected currently by fluorescence, or by labelled secondary antibodies. The resulting spots can be quantified by a microarray quantification software

(Lerou and Daley 2005). The importance of these cells for biomedical research and future therapeutic applications is potentially considerable but remains to be fully investigated. In order to improve our understanding of mechanisms that regulate self-renewal and differentiation, the use of proteomic technologies could reveal to be useful tool to study post-translational regulation and protein quantification, opening new prospective scenarios in the area of cell therapy.

At present, an increasing number of proteomic studies have been undertaken to define the characteristics of SCs and of their microenvironment, in an attempt to develop a proteome profiling of primary stem cells, stem cell lines, and their differentiated derivatives (Baharvand et al. 2007).

One of the first comprehensive map of proteins expressed in hESCs was published by Baharvand et al. (2006), who showed a similar protein expression pattern in three investigated hESC lines. Among the proteins particularly abundant, the authors reported chaperones, heat shock proteins, ubiquitin/proteasome, and oxidative stress responsive proteins underscoring the ability of these cells to resist oxidative stress and increase the life span. Moreover, in this study several previously identified mouse ESC- and stemness-specific proteins, such as hepatoma-derived growth factor, guanine nucleotide-binding protein (G-protein) beta, and CRABP1 (Nagano et al. 2005), were reported.

A comparative analysis of the transcriptome and proteome of hESCs at different stages of differentiation (Fathi et al. 2009) permitted to identify a large number of proteins involved in various biological processes, such as metabolism, protein synthesis, processing and transport, and moreover an abundance of nuclear proteins (Baharvand et al. 2007), probably due to the high differentiation potential of stem cells.

Recently, another type of approach with top-down quantitative proteomic analysis was applied to hESCs (Collier et al. 2010). As a result, 62 intact protein precursors were detected, 11 of which were unambiguously identified by studying intact masses, MS/MS fragmentation data, and the presence of different types of PTMs residing on the whole protein.

A key area in ESC research is the identification of cell surface markers. A multitude of approaches employed to define new markers using membrane proteomes and different sample preparation procedures evaluated to adapt for each individual system have been developed (Ahn et al. 2008a). To solve problems related to solubility and low protein abundance that render the notoriously difficult proteome analyses of cell membranes, especially integral membrane proteins, various modified SDS-PAGE protocols have been developed in the last several years and were recently reviewed (Dormeyer et al. 2008b).

Due to limited amounts of available samples, generally the objective of these studies is to optimize sample preparation procedures for MS-analysis. One of the first proteomic analyses of hESC surface markers was performed by Foster et al. (2005) who reported expression changes of various integral membrane or membrane-anchored proteins and membrane-associated proteins in mesenchymal cells during osteoblast differentiation process. Changes in the proteome of cell lysates from mouse and human ESCs during the differentiation process have been analyzed (Van Hoof et al. 2006). Notably, in comparing the proteome profile of human ESC lines with a heterogeneous pool of their differentiated derivatives, the authors obtained a list of proteins identified in hESCs but not in differentiated HES-2 cells. These proteins included cell surface proteins, transcription factors, such as Oct4 and UTF1, telomerase-associated proteins, such as RIF1, and telomere end-binding protein and other known ESC markers (e.g. alkaline phosphatase, ALPL) that are essential for maintaining the undifferentiated state.

Interestingly, the same membrane proteins were reported in undifferentiated hESC lines by Dormeyer et al. (2008a). Using a new strategy optimized for application to the relatively small number of stem cells, the authors were able to provide a plasma membrane protein signature for hESCs (HUES-7 line) and hECCs (NT2/D1 line) showing similarities and differences between these cell types. In addition to the known stemness-associated cell surface markers such as ALP, CD9, and CTNNB, a large number of receptors, transporters, signal transducers and cell–cell adhesion proteins were identified.

In the same year, Harkness et al. (2008) employed hESC populations obtained from two different but standard culture conditions, feeder-containing and feeder-free cultures, in an attempt to identify a common proteome profile of hESC independent of culture conditions. The authors reported a list of transmembrane or membrane-associated proteins, of which 157 were present in both culture conditions, including receptors and transport proteins, CD antigens and adhesion proteins. In particular, some surface marker molecules not previously observed in hESCs at proteomic level, including Nodal modulator 1 and transgelin-2, CD81 and CD222 were identified in this study.

Recently, a SILAC strategy has been used (Prokhorova et al. 2009) to perform a comparative quantitative analysis of the membrane proteomes of undifferentiated vs. differentiating cells of two distinct hESC lines. Among the identified 811 membrane proteins, six displayed significantly higher levels in the self-renewing cells, including the well-known marker CD133/Prominin-1 and novel potential candidates for hESC surface markers: glypican-4, neuroligin-4, ErbB2, receptor-type protein tyrosine phosphatase zeta (PTPRZ), and glycoprotein M6B. A similar strategy was recently applied to study cell surface proteins specific for cardiomyocytes derived in vitro from hESCs (Van Hoof et al. 2010). By using a SILAC approach, a number of proteins associated with cardiac function or disease were observed, including several proteins that play a crucial role in the development of the heart during embryogenesis, e.g. junctophilin-2 and integrin R7.

A proteomic approach has been applied also to study the characteristics of neural stem cells (NSCs). The 2-DE analysis of a stable human foetal midbrain stem cell line during differentiation process revealed changes in the expression of 45 distinct proteins, including transgelin-2, proliferating cell nuclear antigen, peroxiredoxin 1 and peroxiredoxin-4. Among the regulated proteins, NudC, ubiquilin-1, STRAP, stress-70 protein, creatine kinase B, glial fibrillary acidic protein and vimentin (Hoffrogge et al. 2006).

Recently, an 8-plex i-TRAQ labelling strategy permitted the monitoring of eight different samples simultaneously to obtain a protein expression profile in a detailed time course analysis of neural differentiation (Chaerkady et al. 2009). This approach permitted to identify a large number of proteins that have potential roles in the regulation of neurogenesis and pluripotency including alkaline phosphatase and LIN28, which were found to be downregulated during commitment of neural progenitors into the neural lineage, and S-100, tenascin C, neurofilament-3 protein, doublecortin, CAM kinase-like 1 and nestin proteins, which were upregulated in astrocytes.

Another interesting series of proteomic studies were performed to analyse the composition of medium that promotes the growth of hESCs and to identify factors that regulate proliferation and the maintenance of pluripotency. One of the first MS-based analysis of the conditioned medium (CM) from mouse embryonic fibroblast feeder layers, STO cell line, permitted to identify proteins involved in extracellular matrix formation and remodelling, degradation and turnover, synthesis and processing, as well as chaperones and heat shock, and proteins involved in cell growth and differentiation, such as insulin-like growth factor-binding protein 4, pigment epithelium-derived factor and SPARC (Lim and Bodnar 2002). Some years later, an analysis aimed to find proteins common to the CM of three mitotically inactivated fibroblast lines, two of human origin (foetal and neonatal) and one of mouse origin (MEF), revealed a complex network of intracellular and extracellular proteins associated with a wide variety of biological functions, above all involved in the maintenance of hESCs pluripotency, including the Wnt, BMP/TGF-beta1, activin/inhibin, and insulin-like growth factor 1 (IGF-1) pathways (Prowse et al. 2007). In the same year, another proteomic approach was carried out to better understand the factors present in the MEF-CM capable of supporting hESCs (Bendall et al. 2007). This study permitted to detect numerous low-abundance growth factors, prevalently represented by the IGF, specifically IGF-II, and transforming growth factor (TGF) families. Notably, the authors suggested that IGF-II, in cooperation with basic fibroblast growth factor (bFGF), plays a central role in creating a supportive microenvironment in the regulatory niche of hESCs. A subsequent implementation of MS-based methodologies allowed to detect, among the potential growth-regulating proteins secreted into the extracellular space, various low-abundance growth factors present at concentrations $<10^{-9}$ g/ml, significantly improving research to characterize the hESCs secretome (Bendall et al. 2009).

Overall, these findings clearly emphasize the power of proteomic technologies to examine a wide variety of samples offering the possibility of studying protein expression in terms of qualitative and quantitative changes, including post-translational modifications that are essential for explaining protein activity in different cellular processes. However, due to the different protocols adopted, it remains often difficult to draw consistent results from these studies and to create a definitive proteome profile of hESCs. This has induced the stem cell biology and proteomics communities to collaborate for the "Proteome Biology of the Stem Cells Initiative," endorsed by the Human Proteome Organization (HUPO) and the International Society for Stem Cell Research (ISSCR) (Krijgsveld et al. 2008). This promising project intends to focus on the identification of new protein cell surface markers that may be used as fingerprints for stem cell lines or as benchmarks for specific steps of stem cell differentiation. To this aim, the project proposes to evaluate accurately the number and identity of cell lines that should be included in such an initiative, the growth media and culture conditions, the fractionation procedures and proteomics techniques that should be applied to this study, in an attempt to reduce to a minimum biological and methodological variability (Whetton et al. 2008).

Cancer Stem Cell Proteome

Over the past several years, the proteomic research applied to oncology has analyzed several fundamental intrinsic aspects of cancer cells, such as their genetic instability, which may determine the tumour differentiation grade (level of anaplasia), their tendency to metastasise, and their resistance to radio- or chemotherapy, with significant implications in terms of prognosis and therapy response. However, all these factors make it difficult not only for comparisons among specimens of the same cancer type from different individuals but also between neoplastic tissue and normal tissue from the same patient (Qumsiyeh and Li 2001). Moreover, the roles that microenvironmental factors (e.g. distance from a capillary, immune response and hypoxia) play in determining both the differentiation state and proliferation rate of tumour cells cannot be underestimated. All of these potential cancer cell variations contribute to the heterogeneity of tumour masses and can significantly alter the proteome profile. Thus, the protein expression profiles of different tissue regions within a tumour node can vary considerably (Scatena et al. 2008). In addition, the existence inside of cancer cell masses of CSCs, which are responsible for cancer recurrence and metastatic dissemination, need to be considered. To date, there have been a limited number of proteomic studies investigating CSCs. One of the most important obstacles to overcome in CSCs proteome analyses is the extremely small number of CSCs available to study. Notwithstanding, proteomic research is beginning to contribute to the knowledge of CSC behaviour by examining different aspects in order to clarify the mechanisms for regulation of self-renewal, differentiation and extensive proliferation. Research focused on the definition of specific cell surface markers is a key area in CSC proteomic analysis. In the above-mentioned study (Dormeyer et al. 2008a, b), the plasma membrane proteome of hESC line HUES-7, derived from the inner cell mass of blastocyst-stage embryos, and that of its malignant counterpart, hECC line NT2/D1, the undifferentiated SCs of teratocarcinomas, have been examined. A direct comparison of hESC and hECC cells revealed that, even though hESCs and hECCs dedicate similar proportions of proteins to their respective cellular functions and activities, they do not always employ the same proteins. For instance, several Hedgehog and Wnt pathway members, which play a crucial role in stem cell self-renewal and cancer growth, have been found to be differentially expressed between hESCs and hECCs. Consequently, different ligand-binding affinities, tissue distributions and signalling cascade activations were observed. The results from this study showed that FZD2, FZD6 and LRP6 were uniquely identified in hECCs, whereas FZD7 was only identified in hESCs. Moreover, among the differentially expressed Wnt modulator semaphorins, SEMA7A is found only in hECCs. Based on such experimental evidence, the authors proposed that the FZD2, FZD6, FZD7 and LRP6 receptors and the SEMA7A modulator might be interesting candidates for studies of the differential regulation of Wnt signalling in "benign" and "malignant" pluripotent cells. Overall, these results suggested that the proteins expressed exclusively in hECCs could be responsible for cancerogenesis or characteristics of malignant degeneration. However, it is evident that further findings are needed to clarify their potential roles in tumour formation. Additionally, various proteins encoded on chromosome 12p, including GAPDH, LDHB, YARS2, CLSTN3, CSDA, LRP6, NDUFA9 and NOL1, which have shown high expression levels in testicular cancer, were uniquely identified in hECCs. Distinct HLA molecules were also revealed on the surface of hESCs and hECCs, despite their low abundance. Specifically, the authors were able to identify HLA-A in both hESCs and hECCs, HLA-B uniquely in hECCs, and HLA-C uniquely in hESCs. The potential to investigate whether HLA molecules were present or not, or only weakly present, on the surface of hESC and hECC cells, might have an impact on the design of T cell-based immunotherapies. In fact, this knowledge could be useful to better clarify the regulation mechanisms that control both the immunological rejection of transplanted cells in regenerative medicine and the expression of components of antigen-processing machinery, which appear frequently downregulated during the immune-evasion of tumours (Seliger 2008). Another interesting comparative proteomic analysis of ESCs and ECCs, carried out by using 2DE and LC MS/MS, and iTRAQ method for quantitative analysis, permitted to identify changes in the expression levels of various proteins, including beta-galactoside-binding lectin, undifferentiated embryonic cell transcription factor-1, DNA cytosine methyltransferase 3beta isoform-B, melanoma antigen family-A4 and interferon-induced transmembrane protein-1 (Chaerkady et al. 2010). In addition, the authors observed in ECCs an overexpression of several proteins, such as heat shock 27 kDa protein-1, mitogen-activated protein kinase kinase-1, p53-induced protein, nuclear factor of κ-light polypeptide gene enhancer in B-cells inhibitor-like-2 and S100 calcium-binding protein-A4. These proteins have already been related to a malignant phenotype. Recently, a phosphoproteomic analysis to determine whether the STAT3/IL-6/HIF-1α signalling network plays a role in glioblastoma stem cell (GBM-SCs) survival and in GBM-SCs tumourigenic capacity was published (Nilsson et al. 2010). The interest in investigating possible perturbations of this loop in GBM-SCs comes from various experimental data demonstrating the involvement of STAT3, IL-6 and HIF-1α in regulating GBM-SC behaviour. In particular, STAT3 (signal transducer and activator of transcription 3) has been reported to control, by regulation of gene transcription, many cellular processes including proliferation, differentiation and apoptosis (Levy and Darnell 2002; Leslie et al. 2006). The constitutive activation of STAT3 has been observed in many human cancers, including breast, head and neck, prostate, melanoma and thyroid cancer (Bromberg 2002). Even though the precise function of STAT3 in glioblastoma stem cells has not been determined, increasing evidence demonstrates that its inhibition irreversibly abrogates neurosphere formation. This leads to a downregulation of genes associated with the NSC phenotype and the inhibition of cell proliferation (Sherry et al. 2009). Consistent with findings that provide evidence that STAT3 regulates multipotency in these cells and other studies that report the efficacy of using small molecule inhibitors for STAT3 phosphorylation in GBM cells in animal models (Heimberger and Priebe 2008), it has been suggested that STAT3 could be an effective target for the treatment of GBM. To thoroughly analyse these aspects, a quantitative phosphoproteomic approach to study GSC11 cell responses to STAT3 phosphorylation inhibition by WP1193 treatment and IL-6 stimulation under normoxic and hypoxic conditions generated a large proteomic data set. Alterations in the IL-6/STAT3/HIF-1α loop were revealed, and data about the effects of oxygen concentration, STAT3 phosphorylation inhibition and IL-6 stimulation on cell cultures were also produced.

An interesting approach to study tumour-initiating cells consists in isolating CSCs from tumour tissue and in propagating them using stem cell culture conditions. By isolation of CSCs on the basis of cell surface markers, differential profiles of CD133+ and CD133− cells isolated from the hepatocellular carcinoma cell line Huh-7 were analyzed (Ma et al. 2008). The results from this study indicate that aldehyde dehydrogenase (ALDH), when expressed along with CD133, can specifically characterize the liver CSC population. In addition, isoforms ALDH1A2 and ALDH3A1 seem to be preferentially expressed in the CD133+ subfractions. In another study, proteins differentially expressed between CD133+ cells and CD133− cells were isolated from the same Huh-7 cell line in an attempt to elucidate specifically activated signalling pathways and the molecular mechanism of CSCs (Lee et al. 2010b). Among the identified proteins, the 23-kDa actin-binding protein transgelin, which is a direct target of TGF-β signalling, was highly expressed in CD133+ cells compared to CD133− cells. Similarly, elevated levels of transgelin were also observed also in tumourigenic cells that originated from colorectal and prostate cancers. This overexpression seems to correlate with the increased invasive potential of CSCs. Notably, CXCR4, a receptor of stromal cell-derived factor-1, another well-known mediator of cell migration, was reported to be highly expressed in CD133+ cells. However, there was little to no expression of CXCR4 observed in CD133− cells.

In a more recent study (Fang et al. 2010), CSCs were isolated primarily by enrichment using the CD133 surface marker, followed by confirmation of their tumourigenicity in immunodeficient mice. In this study, a mass spectrometry-based proteomic approach was applied to identify cell surface-associated proteins expressed on colon tumour spheres. Interestingly, the colon CSCs isolated and propagated under serum-free stem cell culture conditions, retained the expression of well-known cell surface markers, including CD133, CD166, CD44 and EpCAM, as well as other stem cell-associated proteins such as NES, BMI-1 and MSI-1. In addition, novel cell surface markers associated with CD133+ colon CSCs were identified, including CEACAM5, biglycan and cadherin 17. The roles of these cell surface molecules were previously documented in various neoplastic processes, and their higher expression levels in tumour sphere culture compared with the epithelial component of the original tumour suggest a potential role as additional colon CSC markers and as new therapeutic targets. Besides indicating that neoplastic spheroid cells can be cultured maintaining all the phenotypic heterogeneity and characteristics of CSCs identified in freshly isolated tumours, this study provides an interesting in vitro tumour model for understanding the biological properties of CSC populations. It also effectively tests the anti-CSC activity of candidate drugs and, thus, enables the design of new therapeutic strategies.

To detect proteins that may be responsible for the self-propagating and tumourigenic properties of breast CSCs, the differential expression profiles between side population (SP) cells (measured by Hoechst 33342 dye efflux), which are known to be enriched in CSCs, and non-side population cells, which are depleted of CSCs, were examined (Steiniger et al. 2008). In analyzing two breast cancer cell lines, MCF7 and MDA-MB-231, the authors observed an upregulation of several important proteins involved in cell cycle control and differentiation in the CSC-containing side population. Notably, high levels of thymosin beta 4 (TB4), whose overexpression has been associated with increased invasiveness and metastasis, and whose role has been proven in promoting the tumourigenic properties of colorectal CSCs, were also reported (Ricci-Vitiani et al. 2010). In SP cells, the downregulation of pyruvate kinase M2 isoform and peroxiredoxin-6 were observed. Interestingly, PKM2 levels have been consistently reported to be altered in a variety of tumour types. Rapidly growing cancer cells have high PKM2 activity, which can be controlled by tyrosine kinase signalling pathways. This allows tumour cells to adapt to variations in environmental nutrient concentrations (Christofk et al. 2008). Regulation of PKM2 activity could be an interesting example of how growth signalling pathways can play a determinant role in influencing metabolic pathways in cells, by mediating long- and short-term changes in their cell metabolism, in general, and by controlling their glycolytic metabolism, in particular. Such data shows that CSC metabolism is notably different than cancer cell metabolism, as recently reviewed (Scatena et al. 2010). It is evident that the field of oncoproteomics, by also investigating the complexity of cancer cell metabolism, could considerably contribute to the definition of CSC bioenergetics, which could have important biological and clinical implications, not only in terms of therapy but also in terms of diagnosis and prognosis.

Typical "Stemness" Signalling Pathways

In addition to directly examining the CSCs proteome, oncoproteomic research has reported often altered expression levels of several proteins that are actually considered characteristic of stemness. It is well-known that self-renewal of human normal and malignant human stem cells involves a network of regulatory mechanisms including various signalling pathways, the presence of typical cell surface proteins, various drug resistance mechanisms, telomerase, oncogenes and oncosuppressors. In several proteomic studies were reported examples of dysregulation of pathways that are involved in self-renewal and differentiation and that are typically, but not specifically, involved in CSC biology. One important example is the Wnt/beta-catenin pathway, which plays a crucial role in directing embryonic formation. However, the pathway is also post-embryonically involved in regulating the proliferation and differentiation of a variety of stem cells and their regenerative responses during tissue repair. Aberrant activations of this pathway have been frequently observed in many diseases processes, including human cancers (Beachy et al. 2004).

To investigate alterations in cellular pathways, tumour profiling and marker discovery in colorectal cancer (CRC), an antibody microarray approach specific for cell signalling in soluble protein extracts from paired tumour/normal biopsies were used (Madoz-Gurpide et al. 2007). In addition to highlighting a series of potential markers preferentially expressed in CRC tumours, such as cytokeratin 13, calcineurin, CHK1, clathrin light chain, MAPK3, phospho-PTK2/focal adhesion kinase (Ser-910) and MDM2, many alterations in signalling pathways in CRC were observed. These included a significant upregulation of different components of the epidermal growth factor receptor and Wnt/beta-catenin pathway and the downregulation of p14(ARF). Mahmoudi et al. (2009) examined the complex series of biochemical events of the Wnt-pathway that lead to the stabilization of the key signalling molecule beta-catenin and, consequently, inappropriate activation of the TCF4/beta-catenin transcriptional programme and tumourigenesis in CRC cells. These authors identified Traf2- and Nck-interacting kinase (Tnik) as a novel protein interacting with Tcf4. This protein is a specific activator of the Wnt transcriptional programme and, thus, represents an attractive candidate for drug targeting in colorectal cancer. To understand the complex networks that exist between the signalling pathways related to the control of cell growth, a proteomic approach was carried out (Lee et al. 2007) in an attempt to investigate proteins interacting with the catalytic subunit of protein phosphatase 2A (PP2A). PP2A is a major cytoplasmic serine/threonine phosphatase and has a wide range of substrates that are involved in the regulation of several different signalling pathways such as the ERK and the Wnt/beta-catenin signalling pathways. Among the identified proteins are not only those previously known to interact with PP2A, such as Axin and CaMK IV, but also several new candidate proteins, such as tuberous sclerosis complex 2, RhoB, R-Ras and Nm23-H2. Further characterization of the roles of these proteins, which seem to be involved in multiple cellular processes, could help to elucidate the complex signalling crosstalk related to the control of cell growth. Considering the deregulated activity of such signalling pathways in many cancers, Wnt-pathway is an attractive target for anticancer therapies. Towards that goal, a iTRAQ quantitative chemical proteomic approach was used to search for novel modulators of the Wnt signalling pathway that would highlight the importance of axin as a key regulatory node in the Wnt signalling cascade (Huang et al. 2009). In particular, they identified a low molecular mass compound, XAV939, that can prolong the half-life of axin and promote the degradation of beta-catenin by inhibiting tankyrase (TNKS). This study represents an interesting proteomic investigation of the molecular mechanisms that controls axin protein homeostasis and Wnt pathway signalling and it could provide new avenues for targeted Wnt pathway therapies.

As demonstrated by studies on the Wnt-pathway, proteomic-based approaches have often been used to elucidate complex interaction mechanisms of different signal transduction pathways. In a recent paper, the proteomic analysis of surgical glioma samples was utilized to identify patterns of coordinate activation among glioma-relevant signal transduction pathways (Brennan et al. 2009). They compared their data with the genomic and expression data from glioblastoma (GBM) samples from The Cancer Genome Atlas (TCGA). Their results showed a predominance of EGFR activation, PDGFR activation or loss of the RAS regulator NF1 in the GBM samples. The EGFR signalling class shows prominent Notch pathway activation, which has been observed in various types of tumours and correlated with several aggressive forms of cancers. A critical role for the Notch pathway in the maintenance of brain tumour stem cells has recently emerged (Wang et al. 2009). Experimental evidence has shown that radiation induces Notch activation, and Notch inhibition by gamma-secretase inhibitors (GSIs) or Notch1/2-specific shRNA renders glioma stem cells more sensitive to radiation at clinically relevant doses. This radioprotective role for Notch has been shown to involve the regulation of the PI3K/Akt pathway and Mcl-1, a molecule that directly regulates the apoptosis signalling cascade (Wang et al. 2010).

From a therapeutic point of view, the problem of radioresistance in anticancer therapy is well-known. Tumour cells often seem to respond to radiotherapy and then cause recurrences, suggesting insufficient killing of tumorigenic cells. Within the last few decades, experimental and clinical findings have provided evidence that CSCs are more resistant to current chemotherapies than non-stem cells and that a higher number of CSCs correlates with higher radioresistance (Baumann et al. 2008). From an oncoproteomic point of view, it is reasonable to expect that drug radioresistance reveals a global changes in expression levels of proteins involved in various intracellular pathways. Notably, Zhou et al. (2008) compared differences in the proteomes of a tumour necrosis factor (TNF)-alpha resistant MCF-7 breast cancer cell line, MCF-7-MEK5 (in which TNF-alpha resistance is mediated by MEK5/Erk5 signalling) and its parental TNF-alpha-sensitive MCF-7 cell line, MCF-7-VEC, to study the mechanisms that underlie resistance to the chemotherapy-sensitizing TNF-alpha. This study demonstrated that MEK5 overexpression promotes a TNF-alpha resistance phenotype associated with distinct proteomic changes, such as the upregulation of vimentin, glutathione-S-transferase P and creatine kinase B-type, and the downregulation of keratin 8, keratin 19 and glutathione-S-transferase Mu 3 in MCF-7-MEK5, as compared to MCF-7-VEC cells. Another recent study examined differences in the proteome profiles of parental and radiation-resistant prostate carcinoma cell lines (IRR cells), which were derived from the parental after repetitive exposure to ionizing radiation (Skvortsova et al. 2008). The identified proteins, which were regulated in the radioresistant prostate carcinoma cells, are involved in the regulation of intracellular routes that control cell survival, growth, proliferation, invasion, motility and DNA repair. These data suggest that the development of radioresistance is accompanied by multiple mechanisms, including activation of cell receptors and related downstream signal transduction pathways such as Ras/MAPK and PI3K/Akt and Jak/STAT. However, the molecular mechanisms by which cancer cells overcome the cytotoxic effects of radiation therapy and the precise roles of the proteins that contribute to the development of a more aggressive phenotype and various drug resistance mechanisms, such as ATP-binding cassette transporters, remain to be clarified. Other alterations in protein expression levels associated with anticancer drug-resistances were investigated in a squamous cell lung carcinoma (Keenan et al. 2009). The authors reported a list of 24 proteins, several of which showed correlations with drug resistance, including NDPK, RPA2, CCT2, HSP70, Annexin A1, HNRPK, H1, aldehyde dehydrogenase (ALDH), stomatin and CCT3.

Proteins related to chemoresistance were also identified in the ovarian cancer cell line SKOV3 (Lee et al. 2010a). These authors performed comparative analyses of whole proteomes between paclitaxel-resistant SKpac sublines and paclitaxel-sensitive parental SKOV3 cells. Of the identified proteins, high levels of ALDH1A1 and Annexin A1 were related with chemoresistant ovarian cancer cells, whereas the downregulation of hnRNP A2 and GDI 2 was the most significant finding in the SKpac cells and chemoresistant ovarian cancer tissues. Another recently published paper (Dai et al. 2010) examined the same ovarian cancer cell line SKOV3 but focused on comparative analyses of 2-D DIGE maps of mitochondrial proteins from platinum-resistant cell lines and their corresponding parental cell lines. Among the 236 differentially expressed spots, five mitochondrial proteins including ATP-α, PRDX3, PHB, ETF and ALDH which participate in the electron transport respiratory chain, were reported to be downregulated in drug-resistant cells.

Other important signalling pathways that control stem cell self-renewal, including polycomb ring finger oncogene BMI-1, and phosphatase and tensin homolog (PTEN), have already been object of various oncoproteomic studies. BMI-1, a member of the polycomb gene family, is a transcription repressor that regulates p16 and p19, which are cell cycle inhibitor genes. Significant BMI-1 overexpression in carcinogenesis has been shown in many types of cancer. Wiederschain et al. (2007) performed a proteomic and gene expression analysis in human medulloblastoma DAOY cells. They identified a number of cancer-relevant pathways that might be controlled by Bmi-1 and Mel-18 and also showed that these Polycomb proteins regulate a set of common gene targets.

PTEN controls stem cell growth by inhibiting proliferation and survival via the phosphatidylinositol-3-OH kinase (PI(3)K) signalling pathway. PTEN deletions or inactivating mutations have been identified in diverse cancers. A multiplex tissue immunoblotting method that allows for the simultaneous quantification of multiplex markers was used to show that quantitative analysis of PTEN expression could provide survival information (Chung et al. 2009). These authors also illustrated the capacity of PTEN/phosphorylated (p)-AKT and PTEN/p-mTOR to stratify patients better than PTEN alone by a univariate analysis. As expected, decreased PTEN expression was observed in patients with increasing depths of invasion, whereas expressions of p-AKT and p-mTOR were significantly increased in extrahepatic cholangiocarcinoma. To search for PTEN-interacting proteins that might be crucial in the regulation of PTEN, a proteomic-based approach was performed (Ahn et al. 2008b). Analyzing PTEN-expressing NIH 3T3 cell lysates, the authors identified an E3 ubiquitin-protein ligase Nedd4 (neural precursor cell-expressed, developmentally down-regulated gene 4) whose levels were down-regulated by PTEN. Nedd4 expression was also reported to decrease with a PI3K (phosphoinositide 3-kinase) inhibitor treatment, LY294002. This result suggested that the regulation is dependent on the phosphatase/kinase activity of the PTEN-PI3K/Akt pathway. Other lines of experimental evidence support an important function for PTEN during oncogenesis and chemoresistance, which demonstrates that loss of PTEN renders different breast cancer cells significantly sensitive to growth inhibition by the PI3K inhibitor LY294002 (Stemke-Hale et al. 2008). From a therapeutic point of view, knowledge of the molecular mechanisms that are the basis of the pharmacological action of these molecules is essential. It is also important that the combination of classical chemotherapy treatments with LY294002 was reported to lead to the effective chemosensitisation in most cell lines tested. Thus, the cells were protected from the cytotoxicity induced by high concentrations of chemotherapy.

Clinical studies have reported a link between the expression levels of a family of integral membrane proteins, the tetraspanins, and tumour progression and metastasis in many cancers. On this basis, a proteomic approach aimed to examine the role of the tetraspanins in organizing multi-molecular complexes with other membrane proteins was developed (Le Naour et al. 2006). These molecules possess numerous properties that implicate their involvement in a large variety of physiological processes such as cell adhesion, cell migration, immune cell activation, cell proliferation and differentiation. However, they are also involved in pathological conditions such as viral infection and metastasis (Hemler 2005). In this study, tetraspanin complexes were isolated from human colon cancer consisting of three cell lines derived from a primary tumour and two metastases (hepatic and peritoneal). The proteomic analysis permitted the identification of a molecular network of interactions that involved several categories of proteins including adhesion molecules and molecules with Ig domains (integrins $\alpha3\beta1$, $\alpha6\beta1$, $\alpha6\beta4$, CD44 and EpCAM), membrane proteases (ADAM10, TADG-15 and CD26), and signalling molecules (heterotrimeric G-protein subunits) as well as a protein involved in membrane fusion, (syntaxin-3). A comparative analysis of the three cell lines showed that some proteins were identified in all cells, whereas others were differentially detected. The laminin receptor Lutheran/B-cell adhesion molecule (Lu/B-CAM) was expressed only on the primary tumour cells, whereas CD26/dipeptidyl peptidase IV and tetraspanin Co-029 were observed only in metastatic cells. The presence of several transmembrane proteases in the tetraspanin web shed new light on the role of tetraspanin complexes in regulating proteolytic activities at the cell surface. As well-known, all the extracellular proteolytic processes such as the degradation of extracellular matrix components, the regulation of chemokine activity, and the release of membrane-anchored growth factors, receptors and adhesion molecules strongly influence cell growth and motility.

Conclusion

From a pathophysiological point of view, the possibility to apply proteomic technologies employing mass spectrometry and protein chip platforms to find more specific markers or combinatorial markers which may differentiate CSCs from normal cancer cells could have significant and rapid clinical applications in prognosis, diagnosis, and therapy of various types of cancer. However, at present, despite increasing attention proteomic research turns to the standardization of operation procedures for sample processing and data manipulations, also in CSCs analysis, it remains quite difficult to draw consistent conclusions from individual studies. Notwithstanding this, if supported by experimental protocols well designed and correctly interpreted, proteomic research may very well contribute not only to the understanding of the CSC pathophysiology, by the identification of a typical protein expression profile of CSC surface markers, but also to supporting new therapeutic approaches for the treatment of cancer by providing novel targets for overcoming drug resistance of which CSCs seem to be chiefly responsible.

References

Ahn SM, Goode RJ, Simpson RJ (2008a) Stem cell markers: insights from membrane proteomics? Proteomics. 8:4946–57.
Ahn Y, Hwang CY, Lee SR et al (2008b) The tumour suppressor PTEN mediates a negative regulation of the E3 ubiquitin-protein ligase Nedd4. Biochem J. 412:331–8.
Al-Hajj M, Wicha MS, Benito-Hernandez A et al (2003) Prospective identification of tumorigenic breast cancer cells. Proc Natl Acad Sci USA 100:3983–8.
Baharvand H, Fathi A, van Hoof D, Salekdeh GH (2007) Concise review: trends in stem cell proteomics. Stem Cells 25:1888–903.
Baharvand H, Hajheidari M, Ashtiani SK, Salekdeh GH (2006) Proteomic signature of human embryonic stem cells. Proteomics 6:3544–9.
Baumann M, Krause M, Hill R (2008) Exploring the role of cancer stem cells in radioresistance. Nat Rev Cancer 8:545–54.
Beachy PA, Karhadkar SS, Berman DM (2004) Tissue repair and stem cell renewal in carcinogenesis. Nature 432:324–31.
Bendall SC, Hughes C, Campbell JL et al (2009) An enhanced mass spectrometry approach reveals human embryonic stem cell growth factors in culture. Mol Cell Proteomics 8:421–32.
Bendall SC, Stewart MH, Menendez P et al (2007) IGF and FGF cooperatively establish the regulatory stem cell niche of pluripotent human cells in vitro. Nature 448:1015–21.
Bonnet D and Dick JE (1997) Human acute myeloid leukemia is organized as a hierarchy that originates from a primitive hematopoietic cell. Nat Med. 3:730–7.
Brennan C, Momota H, Hambardzumyan D et al (2009) Glioblastoma subclasses can be defined by activity among signal transduction pathways and associated genomic alterations. PLoS One 4:e7752.
Brimble SN, Zeng X, Weiler DA, et al (2004) Karyotypic stability, genotyping, differentiation, feeder-free maintenance, and gene expression sampling in three human embryonic stem cell lines derived prior to August 9, 2001. Stem Cells Dev. 13:585–97.
Bromberg J (2002) Stat proteins and oncogenesis. J Clin Invest 109:1139–1142.
Chaerkady R, Kerr CL, Kandasamy K et al (2010) Comparative proteomics of human embryonic stem cells and embryonal carcinoma cells. Proteomics 10:1359–73.
Chaerkady R, Kerr CL, Marimuthu A et al (2009) Temporal analysis of neural differentiation using quantitative proteomics. J Proteome Res. 8:1315–26.
Christofk HR, Vander Heiden MG, Wu N et al (2008) Pyruvate kinase M2 is a phosphotyrosine binding protein. Nature 452:181–186.
Chung JY, Hong SM, Choi BY et al (2009) The expression of phospho-AKT, phospho-mTOR, and PTEN in extrahepatic cholangiocarcinoma. Clin Cancer Res. 15:660–7.
Collier TS, Sarkar P, Rao B, Muddiman DC (2010) Quantitative top-down proteomics of SILAC labeled human embryonic stem cells. J Am Soc Mass Spectrom. 21:879–89.
Dai Z, Yin J, He H et al (2010) Mitochondrial comparative proteomics of human ovarian cancer cells and their platinum-resistant sublines. Proteomics 10:3789–99.
Dalerba P, Dylla SJ, Park IK, et al (2007) Phenotypic characterization of human colorectal cancer stem cells. Proc Natl Acad Sci USA 104:10158–63.
Dormeyer W, van Hoof D, Braam SR et al (2008a) Plasma membrane proteomics of human embryonic stem cells and human embryonal carcinoma cells. J Proteome Res. 7:2936–51.

Dormeyer W, van Hoof D, Mummery CL et al (2008b) A practical guide for the identification of membrane and plasma membrane proteins in human embryonic stem cells and human embryonal carcinoma cells. Proteomics 8:4036–53.

Fang DD, Kim YJ, Lee CN et al. (2010) Expansion of CD133(+) colon cancer cultures retaining stem cell properties to enable cancer stem cell target discovery. Br J Cancer 102:1265–75.

Fathi A, Pakzad M, Taei A et al (2009) Comparative proteome and transcriptome analyses of embryonic stem cells during embryoid body-based differentiation. Proteomics 9:4859–70.

Foss EJ, Radulovic D, Shaffer SA et al (2007) Genetic basis of proteome variation in yeast. Nat Genet. 39:1369–75.

Foster LJ, Zeemann PA, Li C et al (2005) Differential expression profiling of membrane proteins by quantitative proteomics in a human mesenchymal stem cell line undergoing osteoblast differentiation. Stem Cells 23:1367–77.

Harkness L, Christiansen H, Nehlin J et al (2008) Identification of a membrane proteomic signature for human embryonic stem cells independent of culture conditions. Stem Cell Res 1:219–27.

Heimberger AB, Priebe W (2008) Small molecular inhibitors of p-STAT3: novel agents for treatment of primary and metastatic CNS cancers. Recent Pat CNS Drug Discov. 3:179–88.

Hemler ME (2005) Tetraspanin functions and associated microdomains. Nat Rev Mol Cell Biol 10:801–811.

Hoffrogge R, Mikkat S, Scharf C et al (2006) 2-DE proteome analysis of a proliferating and differentiating human neuronal stem cell line (ReNcell VM). Proteomics 6:1833–47.

Huang SM, Mishina YM, Liu S et al (2009) Tankyrase inhibition stabilizes axin and antagonizes Wnt signalling. Nature 461:614–20.

Keenan J, Murphy L, Henry M et al (2009) Proteomic analysis of multidrug-resistance mechanisms in adriamycin-resistant variants of DLKP, a squamous lung cancer cell line. Proteomics 9:1556–66.

Krijgsveld J, Whetton AD, Lee B et al (2008) Proteome biology of stem cells: a new joint HUPO and ISSCR initiative. Mol Cell Proteomics 7:204–5.

Le Naour F, André M, Greco C et al (2006) Profiling of the tetraspanin web of human colon cancer cells. Mol Cell Proteomics 5:845–57.

Lee DH, Chung K, Song JA et al (2010a) Proteomic identification of paclitaxel-resistance associated hnRNP A2 and GDI 2 proteins in human ovarian cancer cells. J Proteome Res. 9:5668–76.

Lee EK, Han GY, Park HW et al (2010b) Transgelin promotes migration and invasion of cancer stem cells. J Proteome Res. 9:5108–17.

Lee WJ, Kim DU, Lee MY, Choi KY (2007) Identification of proteins interacting with the catalytic subunit of PP2A by proteomics. Proteomics 7:206–14.

Lerou PH and Daley GQ (2005) Therapeutic potential of embryonic stem cells. Blood Rev. 19:321–31.

Leslie K, Lang C, Devgan G et al (2006) Cyclin D1 is transcriptionally regulated by and required for transformation by activated signal transducer and activator of transcription 3. Cancer Res 66:2544–2552.

Levy DE, Darnell JE Jr. (2002) Stats: Transcriptional control and biological impact. Nat Rev Mol Cell Biol 3:651–662.

Li C, Heidt DG, Dalerba P et al (2007) Identification of pancreatic cancer stem cells. Cancer Res 67:1030–7.

Lim JW and Bodnar A (2002) Proteome analysis of conditioned medium from mouse embryonic fibroblast feeder layers which support the growth of human embryonic stem cells. Proteomics 2: 1187–203.

Lottaz C, Beier D, Meyer K et al (2010) Transcriptional profiles of CD133+ and CD133- glioblastoma-derived cancer stem cell lines suggest different cells of origin. Cancer Res. 70:2030–40.

Ma S, Chan KW, Lee TK et al (2008) Aldehyde dehydrogenase discriminates the CD133 liver cancer stem cell populations. Mol Cancer Res. 6:1146–53.

Madoz-Gurpide J, Canamero M, Sanchez L et al (2007) A proteomics analysis of cell signaling alterations in colorectal cancer. Mol Cell Proteomics 6:2150–64.

Mahmoudi T, Li VS, Ng SS et al (2009) The kinase TNIK is an essential activator of Wnt target genes. EMBO J. 28:3329–40.

Nagano K, Taoka M, Yamauchi Y et al (2005) Large-scale identification of proteins expressed in mouse embryonic stem cells. Proteomics 5:1346–61.

Nilsson CL, Dillon R, Devakumar A et al (2010) Quantitative phosphoproteomic analysis of the STAT3/IL-6/HIF1alpha signalling network: an initial study in GSC11 glioblastoma stem cells. J Proteome Res. 9:430–43.

O'Brien CA, Pollett A, Gallinger S, Dick JE (2007) A human colon cancer cell capable of initiating tumour growth in immunodeficient mice. Nature 445:106–10.

Patrawala L, Calhoun T, Schneider-Broussard R et al (2006) Highly purified CD44+ prostate cancer cells from xenograft human tumors are enriched in tumorigenic and metastatic progenitor cells. Oncogene 25:1696–708.

Prokhorova TA, Rigbolt KT, Johansen PT et al (2009) Stable isotope labeling by amino acids in cell culture (SILAC) and quantitative comparison of the membrane proteomes of self-renewing and differentiating human embryonic stem cells. Mol Cell Proteomics 8:959–70.

Prowse AB, McQuade LR, Bryant KJ et al (2007) Identification of potential pluripotency determinants for human embryonic stem cells following proteomic analysis of human and mouse fibroblast conditioned media. J Proteome Res. 6:3796–807.

Qumsiyeh MB, Li P (2001) Molecular biology of cancer: Cytogenetics. In: De Vita VT, Hellmann S, Rosenberg SA (eds) Cancer: Principles and Practice of Oncology, 6th edn. JB Lippincott Company, Philadelphia, pp. 77–90.

Ricci-Vitiani L, Collinari C, di Martino S et al (2010) Thymosin {beta}4 targeting impairs tumorigenic activity of colon cancer stem cells. FASEB J 24:4291–301.

Scatena R, Bottoni P, Giardina B (2008) Modulation of cancer cell line differentiation: a neglected proteomic analysis with potential implications in pathophysiology, diagnosis, prognosis, and therapy of cancer. Proteomics Clin. Appl. 2:229–237.

Scatena R, Bottoni P, Pontoglio A, Giardina B (2010) Revisiting the Warburg effect in cancer cells with proteomics. The emergence of new approaches to diagnosis, prognosis and therapy. Proteomics Clin Appl 4:143–158.

Seliger B (2008) Molecular mechanisms of MHC class I abnormalities and APM components in human tumors. Cancer Immunol Immunother. 57:1719–26.

Sherry MM, Reeves A, Wu JK, Cochran BH (2009) STAT3 is required for proliferation and maintenance of multipotency in glioblastoma stem cells. Stem Cells 27:2383–92.

Singh SK, Hawkins C, Clarke ID, et al (2004) Identification of human brain tumour initiating cells. Nature 432:396–401.

Skvortsova I, Skvortsov S, Stasyk T et al (2008) Intracellular signaling pathways regulating radioresistance of human prostate carcinoma cells. Proteomics 8:4521–33.

Sperger JM, Chen X, Draper JS et al (2003) Gene expression patterns in human embryonic stem cells and human pluripotent germ cell tumors. Proc Natl Acad Sci USA 100:13350–55.

Spooncer E, Brouard N, Nilsson SK, et al (2008) Developmental fate determination and marker discovery in hematopoietic stem cell biology using proteomic fingerprinting. Mol Cell Proteomics 7:573–81.

Steiniger SC, Coppinger JA, Krüger JA et al (2008) Quantitative mass spectrometry identifies drug targets in cancer stem cell-containing side population. Stem Cells 26:3037–46.

Stemke-Hale K, Gonzalez-Angulo AM, Lluch A et al (2008) An integrative genomic and proteomic analysis of PIK3CA, PTEN, and AKT mutations in breast cancer. Cancer Res. 68:6084–91.

Unlu M, Morgan ME, Minden JS (1997) Difference gel electrophoresis: A single gel method for detecting changes in protein extracts. Electrophoresis 18:2071–2077.

Unwin RD, Smith DL, Blinco D et al (2006) Quantitative proteomics reveals posttranslational control as a regulatory factor in primary hematopoietic stem cells. Blood. 107:4687–94.

Van Hoof D, Dormeyer W, Braam SR et al (2010) Identification of cell surface proteins for antibody-based selection of human embryonic stem cell-derived cardiomyocytes. J Proteome Res. 9:1610–8.

Van Hoof D, Passier R, Ward-Van Oostwaard D et al (2006) A quest for human and mouse embryonic stem cell-specific proteins. Mol Cell Proteomics. 5:1261–73.

Wang J, Wakeman TP, Lathia JD et al (2010) Notch promotes radioresistance of glioma stem cells. Stem Cells 28:17–28.

Wang Z, Li Y, Banerjee S et al. Emerging role of Notch in stem cells and cancer. Cancer Lett 2009, 279:8–12.

Whetton AD, Williamson AJ, Krijgsveld J et al (2008) The time is right: proteome biology of stem cells. Cell Stem Cell. 2:215–7.

Wiederschain D, Chen L, Johnson B et al (2007) Contribution of polycomb homologues Bmi-1 and Mel-18 to medulloblastoma pathogenesis. Mol Cell Biol. 27:4968–79.

Yang ZF, Ngai P, Ho DW, et al (2008) Identification of local and circulating cancer stem cells in human liver cancer. Hepatology 47:919–28.

Zhou C, Nitschke AM, Xiong W et al (2008) Proteomic analysis of tumor necrosis factor-alpha resistant human breast cancer cells reveals a MEK5/Erk5-mediated epithelial-mesenchymal transition phenotype. Breast Cancer Res. 10:R105.

Chapter 15
Cancer Stem Cells: An Innovative Therapeutic Approach

Roberto Scatena, Patrizia Bottoni, Alessandro Pontoglio, Salvatore Scarà, and Bruno Giardina

Background

Cancer stem cells (CSCs) are a peculiar subpopulation of cancer cells that play an important role in the pathophysiology of cancer with dramatic clinical implications in terms of prognosis and therapy (Wang and Dick 2008; Zhou et al. 2009).

From a pharmacological point of view, these cells show intriguing structural and functional aspects that may represent new and interesting targets that could dramatically influence cancer therapy (Tang et al. 2007; Mittal et al. 2009). This consideration justifies the strong interest in pharmacological research regarding this particular subpopulation of cancer cells. More than 30 companies are using CSC research in drug discovery activities, including drug pipelines (preclinical to phase III). Moreover, interesting diagnostic approaches are being developed for the detection of CSCs. A growing number of academic research teams from different countries have shifted their research toward different aspects of the pathophysiology of CSCs. Several patents referring to CSCs have been presented.

This burst of pharmacological research is directed toward different potential targets of CSC pathophysiology, such as the following:

(a) Cell surface proteins [CD133, CD44/CD24, IL-3, EpCAM and C-X-C chemokine receptor type 4 (CXCR-4), which is also known as fusion or CD184].
(b) Peculiar signaling pathways generally related to self-renewal mechanisms (e.g., Hedgehog, Notch, and Wnt).
(c) Structural and/or functional components of the stem cell niche.
(d) Various detoxifying mechanisms [ABC transporters, aldehyde dehydrogenase (ALDH)].
(e) Telomerase and pathways related to cellular senescence.

R. Scatena (✉) • P. Bottoni • A. Pontoglio • S. Scarà • B. Giardina
Department of Laboratory Medicine, Catholic University,
Largo A. Gemelli 8, 00168 Rome, Italy
e-mail: r.scatena@rm.unicatt.it

(f) Oncogenes and oncosuppressors (p16INK4 – Rb).
(g) Cell differentiation-inducing pathways.
(h) Various microRNAs.

Some clinical studies have been published with interesting and intriguing results. This burst of pharmacological research into CSCs is significantly expanding our understanding of the pathophysiology of the disease, emphasizing concepts and molecular mechanisms that have been partially neglected, facilitating the understanding of a global vision of complex cancer cell biology and leading to significant progress in cancer therapy. A more accurate definition of the molecular mechanisms underlying cancer stem cells could represent a fundamental preventive measure to reduce the potential incidence of neoplastic transformation of transplanted normal stem cells.

CSC Inhibitors and Potential Targets

To selectively kill this particular subpopulation of cancer-maintaining cells that may be responsible for disease recurrence and metastatic dissemination, researchers have adopted different strategies to identify drug molecules that selectively target CSCs. Many of these molecules have been shown to kill the bulk of cancer cells without a particular selectivity for CSCs/tumor-initiating cells. For example, different tyrosine kinase inhibitors, free or conjugated with targeting monoclonal antibodies, have been tested (Zhou et al. 2009; Levitzki 2002). To outline the status of this particular anticancer therapeutic approach, we will emphasize only the pharmacological research that is specifically designed to target CSCs/tumor-initiating cells and is in preclinical or clinical phase trials (Table 15.1).

Potential CSC Surface Markers

The discovery of CSCs was originated in acute myeloid leukemia (AML). This discovery was possible because of the detailed characterization and isolation of specific hematopoietic cell surface antigens by flow cytometry (Bonnet and Dick 1997). Following their isolation, the characteristic stem cell-like properties and carcinogenicity of these cells was identified in the now classic xenotransplantation assay using severe combined immune-deficient (SCID) or nonobese diabetic (NOD)/SCID mice as recipients. This approach assessed the ability of leukemic cells to initiate disease in vivo (Dick 2008; Gupta et al. 2009a, b; Shackleton et al. 2009). Interestingly, these cells, $CD34^+CD38^-$, represented less than 1% of the total blast population. It quickly became evident that these markers were also present in normal hematopoietic stem cells, making it important to highlight markers or some pattern of markers to selectively identify and target these tumor stem cells (Blair et al. 1997).

Table 15.1 CSC inhibitors in preclinical or clinical phase trials

Cell surface markers	mAb anti-CD123	7G3
	mAb anti-CD44	A3D8
		H90
		mAb p245
	Gemtuzumab ozogamicin	mAb to CD33 +N-acetyl-calicheamicin 1,2-dimethyl hydrazine dichloride
	Bivatuzumab mertansine	Anti-CD44v6 +DM1 (mertansine)
	EpCAM	MT110 (EpCAM/CD3-bispecific BiTE antibody)
		MT201 (Adecatumumab)
Typical CSC signaling pathways	TKIs	Lapatinib
		Dasatinib
		Imatinib
	Wnt signaling pathway	Small-molecule inhibitors
		Drugs	NSAIDs	NO-ASA
				Celecoxib
		Natural Compounds	Vitamin A	Dab2 inhibitor
			Vitamin D	Dkk-1 and Dkk-4 inhibitor
			Polyphenols	Resveratrol, quercetin, curcumin
				Epigallocatechin-3-gallate
		Molecular-targeted agents	Beta-catenin/TCF-antagonists (ICG-001)
			Transcriptional co-activator modulators
			PDZ domain of Dv1 binders (NSC668036)
			Other mechanism-based inhibitors

(continued)

Table 15.1 (continued)

	Biologic inhibitors	
		mAbs against WNT1 and WNT2
		Small interfering RNA (siRNA)
		Therapeutic proteins (WIF1, SFRPs)
Hedgehog signaling pathway	Vismodegib (GDC-0449)	
	IPI-926	
	LDE225	
	BMS-863923/ XL139	
Notch signaling pathway	γ-secretase inhibitors	MK-0752
		RO4929097
		PF-03084014
	mAb	Anti-DLL4 (OMP-21M18)
	MALM protein Tr4	
PI3Ks signaling pathway	CAL-101	
	XL-147	
	BGT-226	
	BEZ-235	
	mAb Trastuzumab	

Telomerase inhibitors	Imetelstat
CSC Niche-targeted drugs	Cediranib (VEGFRs inhibitor) Sunitinib (VEGFRs and PDGF-Rs inhibitors)
Drug transporter inhibitors	Dofequidar fumarate (ABCB1/P-gp, ABCC1/MDR inhibitor) Vandetanib (ABCC1- and ABCG2 inhibitor) Salinomycin (MDR gp170 inhibitor)
Differentiation therapy	ATRA Histone deacetylase inhibitors (HDIs): SAHA/Vorinostat PPAR-alpha and -gamma ligands

Some early studies showed that the interleukin-3 receptor alpha chain (CD123) was able to distinguish leukemic stem cells (LSCs) from normal (hematopoietic stem cells) HSCs (Jordan et al. 2000; Jin et al. 2009). From these original observations, a series of molecules were developed and are under evaluation in an attempt to selectively target these cancer-initiating/-maintaining cells. For example, the anti-interleukin-3 (IL-3) receptor alpha chain (CD123)-neutralizing antibody (7G3) was targeted against AML stem cells. This molecule seems to impair the homing of these cells to bone marrow and to activate the innate immunity of tumor-transplanted NOD/SCID mice. Specifically, 7G3 inhibited the IL-3-mediated intracellular signaling in isolated AML CD34(+)CD38(−) cells in vitro and reduced their survival (Jin et al. 2009).

Another important marker of CSCs is CD44. This cell surface glycoprotein, characterized by multiple isoforms, is a receptor for hyaluronic acid, osteopontin, collagens, and matrix metalloproteinases (MMPs). CD44 primarily acts as an adhesion molecule involved in signaling, migration and homing. Interestingly, a sialofucosylated isoform of CD44, called HCELL, is found on human hematopoietic stem cells, where it functions as a "bone-homing receptor." Other biological activities have been described, including lymphocyte activation, recirculation and homing, hematopoiesis and tumor metastasis (Zhou et al. 2009; O'Sullivan and Thomas 2004). Some studies have been published regarding the potential therapeutic activity of this receptor. By utilizing two activating monoclonal antibodies (mAbs) anti-CD44, named A3D8 and H90, the terminal differentiation of leukemic blasts in AML-M1/2 can be induced to AML-M5 subtypes, which are the most frequent clinical types (Charrad et al. 2002). Moreover, the same authors showed that these mAbs can induce terminal differentiation and a loss of proliferative capacity in THP-1, NB4 and HL60 cells, which are well-known models of AML-M5 (monoblastic subtype), AML-M3 (promyelocytic subtype) and AML-M2 (myeloblastic subtype), respectively (Charrad et al. 2002; Gadhoum et al. 2004).

Recently, an activating mAb directed to the adhesion molecule CD44 in NOD/SCID mice transplanted with human AML markedly reduced the leukemic repopulation. The mechanisms underlying this eradication seem to include interference with transport to the stem cell-supportive microenvironmental niches and an alteration of the AML-LSC fate. Importantly, the results seem to stress the role of CD44 as a key regulator of leukemic stem cell functions in general and their interaction with niches in particular (Jin et al. 2006). CD44 has been confirmed as a positive marker of tumor-initiating cells in different types of tumors, including breast cancers (Al-Hajj et al. 2003). Interestingly, in vivo CD44 targeting by small interfering RNA (siRNA) and by specific antibodies results in antitumor activity in xenografts of colon cancer and human acute leukemia, respectively (Jin et al. 2006; Subramaniam et al. 2007). Recently, Marangoni et al. (2009) showed that targeting CD44 with the mAb p245 in an experimental model of human breast cancer xenografts may significantly inhibit tumor growth and postchemotherapy tumor recurrence in both estrogen receptor positive (ER+) and basal-like breast cancer. In addition, their results showed that the effect of the p245 mAb was associated with the induction of cytokines known to have antiproliferative activity.

Recently, two communications presented at the American Association of Cancer Research (AACR) 101st Annual Meeting in Washington, DC (2010) demonstrated the ability of the technology that uses the biochemical properties of hyaluronic acid (HA) to enhance the delivery and retention of chemotherapeutic drugs and biologics at the site of the tumor. Specifically, the HyACT doxorubicin formulation (HA-doxorubicin) has been shown to be up to 40 times more potent than doxorubicin alone at killing putative breast cancer stem cells (Entimov and Brown 2010a). Similarly, in human colorectal cancer cells, HyACT formulations of the drug irinotecan (HA-irinotecan) showed up to a 50-fold increase in potency against stem cell-like populations (Entimov and Brown 2010b).

Other companies also adopted the CSC surface markers as a guide for targeting different cytotoxic drugs to cancer cells in general and/or tumor-initiating cells in particular. One drug that has been utilized to selectively target CSCs is gemtuzumab ozogamicin. This drug is an mAb to CD33 and has been linked to the cytotoxic agent N-acetyl-calicheamicin 1,2-dimethyl hydrazine dichloride, which is a potent enediyne antitumour antibiotic from the class of calicheamicins. This drug is classically indicated to treat AML. In fact, the CD33 molecule is expressed by approximately 90% of AMLs but not by CD34(+) bone marrow-resident hematopoietic stem cells. In this conjugate, the antibody binds to and is internalized by tumor cells expressing the CD33 antigen (a sialic acid-dependent glycoprotein commonly found on the surface of leukemic blasts), thereby delivering the attached calicheamicin to CD33-expressing tumor cells. This molecule is a potent intercalating agent and is only released in an intracellular environment (lower pH) (Bross et al. 2001).

Gemtuzumab is not free from toxic effects such as shivering, fever, nausea, and vomiting. This drug has also been linked to severe myelosuppression (by suppressing the activity of bone marrow), respiratory system disorders, tumor lysis syndrome and type III hypersensitivity with an increased risk of veno-occlusive disease in the absence of bone marrow transplantation. Intriguingly, the onset of thrombosis can also be delayed and can occur with an increased frequency following bone marrow transplantation (Clarke and Marks 2010). In June 2010, gemtuzumab ozogamicin was withdrawn from the market at the request of the Food and Drug Administration (US) because a postapproval clinical trial raised new questions about the drug's safety and effectiveness. The trial showed that adding this drug to existing chemotherapy for the treatment of AML provided no benefit and even showed a higher death rate (Halsen and Krämer 2010).

The development of bivatuzumab mertansine, a drug analogous to gemtuzumab, consists of the anti-CD44v6 antibody linked to the DM1 cytotoxic agent mertansine and was discontinued due to the occurrence of skin toxicity in phase I clinical trials in patients with advanced carcinomas (Koppe et al. 2004). CD44v6 is expressed in various carcinomas, including squamous cell carcinomas and some adenocarcinomas. However, some data indicate that the CD44v6 antigen is also expressed on normal proliferating epidermal cells (Rupp et al. 2007).

The epithelial cell adhesion molecule (EpCAM) is a protein that is encoded by the EPCAM gene in humans. EpCAM has also been designated as tumor-associated calcium signal transducer 1 (TACSTD1) and CD326. This particular glycosylated adhesion molecule (30–40 kDa) is a pan-epithelial differentiation antigen that is expressed in a variety of human epithelial tissues, cancers, and stem cells. EpCAM contains an extracellular domain with epidermal growth factor (EGF) and thyroglobulin repeat-like domains, a single transmembrane domain and a short, 26-amino acid intracellular domain called EpICD. EpCAM functions as a homotypic calcium-independent cell adhesion molecule, and it is intricately linked with the cadherin–catenin pathway and the fundamental Wnt pathway responsible for intracellular signaling and polarity. Importantly, EpCAM in normal cells is predominantly located in intercellular spaces where epithelial cells form very tight junctions. EpCAM has been speculated to be sequestered on normal epithelia, whereas it is homogeneously distributed in cancer tissue. Moreover, the high expression level of EpCAM on cancer-initiating and normal stem cells and its positive autoregulation may ensure that the protein can provide a sustained proliferative signal to such cells (Munz et al. 2009). The overexpression of EpCAM has been shown to promote the proliferation, migration, and invasiveness of breast cancer cells. The expression of EpCAM is associated with decreased survival in a number of cancer indications, including breast, gallbladder, bile duct, ovarian and ampullary pancreatic cancer. As a result, this molecule is considered by some authors to be a valuable marker for cancer stem cells (Gires et al. 2009).

Based on these aspects, EpCAM has been adopted for antibody-based immunotherapeutic approaches. Specifically, a series of so-called BiTE antibodies that are designed to direct the body's cytotoxic T cells against tumor cells were developed. These bioengineered antibodies have been shown to induce an immunological synapse between a T cell and a tumor cell similar to those observed during physiological T-cell attacks. These synapses mediate the delivery of cytotoxic proteins called perforins and granzymes from the T cells into tumor cells (Brischwein et al. 2006). A preliminary approach with MT110 (an EpCAM/CD3-bispecific BiTE antibody) showed that T cells induced by extremely low doses of MT110 can lyse cancer stem cells from human colorectal cancer patients in vitro (Osada et al. 2010; Munz et al. 2009). Moreover, tumors grown in SCID mice with a 5,000-fold excess of a tumor-forming cell dose are prevented by MT110 treatment (Amann et al. 2009). MT110 is a recombinant, bispecific, single-chain antibody that consists of four immunoglobulin variable domains assembled into a single polypeptide chain. Two of the variable domains form the binding site for EpCAM, a cell surface antigen expressed on most solid tumors. The other two variable domains form the binding site for the CD3 complex on T cells (Baeuerle et al. 2009).

Adecatumumab (MT201) serves as an additional example. This biotechnology product is a recombinant human mAb of the IgG1 subclass mediating antibody-dependent cellular cytotoxicity (ADCC) and complement-mediated cytotoxicity (CDC) against EpCAM-positive cancer cells in general and cancer stem cells in particular (Schuler et al. 2008).

CSC Signaling Pathways

As previously mentioned, CSCs are characterized by a series of signaling pathways that are typical but are not specific for these "tumor stem-like cells."

The targeting of these particular pathways could induce a better therapeutic response and might reduce the possibility of recurrences.

Tyrosine kinase inhibitors (TKIs). TKIs are capable of modulating particular cellular signaling pathways with important repercussions on the cellular pathophysiology (Agrawal et al. 2010). These molecules have revolutionized the therapeutic approach to cancer, particularly leukemias. In fact, several pathways involved in oncogenesis are driven by tyrosine kinases (TKs). TKs seem to govern a multitude of cellular activities, including growth, survival, proliferation and, most importantly, differentiation and apoptosis. However, this subclass of protein kinases has not been considered a primary target for CSCs because they lack sufficient selectivity for this peculiar cell type.

Originally, quiescent stem cells of hematological tumors were postulated to be refractory to TKIs (Naka et al. 2010). However, lapatinib has been specifically adopted to target leukemia stem cells and/or CSCs based on the idea that the HER-2 pathway may be important for their survival. Interestingly, in a phase II clinical study on patients with HER-2-positive locally advanced breast cancer, biopsies showed that the number of tumorigenic $CD44^+/CD24^{-/low}$ cells typically increased following conventional chemotherapy, whereas no increase in the proportion of these tumorigenic cells was observed in the lapatinib-treated patients (Mustjoki et al. 2010). This study showed several potential limitations, but it is one of the first clinical studies published in which targeting the stem cell self-renewal properties of residual cells with TKIs in combination with conventional chemotherapy provided a specific approach to prevent cancer recurrence and improve long-term survival.

Importantly, further studies on TKI on cancer stem cells are in development for breast (Wicha 2009; Roesler et al. 2010), lung (Diaz et al. 2010), prostate (Mimeault et al. 2010), and gastrointestinal stromal tumors (Croom and Perry 2003) as well as glioblastoma (Griffero et al. 2009).

Other proteins belonging to more specific pathways activated in stem cells have been preferentially studied for therapeutic purposes. Some of the well-known pathways typically involved in stem cell self-renewal, including Wnt, Notch, Hedgehog (Hh), BMP, Bmi1 and Pten (which were previously identified as relevant in cancer and developmental biology), are now of increased interest due to their potential role in CSCs. These signaling pathways are commonly accepted to cause neoplastic proliferation when dysregulated by mutations.

Wnt signaling pathways. Cell-signaling cascades activated by Wnt proteins have been well conserved throughout evolution. In addition to regulating cellular processes, including proliferation, differentiation, motility and survival and/or apoptosis, the Wnt signaling pathways play key roles in embryonic development and the maintenance of homeostasis in mature tissues. Among the described Wnt signaling pathways, the Wnt/β-catenin signaling pathway is the best characterized from a physiological and pathological point of view. Wnt proteins are secreted molecules that regulate proliferation and patterning during development. The binding of Wnts to frizzled receptors causes β-catenin to accumulate and translocate into the nucleus, where it binds to the LEF/TCF transcription factors and activates the transcription of genes that promote proliferation. Mutations that activate the Wnt pathway have been implicated in a wide variety of cancers, including those of the colon, prostate, ovary and breast. The expression of stabilized β-catenin promotes the self-renewal of central nervous system (CNS) stem cells and keratinocyte stem cells, and it leads to tumorigenesis in the CNS and skin. Wnt signaling activates the same downstream pathways in colorectal cancer cells. The self-renewal of hematopoietic stem cells is also promoted by Wnt signaling. Importantly, the ectopic expression of axin, a negative regulator of Wnt signaling, inhibited the proliferation of hematopoietic stem cells, promoted apoptosis in vitro and reduced the ability of these cells to reconstitute in irradiated mice (Reya and Clevers 2005; Cantley and Carpenter 2008).

Inhibitors of the Wnt/β-catenin signaling pathway can be grouped into two classes: small-molecule inhibitors and biologic inhibitors. Small-molecule inhibitors include existing drugs, such as nonsteroidal anti-inflammatory drugs (NSAIDs) and molecular-targeted agents (e.g., the CBP/β-catenin antagonist ICG-001). Biological inhibitors include antibodies, RNA interference (RNAi), and recombinant proteins (Takahashi-Yanaga and Kahn 2010).

As mentioned previously, a number of existing drugs and natural compounds have been identified as inhibitors and/or modulators of the Wnt/β-catenin signaling pathway. Recently, both vitamin A and D have been suggested to induce Wnt/β-catenin inhibitory proteins, such as Disabled-2 (Dab2) by retinoic acids and Dickkopf-1 and −4 (Dkk-1 and Dkk-4) by vitamin D (Roccaro et al. 2008; Redova et al. 2010). In addition, polyphenols, a group of chemicals found in plants (such as quercetin, epigallocatechin-3-gallate, curcumin, and resveratrol), have been implicated as inhibitors of the Wnt/β-catenin signaling pathway, although the mechanism of action for these agents is unclear.

More recently, small-molecule inhibitors have been identified via high-throughput screening (Emami et al. 2004; Takahashi-Yanaga and Kahn 2010; Vanamala et al. 2010). These targeted agents, most of which are in the preclinical phase, can be classified into four groups: β-catenin/TCF-antagonists, transcriptional co-activator modulators, PDZ domain of Dvl binders, and other mechanism-based inhibitors. Importantly, the so-called β-catenin/TCF interaction antagonists are not highly selective for disrupting the β-catenin/TCF complex because they also interact with adenomatous polyposis coli (APC) (Reya and Clevers 2005; Takahashi-Yanaga and Kahn 2010) .

The protective effects of NSAIDs such as aspirin toward colon cancer are well known. Some authors have suggested that the mechanism could be related to NSAID-related inhibition of the Wnt pathway due to the increased phosphorylation of protein phosphatase 2A (PP2A) inhibiting PP2A enzymatic activity (Bos et al. 2006). Intriguingly, this particular chemopreventive effect for colon cancer has led to a push to consider a potential therapeutic role of this class of drug on CSCs.

An indirect confirmation of this hypothesis could be derived from the studies of Deng et al. (2009) and Wang et al. (2006), which showed that the Wnt/beta-catenin pathway is a key modulator of aspirin proliferation inhibition and apoptosis induction in mesenchymal stem cells. More recently, a nitric oxide-donating acetylsalicylic acid (NO-ASA) was shown to have an antineoplastic effect in Wnt/β-catenin-active cancers such as chronic lymphocytic leukemia (CLL). Specifically, NO-ASA induced apoptosis in CLL cells of a xenograft mouse model with an LC_{50} of $8.72 + 0.04$ μM, whereas healthy blood cells were not affected. Furthermore, the compound induced caspase 9, caspase 3, and PARP cleavage. Additionally, the cleavage of β-catenin and the downregulation of β-catenin/Lef-1 targets were observed. In conclusion, NO-ASA demonstrated strong antitumor efficacy with a tumor inhibition rate of approximately 80% in these experimental settings (Razavi et al. 2011).

With regards to the more specific role of COX-2 inhibitors, some studies have utilized these drugs to ameliorate targeting of cancer stem cells. For example, treatment with 30 μM of celecoxib effectively inhibited in vitro cell proliferation and colony formation and increased the ionizing radiotherapy-induced apoptosis in treated medulloblastoma (MB)-CD133(+) cells. Furthermore, an in vivo study demonstrated that celecoxib significantly enhanced radiosensitivity in MB-CD133(+)-transplanted grafts. Notably, xenotransplantation analysis demonstrated that the treatment of celecoxib could further suppress the expression of angiogenic and stemness-related genes in treated MB-CD133(+) grafts in SCID mice (Chen et al. 2010). Similarly, Singh et al. (2010) showed that a COX-2-transfected MCF7 breast cancer cell line was able to generate long-term tumorosphere cultures, even though the transfection efficiency was only one in a million cells. Moreover, some high-expressing COX-2 cells also showed high expression of OCT4, supporting the hypothesis that these cells could be cancer stem-like cells. Intriguingly, celecoxib inhibited the growth of tumorosphere cultures and the ability of tumorosphere-derived cells to form colonies in vitro, indicating an active role of COX-2 in these processes. However, celecoxib failed to eradicate tumorosphere-initiating cells.

A study by Redova et al. (2010) investigated the possible modulation of all-transretinoic acid (ATRA)-induced cell differentiation by LOX/COX inhibitors (caffeic acid, an inhibitor of 5-lipoxygenase and celecoxib, an inhibitor of cyclooxygenase-2) in two established neuroblastoma cell lines, SH-SY5Y and SK-N-BE(2). The higher sensitivity of the SK-N-BE(2) cell line to the combined treatment with ATRA and LOX/COX inhibitors suggested that CSCs are a primary target for this therapeutic approach. In addition, Kang et al. (2007) reported on the effect of celecoxib on an experimental model of glioblastoma multiforme, a typical neoplasia in which CSCs seem to play a significant pathogenic role. In this study, celecoxib enhanced U-87MG cell radiosensitivity by significantly reducing the clonogenic survival of irradiated cells. The median survival of control mice intracranially implanted with U-87MG cells was 18 days. This COX-2 inhibitor significantly extended the median survival of irradiated mice from 34 to 41 days with extensive tumor necrosis compared with irradiation alone. Importantly, the tumor microvascular density was also significantly reduced in combined celecoxib and irradiated tumors compared with irradiated tumors alone. Interestingly, resveratrol (3,4′,5-tri-hydroxy-trans-stilbene), a bioflavonoid with antioxidant properties that is a constituent of a wide variety of plant species, including grapes, also showed some anticancer activities primarily related to a Wnt cell-signaling alteration caused by COX-2 inhibition (Roccaro et al. 2008; Vanamala et al. 2010).

With regards to molecularly targeted drugs, ICG-001 is a small molecule that downregulates beta-catenin/T-cell factor signaling by specifically binding to the cyclic AMP response element-binding protein. ICG-001 seems to selectively induce apoptosis in colon cancer cells but not in normal colon cells, reducing the in vitro growth of these pathological cells. In addition, ICG-001 is efficacious in the Min mouse and nude mouse xenograft models of colon cancer (Emami et al. 2004). A recent study on the molecular mechanisms of neurodegeneration in mice showed that treatment with ICG-001 could cause degeneration of hippocampal neurons, whereas treatment with a JNK-specific inhibitor does not show any effect. These results seem to indicate that degeneration occurs via apoptotic processes. In this study, the inhibition of Wnt signaling reduced IGF-1 expression, and the addition of IGF-1 blocked degeneration, suggesting that the downregulation of IGF-1/Akt signaling is partially responsible for the phenomenon (Kim et al. 2010).

Another interesting molecularly targeted drug is an organic molecule (NSC 668036) from the National Cancer Institute small-molecule library that binds the Dishevelled (Dvl) PDZ domain. This Dvl PDZ domain is believed to play an essential role in the canonical and noncanonical Wnt signaling pathways (Chen and Deng 2009).

With regards to biological Wnt inhibitors, mAbs against WNT1 and WNT2, siRNA and therapeutic proteins (WIF1, SFRPs) are in the preclinical phase (Takahashi-Yanaga and Kahn 2010). He et al. (2004) investigated the effects of Wnt-1 signaling inhibition by mAb and RNAi in a variety of human cancer cell lines, including non-small-cell lung cancer, breast cancer, mesothelioma, and sarcoma. The results showed that incubation of a monoclonal anti-Wnt-1 antibody induced apoptosis and caused downstream protein changes in cancer cells overexpressing Wnt-1. In contrast, apoptosis was not detected in cells lacking or having minimal Wnt-1 expression. The RNAi targeting of Wnt-1 in cancer cells overexpressing Wnt-1 demonstrated similar downstream protein changes and the induction of apoptosis. Importantly, the antibody also suppressed tumor growth in vivo.

Similar results were obtained by You et al. (2004) targeting Wnt-2 signaling in human melanoma cells. The authors developed a mAb against the NH(2) terminus of the human Wnt-2 ligand that induced apoptosis in human melanoma cells overexpressing this protein. Importantly, this antibody does not induce apoptosis in normal cells lacking Wnt-2 expression. Wnt-2 siRNA treatment in these cells yielded similar apoptotic effects and downstream changes. Downregulation of an inhibitor of survivin, a member of the apoptosis protein family, was observed in both the Wnt-2 antibody-treated and siRNA-treated melanoma cell lines, suggesting that the antibody induces apoptosis by inactivating survivin. In an in vivo study, this monoclonal anti-Wnt-2 antibody suppressed tumor growth in a xenograft model (You et al. 2004). With regards to protein-based therapeutic approaches for Wnt inhibition, the secreted frizzled-related proteins (SFRPs) function as negative regulators of

Wnt signaling and have important implications in tumorigenesis. Frequent promoter hypermethylation of SFRPs has been identified in human cancers. The restoration of SFRP function attenuates Wnt signaling and induces apoptosis in a variety of cancer types. Wnt signaling is known to inhibit apoptosis through the activation of beta-catenin/Tcf-mediated transcription. Recently, He et al. (2004) identified aberrant Wnt activation as a result of Dvl overexpression in malignant mesotheliomas. The authors reported that silencing SFRP4 was correlated with promoter hypermethylation in β-catenin-deficient mesothelioma cell lines. Re-expression of SFRP4 in these β-catenin-deficient mesothelioma cell lines blocked Wnt signaling, induced apoptosis, and suppressed growth. Interestingly, knocking down SFRP4 with siRNA in cell lines expressing both SFRP4 and β-catenin stimulated Wnt signaling, promoted cell growth, and inhibited chemodrug-induced apoptosis (He et al. 2005).

According to Takahashi-Yanaga and Kahn (2010), the Wnt signaling cascade also has a significant functional role in normal somatic stem cells, in the homeostasis of normal differentiated cells and, thereby, in tissue maintenance. As a result, this particular approach, like all other approaches that influence signaling pathways preferentially active in CSCs, should always be studied in terms of the therapeutic index.

The Hedgehog Signaling Pathway. This pathway is one of the key regulators of animal development and is conserved from flies to humans. The pathway takes its name from its peptide ligand, an intercellular signaling molecule called Hedgehog originally found in *Drosophila* fruit flies. Hh is one of the segment polarity gene products in *Drosophila* and is involved in wing development. In addition, this molecule is important during later stages of embryogenesis and metamorphosis. The main components of this signaling pathway are the ligands (secreted Hedgehog proteins that diffuse to their targets), the Patched receptor (PTCH, a 12-pass transmembrane protein) and the intracellular transducing molecules Smoothened (Smo – a second transmembrane protein) and Gli (zinc-finger transcription factors). Mammals have three Hedgehog genes encoding three different receptors. Sonic Hedgehog is the best studied. In vertebrates, this pathway is equally important during embryonic development. In knock-out mice lacking components of the pathway, the brain, skeleton, musculature, gastrointestinal tract, and lungs fail to develop correctly. Importantly, some studies point to a role for Hedgehog signaling in regulating adult stem cells involved in the maintenance and regeneration of adult tissues (primarily muscular and nervous tissues). Moreover, this pathway has also been implicated in the development of some cancers (King et al. 2008). The identification of somatic PTCH mutations in patients with Gorlin syndrome and basal cell nervous syndrome first suggested a role for the Hh pathway in cancer. This hypothesis was confirmed by the observation that these individuals are highly predisposed to developing basal cell carcinoma (BCC), medulloblastoma (MB), and rhabdomyosarcoma (Von Hoff et al. 2009; Yauch et al. 2009; Zibat et al. 2010). Other Hh pathway dysfunctions have been also identified in other human cancers, including breast, pancreatic, gastric, colon, melanoma, lung and prostate cancer (Merchant and Matsui 2010).

Anticancer drugs that specifically target Hedgehog signaling are being actively developed by a number of pharmaceutical companies and are already in the clinical phase. One of the most well-known Hh inhibitors is GDC-0449 (Vismodegib), which is a small, orally administrable molecule that belongs to the 2-arylpyridine class. This drug is currently undergoing phase II clinical trials for the treatment of advanced BCC, metastatic colorectal cancer, ovarian cancer, MB, and other solid tumors (So et al. 2010). Because of its low toxicity and specificity for the Hh pathway, this drug seems to show potential advantages compared with conventional chemotherapy and may be used in combination with other treatments. GDC-0449 acts as a more targeted drug (it is the first systemic Smo-inhibitor) because it can inhibit Hh signaling pathologically activated by point mutations in different hedgehog pathway members in a variety of solid tumors and hematologic malignancies. Moreover, GDC-0449 seems to inhibit abnormal stimulation of the Hh pathway in some cancers related to autocrine or paracrine ligand secretion (Merchant and Matsui 2010). One of the best known clinical studies published on GDC-0449 evaluated the effect of Hedgehog pathway inhibition in advanced basal-cell carcinoma (Doggrell 2010).

The initial phase I/II clinical studies did not specifically target CSCs, but recent clinical studies are being developed to analyze drug effects on this particular subpopulation of cancer cells (Rudin et al. 2009; Doggrell 2010). Specifically, studies are in progress for metastatic pancreatic cancer treated with gemcitabine hydrochloride and the Hedgehog antagonist GDC-0449. Another study looks at the effects of the Pan-Notch Inhibitor RO4929097 on advanced breast cancer. Both studies strictly monitor the stem-like tumor cell population. Similar studies are currently in the recruiting phase, and analysis of the cancer stem cell population during pharmacological treatment is one of the primary goals (Scatena et al. 2011).

Interestingly, the recent phase II clinical study by Von Hoff et al. (2009) analyzed the effects of GDC-0449 in BCC, a cancer that characteristically presents activating mutations in Hedgehog pathway genes [primarily genes encoding the patched homologue 1 (*PTCH1*) and the smoothened homologue (*SMO*)]. Interestingly, 18 of 33 patients showed an objective response to drug treatment (54%). In addition, two patients (6%) had a complete response, and 16 patients (48%) had a partial response. The other 15 patients (45%) had either the stable (11 patients) or progressive (four patients) forms of the disease. Importantly, eight grade 3 adverse events that were thought to be related to the drug under study were reported in six patients (18%). Considering that the drug is selectively targeted toward the typical oncogenic lesion of tumors, these results are encouraging.

Moreover, cancer cells may acquire an intrinsic resistance to the drug, analogous to imatinib. This resistance has been recently studied in MB and appears to be due to an amino acid substitution at a conserved aspartic acid residue of Smo that had no effect on Hh signaling but disrupted the ability of GDC-0449 to bind Smo and suppress this pathway (Yauch et al. 2009). Other drug inhibitors of aberrant Hh signaling activation in cancer are in clinical trials, and some of these are considered to specifically target CSCs. One such drug is IPI-926, a novel, orally available small molecule that inhibits Smo and is able to target a broad range of critical oncology targets from the cancer cell to the cancer microenvironment. Patients with previously untreated metastatic pancreatic cancer were recruited in a phase I/II clinical trial to evaluate IPI-926 activity in combination with gemcitabine, a chemotherapeutic agent (Hidalgo and Maitra 2009).

Other Hh inhibitors, such as LDE225 (a selective orally bioavailable Smo antagonist) and BMS-863923/XL139, are in phase I/II clinical trials for patients with advanced solid tumors. However, the selectivity of these drugs for CSCs has not been reported (Merchant and Matsui 2010).

The Notch Signaling Pathway. The Notch pathway is controlled by Notch proteins located in the membranes of cells. This pathway is found throughout the animal kingdom. The first Notch gene was discovered in *Drosophila*, where its mutation produced notches in the wings. Notch differs from many of the other signaling pathways in that the ligands and their receptors are transmembrane proteins embedded in the plasma membrane of cells. Thus, signaling in this pathway requires direct cell-to-cell contact. The Notch proteins (receptors) are single-pass transmembrane glycoproteins encoded by four genes in vertebrates. The ligands are various single-pass transmembrane proteins that are grouped into families. Often, several versions exist within a family, such as Delta (1, 3, and 4) and Jagged (1 and 2). The activation of this signaling pathway is based on the interaction between a cell bearing the ligand and a cell displaying the Notch receptor. After binding, Notch undergoes cleavage by γ-secretases and metalloproteinases, and the external portion of notch is cleaved away from the cell surface and engulfed by the ligand-bearing cell via endocytosis. The internal portion of the Notch receptor is cut away from the interior of the plasma membrane and travels into the nucleus, where it activates transcription factors that turn the appropriate genes on or off.

The proper development of virtually all organs (e.g., brain, immune system, pancreas, intestine, heart, blood vessels, and mammary glands) depends on adequate Notch signaling. Notch signaling appears to be a mechanism by which one cell tells an adjacent cell which path of differentiation to take. Intriguingly, depending on its physiological role, Notch signaling can act as an oncopromoter (gatekeeper of stem cells) or an oncosuppressor (differentiating factor) (Bolós et al. 2007; Pannuti et al. 2010). Dysregulation of Notch signaling pathways has been observed in melanomas, primary human gliomas, ovarian cancer, gastrointestinal cancer, lymphoblastic leukemia, and breast cancer (Koch and Radtke 2010; Yin et al. 2010). A number of compounds have been tested for their ability to inhibit Notch signaling, and some of these, specifically those inhibiting γ-secretase, are already in clinical trials.

MK-0752 is an orally administered active inhibitor of γ-secretase that blocks cleavage of the Notch receptor and halts Notch signaling. This drug is in phase I/II clinical trials alone and/or in association with other anticancer agents for the treatment of various solid tumors, such as glioblastoma, medulloblastoma (also in pediatric patients), pancreatic and breast cancer, T-cell acute lymphoblastic leukemia/lymphoma (T-ALL), and other leukemias (Bolós et al. 2007; Pannuti et al. 2010).

RO4929097 is also a γ-secretase inhibitor that is in phase I/II clinical trials involving patients with various solid tumors. Several cancers seem to show sensitivity to γ-secretase inhibitors, particularly lung cancer, Kaposi's sarcoma, multiple myeloma, and T-cell acute lymphoblastic leukemia. On the basis of these results, a large series of phase I/II clinical studies are in progress on the effects of these compounds alone or in association with other anticancer agents in various cancers, including pancreas, prostate, lung, breast, ovarian, brain and colon cancer in addition to melanoma, sarcoma and different hematological malignancies (TLL, lymphoma and multiple myeloma) (Luistro et al. 2009; Pannuti et al. 2010). Importantly, some of these studies have various outcomes for the analysis of drug-induced modification of the CSC population.

- Phase I dose-escalation study of the Hedgehog Smoothened antagonist GDC-0449 plus pan-Notch inhibitor RO4929097 administered in patients with advanced breast cancer. The purpose of this study was to attempt to evaluate select pharmacodynamic stem cell differentiation biomarkers in the Hedgehog and Notch signaling pathways (e.g., Gli1/2/3, Ptch1/2, Hes1, Hip1, Hey1, Notch4, Jagged1, Numb, Bmi-1, CD44/CD24, and ALDH) and the percentage of breast cancer stem cells in serial breast tumor biopsies before and after Hedgehog antagonist GDC-0449 or γ-secretase inhibitor RO4929097 when administered alone and after one course of treatment when administered in combination (Scatena et al. 2011).
- Phase II/pharmacodynamic study of the gamma-secretase inhibitor RO4929097 in patients who are progression-free at completion of chemotherapy for advanced non-small-cell lung cancer. The main outcomes were (1) a comparison between tumor Notch and stem cell markers expression in patients with or without genotype polymorphisms, EGFR-activating mutations, response and tumor progression and (2) a comparison between the expression of the Notch pathway and stem cell markers before and after therapy (Scatena et al. 2011).

Similar objectives for the effects of RO4929097 on the CSC population have been implemented for pancreatic cancer and advanced melanoma (Wu et al. 2010).

A different approach to the inhibition of Notch signaling that specifically focused on targeting CSCs consists in the synthesis of an anti-DLL4 (delta-like 4) mAb called OMP-21M18. This humanized mAb is directed against the N-terminal epitope of the Notch ligand DLL4 and has potential antineoplastic activity. The anti-DLL4 mAb OMP-21M18 binds to the membrane-binding portion of DLL4 and prevents its interaction with Notch-1 and Notch-4 receptors, thereby inhibiting Notch-mediated signaling and gene transcription. Because the expression of DLL4 seems to be restricted to the vascular endothelium and the net result is a disruption of tumor angiogenesis, this should damage the CSC microenvironment (Hoey et al. 2009). At present, some phase I/II clinical studies are in progress. Specifically, three studies are planned to evaluate the cytotoxic effect of OMP-21M18 in association with gemcitabine (Advanced or Metastatic Pancreatic Cancer), FOLFIRI (Metastatic Colorectal Cancer) or carboplatin and pemetrexed (Non-Squamous Non-Small Cell Lung Cancer) on the CSC population and changes in CSC biomarker (Wei et al. 2010; Scatena et al. 2011).

PF-03084014, another γ-secretase inhibitor, is also in phase I clinical trials. The inhibition of secondary Notch signaling pathways may result in the induction of apoptosis in tumor cells that overexpress Notch (Deonarain et al. 2009).

A different molecular approach has been taken with Tr4, which is a genetically engineered Mastermind-like (MAML) glutamine-rich nuclear protein. This protein is physiologically essential for Notch signaling activation. The formation of complexes of MAML with the intracellular portion of activated Notch (NICD), the transcription factor CBF1 and DNA results in the activation of the Notch target genes *Hes* and *Hey*. The bioengineered, truncated version of MAML maintains association with the complex, behaving in a dominant negative fashion and leading to the prevention of Notch activation (van der Heijden and Bernards 2010).

Phosphatidylinositol 3-kinases (PI3Ks) signaling pathway. A discussion of signal transduction cannot omit PI3Ks. This signaling pathway has roles in cell proliferation, apoptosis, protein synthesis and metabolism, and it is one of the most commonly dysregulated pathways in human cancer. The PI3K pathways can be activated by amplification or activation mutations of upstream receptor tyrosine kinases and by mutations or deletions downstream in the pathway. Class I PI3Ks are one of the key components of the PI3K/Akt pathway. These are enzymes recruited by activated membrane receptors to convert an extracellular message into an intracellular message (phosphoinositol triphosphate, PIP3). This activity is counterbalanced by a phosphatase (PTEN) that attenuates and/or turns off the signal. The next key component is Akt, a protein kinase that is activated by PIP3. This enzyme acts on various substrates, including the transcription factor FOXO and a protein designated as TSC2. The phosphorylation of FOXO prevents the transcription of genes that regulate the cell cycle and apoptosis, whereas the phosphorylation of TSC2 disrupts cell cycle regulation. Akt also inhibits apoptosis directly by acting on another protein, BAD. BAD downregulates the expression of the tumor suppressor p53 via MDM2 and disrupts another regulatory pathway controlling apoptosis that is mediated by nuclear factor κB (NF-κB). Moreover, Akt regulates other proteins and kinases involved in cellular glucose metabolism. In conclusion, several studies have demonstrated an important role for the PTEN/PI3-K/Akt/beta-catenin pathway in the regulation of normal and malignant stem/progenitor cell populations and suggest that agents that inhibit this pathway could be able to effectively target CSCs (Trumpp and Wiestler 2008; Scatena et al. 2010; Murphy and Fornier 2010).

At present, several drugs targeting this signaling pathway are in various stages of preclinical development in the pharmaceutical industry. Some of these, including CAL-101, XL-147, BGT-226 and BEZ-235, could be specifically targeted against CSCs (Scatena et al. 2010).

Some interesting experimental studies seem to show that ErbB-mediated carcinogenesis might be due to dysregulated receptor function on CSCs and that the clinical efficacy of trastuzumab and lapatinib (specifically in breast cancer) could depend on the selectivity of these drugs for the tumor-initiating and/or -maintaining cells. However, other preclinical studies and clinical phase IV studies seem to indicate a relative insensitivity of Ph1 CML stem cells and the CSCs of some solid tumors to imatinib and other TKIs used as single antitumor treatments (LoRusso et al. 2008).

Interestingly, a phase II clinical study to evaluate the effect of vorinostat and lapatinib on biomarkers of epithelial–mesenchymal transition (EMT) and breast cancer stem cells in patients with advanced solid tumor malignancies and women with recurrent local, regional or metastatic breast cancer is in progress (Deng et al. 2008).

Telomerase Inhibitors

Telomerase is a particular reverse transcriptase found in all eukaryotic cells. Although its expression is widely variable, telomerase is essential for the replication of chromosome ends (telomeres). Interestingly, high levels of telomerase are also found in stem cells. Moreover, recent work has shown that telomerase is one of the most reliable tumor markers for cancer detection because it does not exist in benign tumors. From a pathophysiological point of view, the continued proliferation of tumor cells requires the activation of telomerase to maintain chromosomal stability and to extend lifespan because it elongates telomere length and rewinds the cellular mitotic clock. Conversely, the shortening of telomeres by the inhibition of telomerase activity induces growth arrest (senescence) and apoptosis in tumor cells. The pharmacological inhibition of telomerase increases the susceptibility of tumor cells to apoptosis induced by anticancer agents. Intriguingly, CSCs also show high levels of telomerase activity. Therefore, the so-called telomerase inhibitors are considered to be a potential novel cancer specific therapy, considering that most normal somatic cells express low levels of telomerase (Castelo-Branco et al. 2011).

Imetelstat is one of the most studied telomerase inhibitors. Imetelstat is a 13-mer oligonucleotide N3′–P5′ thiophosphoramidate (NPS oligonucleotide) that is covalently attached to a C16 (palmitoyl) lipid moiety, which increases its potency and improves its pharmacokinetic and pharmacodynamic properties. Imetelstat binds directly and with high affinity to the template region of the RNA component of human telomerase (hTR), which lies in the active or catalytic site of hTERT, the telomerase reverse transcriptase. The binding of imetelstat to hTR results in the direct, competitive inhibition of telomerase enzymatic activity (Brennan et al. 2010; Joseph et al. 2010).

In experimental studies, imetelstat treatment inhibited tumor growth in different neoplasias (multiple myeloma, breast cancer, pancreatic cancer, and human glioblastoma) and significantly reduced the tumor-initiating cell population, as shown by the expression of typical cell markers (i.e., antigen CD138 and/or aldehyde dehydrogenase). Importantly, imetelstat also decreased the expression of genes typically expressed by stem cells (*OCT3/4*, *SOX2*, *NANOG*, and *BMI1*), as revealed by quantitative real-time PCR (Brennan et al. 2010; Joseph et al. 2010; Marian et al. 2010).

A phase II clinical study with imetelstat as a maintenance therapy after initial induction chemotherapy for advanced non-small-cell lung cancer (NSCLC) is ongoing. One aim of this study is the monitoring of the CSC population (Butler et al. 2010).

CSC Niche-Targeted Drugs

Recent reports in stem cell biology suggest a model for tumors in which tumor growth is governed by the generation of cells from tumor cell niches rather than from the population as a whole. Specifically, each niche contains a population of tumor stem cells supported by a closely associated vascular bed composed of mesenchyme-derived cells, the extracellular matrix, and endothelial cells derived from the tumor itself that differentiated from tumor stem-like cells (LaBarge 2010). In this particular pathophysiological setting, vascular endothelial cells, regardless of their origin, play a critical role in the stem cell niche, confirming the hypothesis that CSCs may also rely on signaling interactions with nearby tumor vasculature to maintain their stem-like state. The disruption of such a tumor-maintaining vascular niche by an antiangiogenic therapy could result in a loss of their stem cell-like characteristics, thus preferentially sensitizing CSCs to the effects of chemotherapy (Ramalingam et al. 2010).

Based on this hypothesis, some clinical studies on drugs acting mainly as inhibitors of the vascular endothelial growth factor (VEGF) receptor tyrosine kinase are in progress. One of the first examples was cediranib, currently undergoing phase I clinical trials for the treatment of non-small-cell lung cancer, kidney cancer and colorectal cancer in adults as well as tumors of the central nervous system in children. The use of Recentin in non-small-cell lung cancer did not progress into phase III after failing to meet its primary goal. In 2010, a press release stated that Recentin had failed phase III clinical trials for use in first-line metastatic colorectal cancer when it was compared clinically with the market-leader, Avastin (Zama et al. 2010).

A more targeted drug could be sunitinib (previously known as SU11248), a kinase inhibitor that targets platelet-derived growth factor receptors (PDGF-Rs) and vascular endothelial growth factor receptors (VEGFRs). Sunitinib is an orally available, small-molecule, multi-targeted receptor tyrosine kinase (RTK) inhibitor that was approved by the FDA for the treatment of renal cell carcinoma (RCC) and imatinib-resistant gastrointestinal stromal tumors (GIST). In 2010, sunitinib gained approval from the European Commission for the treatment of unresectable or metastatic well-differentiated pancreatic neuroendocrine tumors (Younus et al. 2010; Neyns et al. 2010).

Sunitinib disrupts cellular signaling by targeting multiple RTKs. These include all receptors for platelet-derived growth factors and vascular endothelial growth factors, which play roles in both tumor angiogenesis and tumor cell proliferation. The simultaneous inhibition of these targets, leading to both reduced tumor vascularization and cancer cell death, could make this drug an effective agent against CSC niches (Shojaei et al. 2010).

Importantly, sunitinib also inhibits KIT (CD117), the RTK that, when improperly activated by mutations, drives the majority of gastrointestinal stromal cell tumors, including RET, CSF-1R and flt3. The fact that sunitinib targets various receptors explains some of its side effects, such as the classic hand–foot syndrome, stomatitis, and other dermatologic toxicities (Fletcher et al. 2010; Phay and Shah 2010; Younus et al. 2010).

ATP-Binding Cassette Drug Inhibitors

The protection of stem cells from damage or death due to toxins is a critical function of an organism because stem cells need to remain intact for the entire life of the organism. One of the principal mechanisms for protecting stem cells is through the expression of multifunctional efflux transporters from the ATP-binding cassette

(ABC) gene family. One of the more reliable stemness markers for both normal and cancer cells is the high expression of the ABC multidrug efflux transporter. Drugs that target these transmembrane proteins should be characterized by a particular selectivity in order to dysregulate the fundamental defense function of CSCs (Katayama et al. 2009).

Some drugs belonging to this class are already in clinical trials. Dofequidar fumarate is an orally active quinoline compound that overcomes multiple drug resistance (MDR) of cancer cells by inhibiting ABCB1/P-gp, ABCC1/MDR-associated protein 1 or both. Phase III clinical trials suggest that dofequidar has efficacy in patients who have not received prior therapy. Recently, Katayama et al.(2009) showed that dofequidar may inhibit the efflux of chemotherapeutic drugs and increase the sensitivity to anticancer drugs in CSC-like side population (SP) cells isolated from various cancer cell lines. Moreover, dofequidar treatment greatly reduced the number of cells in the SP fraction.

Vandetanib is one of the various TKIs (cediranib, gefitinib) that seems not only to be able to inhibit VEGFR and EGFR signaling but also to directly and/or indirectly antagonize ABCC1- and ABCG2-mediated MDR by inhibiting their transport function (Kitazaki et al. 2005; Zheng et al. 2009; Tao et al. 2009; Gupta et al. 2009a, b).

Vandetanib is unlikely to be a substrate of ABCC1 or ABCG2. Vandetanib overcomes ABCC1- and ABCG2-mediated drug resistance by inhibiting the transporter activity independently of the blockade of AKT and ERK1/2 signal transduction pathways (Kitazaki et al. 2005).

Salinomycin is a polyether antibiotic that acts as a highly selective potassium ionophore and is widely used as an anticoccidial drug. Salinomycin was recently shown to act as a specific inhibitor of CSCs. Gupta et al. (2009a, b) used a high-throughput screening approach to determine the anticancer activity of a large array of compounds and identified salinomycin, which was able to selectively target and show toxicity for breast CSCs. Specifically, salinomycin reduced the proportion of CSCs by >100-fold relative to paclitaxel, a commonly used breast cancer chemotherapeutic drug. Moreover, the treatment of mice with salinomycin inhibited mammary tumor growth in vivo and induced increased epithelial differentiation of tumor cells. In addition, global gene expression analyses show that salinomycin treatment results in the loss of expression of breast CSC genes previously identified by analyses of breast tissues isolated directly from patients. The actual mechanism of action of this potassium ionophore in CSCs is still under debate. However, recent reports have shown that salinomycin acts as a potent inhibitor of MDR gp170, as evidenced by drug efflux assays in MDR cancer cell lines overexpressing P-gp (CEM-VBL 10 and CEM-VBL 100; A2780/ADR). Moreover, a conformational P-gp assay provided evidence that the inhibitory effect of salinomycin on P-gp function could be mediated by the induction of a conformational change in the ATP transporter (Massard et al. 2006). Treatment with salinomycin induced the expression of plasma membrane E-cadherin, suggesting that the drug might also eliminate CSCs by inducing differentiation. This effect seems to be related to the suppressive actions of the drug on the metastasis process, which is in turn related to EMT transition inhibition (Riccioni et al. 2010).

Differentiation Therapy

Current anticancer therapies destroy the nontumorigenic bulk of cancer cells but fail to kill CSCs. An alternative approach could be differentiation therapy, which should induce cancer cells and CSCs toward a more differentiated phenotype and therefore cease proliferation (Scatena et al. 2008a, b). Although a number of differentiating agents have been studied over the years, the most thoroughly examined and clinically tested is retinoic acid (RA, vitamin A), specifically all-trans-retinoic acid (ATRA) (Nowak et al. 2009).

ATRA is used to treat acute promyelocytic leukemia (APL) by causing immature blood cells to differentiate. This therapeutic effect depends on the specific pathophysiology of APL. The majority of these leukemia cases show a chromosomal translocation of chromosomes 15 and 17, which causes genetic fusion of the retinoic acid receptor (*RAR*) gene to the promyelocytic leukemia (*PML*) gene. This fusion protein, PML-RAR, is responsible for preventing the differentiation of immature myeloid cells, which is thought to cause leukemia. ATRA acting on PML-RAR lifts this block and induces immature promyelocytes to differentiate. Treatment with ATRA could be considered the first example of treating tumor-initiating cells or tumor maintenance cells. Interestingly, ATRA was able to differentiate other cancer cells (i.e., Kaposi's sarcoma, head and neck squamous cell carcinoma, ovarian carcinoma, neuroblastoma and melanoma as well as bladder, breast and thyroid cancer) that do not express the PML-RAR protein. One hypothesis is that a mechanism related to its physiological function as regulator of differentiation at various stages of vertebrate embryogenesis, partially related to the stimulation of its specific nuclear receptor (RAR), is responsible for the effects in these cancers (Rosato and Grant 2004).

However, the original class of differentiating agents was defined as histone deacetylase inhibitors (HDIs) (Atadja 2011). These drugs inhibit histone deacetylase (HDAC), thus regulating histone acetylation and modulating the transcriptional activity of certain genes. Specifically, the HDI suberoylanilide hydroxamic acid (SAHA) was initially identified as a result of its ability to induce differentiation in cultured murine erythroleukemia cells. Studies have shown that SAHA can induce morphological changes (including the flattening and enlargement of cytoplasm), decrease the nuclear-cytoplasmic ratio and induce milk fat globule protein, milk fat membrane globule protein and lipid droplets in the breast cancer MCF7 cell line, suggesting that the SAHA-mediated inhibition of HDAC can induce differentiation (Bottoni et al. 2005; Marks 2007; Martínez-Iglesias et al. 2008). However, for all of these so-called differentiating agents, cell pseudo-differentiation is more appropriate for describing SAHA actions than actual cell differentiation.

At present, SAHA is marketed for the treatment of cutaneous T-cell lymphoma (CTCL) when the disease persists, worsens or recurs during or after classical anticancer treatments. Interestingly, this class of epigenetic drugs has lost the characteristic of being a differentiating agent in favor of a more generic antineoplastic action that, from a molecular point of view, has not been fully characterized. In some cancer cells, overexpression of HDACs occurs or there is an aberrant recruitment of HDACs to oncogenic transcription factors causing hypoacetylation of core nucleosomal histones.

SAHA/vorinostat inhibits the enzymatic activity of histone deacetylases HDAC1, HDAC2, HDAC3 (Class I), and HDAC6 (Class II) at nanomolar concentrations. These enzymes catalyze the removal of acetyl groups from the lysine residues of proteins, including histones and transcription factors. The hypoacetylation of histones is associated with a condensed chromatin structure and the repression of gene transcription. The inhibition of HDAC activity allows for the accumulation of acetyl groups on the histone lysine residues, resulting in an open chromatin structure and transcriptional activation. In vitro, these epigenetic modifications may induce cell cycle arrest and/or apoptosis in proliferating cells (Bottoni et al. 2005; Marks 2007; Martínez-Iglesias et al. 2008). The evaluation of potential side effects due to a nonspecific modification of epigenetic program in normal cells warrants further attention.

Intriguingly, these particular mechanisms of action could also be effective in targeting CSCs because abruptly disrupting gene expression related to stemness could impair the reservoir ability of tumor-initiating cells. Moreover, the particular liposolubility of these molecules could permit them to reach organs and/or regions of the organism in which classic therapeutic regimens do not show particular efficacy due to drug distribution problems (i.e., brain tumors).

In addition, PPAR alpha and gamma ligands have been shown to be differentiating agents for various types of cancer (Scatena et al. 2008a, b; Khanim et al. 2009). At present, phase II clinical studies are in progress for these new indications (Khanim et al. 2009; Murray et al. 2010).

The capability of drugs to induce differentiation in CSCs has not yet been considered.

Conclusions

This chapter cannot consider all of the molecules under investigation to selectively destroy CSCs; thus, we have focused on promising drugs or therapeutic approaches that are already in clinical phase trials or represent innovative preclinical approaches potentially useful to target CSCs. Pharmacological research is studying a therapeutic approach to CSCs, some by researching new targeted molecules and others by utilizing well-known drugs addressed against this new target.

Characterizing the pathogenesis of these intriguing cancer cells (i.e., real CSCs or "tumor cells partially resembling stem cells") is expanding the knowledge of the pathophysiology of the disease, emphasizing the concepts and molecular mechanisms that have been partially neglected and facilitating the understanding of a global vision of complex cancer cell biology.

Utilizing this new therapeutic approach, pharmacological research aims to destroy proliferating cancer cells and to kill or limit the potential of cancer cell reservoirs.

Specifically, future research could clarify the real therapeutic index of these innovative strategies against cancer by evaluating the studies currently in progress. At present, the results of pharmacological research against CSCs could be considered promising, even if these data seem to give an optimistic vision of the next future of chemotherapy.

Importantly, the CSC hypothesis is still debated (Bjerkvig et al. 2005). Some authors strongly criticize the idea of stem cells with malignant features. Other authors prefer to use the term "cancer-initiating cells" (perhaps more accurately "cancer-originating or maintaining cells"), whereas others prefer to use the term "stem-like" cancer cells or "tumor stem-like cells." The latter terms are probably the most appropriate because they imply both a stochastic (clonal) and hierarchical (stem cell) model and permit a better understanding of some intriguing aspects of cancer pathophysiology, particularly:

- The relative dormancy
- The efficient DNA repair
- The high expression of MDR-type membrane transporters.
- The protective role of hypoxic niche environments.

All of these factors determine the marked resistance toward classical antitumour regimens and the high incidence of recidivism.

The fundamental task now, and not only from a pharmacological point of view, is the accurate identification/targeting of these CSCs. Such attempts must consider that these are tumor stem-like cells with only some aspects typical of stem cells. This sharing of certain structural and functional characteristics from one side should permit more selective therapeutic targeting but may expose normal stem cells to iatrogenic insult with potentially dangerous side effects.

At present, targeting CSCs via surface markers (i.e., CD133, CD34, and CD24) has produced interesting but debated results. More promising data have come from studies with drugs that target different stem cell-signaling pathways (TKIs, Hh inhibitors). In our opinion, however, an interesting approach to killing cancer cells that have acquired stemness through the selective pressures of a microenvironment could be the targeting of the niche with an antiangiogenic approach that curtails the nutrient supply for tumor cells and alters the selective environment that promotes stemness and thereby dormancy. Moreover, these data suggest the importance of analyzing a further intriguing aspect of CSCs: cell metabolism. In fact, the peculiar functional characteristics of these cells must be associated with a unique metabolism that should be completely different from that of proliferating cancer cells. This unique metabolism, together the intriguing genetic plasticity could represent further selective and significant targets for the identification and extermination of the malignant cells determining cancer recidivism.

References

Agrawal M, Garg RJ, Cortes J, Quintás-Cardama A (2010) Tyrosine kinase inhibitors: the first decade. Curr Hematol Malig Rep 5:70–80.

Al-Hajj M, Wicha MS, Benito-Hernandez A et al (2003) Prospective identification of tumorigenic breast cancer cells. Proc Natl Acad Sci USA 100:3983–88.

Amann M, D'Argouges S, Lorenczewski G et al (2009) Antitumor activity of an EpCAM/CD3-bispecific BiTE antibody during long-term treatment of mice in the absence of T-cell anergy and sustained cytokine release. J Immunother 32:452–64.

Atadja PW (2011) HDAC inhibitors and cancer therapy. Prog Drug Res 67:175–95.

Baeuerle PA, Kufer P, Bargou R (2009) BiTE: Teaching antibodies to engage T-cells for cancer therapy. Curr Opin Mol Ther 11:22–30.

Bjerkvig R, Tysnes BB, Aboody KS et al (2005) Opinion: the origin of the cancer stem cell: current controversies and new insights. Nat Rev Cancer 5:899–904.

Blair A, Hogge DE, Ailles LE et al (1997) Lack of expression of Thy-1 (CD90) on acute myeloid leukemia cells with long-term proliferative ability in vitro and in vivo. Blood 89:3104–12.

Bolós V, Grego-Bessa J, de la Pompa JL (2007) Notch signaling in development and cancer. Endocr Rev 8:339–63.

Bonnet D, Dick JE (1997) Human acute myeloid leukemia is organized as a hierarchy that originates from a primitive hematopoietic cell. Nat Med 3:730–7.

Bos CL, Kodach LL, van den Brink GR et al (2006) Effect of aspirin on the Wnt/beta-catenin pathway is mediated via protein phosphatase 2A. Oncogene 25:6447–56.

Bottoni P, Giardina B, Martorana GE et al (2005) A two-dimensional electrophoresis preliminary approach to human hepatocarcinoma differentiation induced by PPAR-agonists. J Cell Mol Med 9:462–7.

Brennan SK, Wang Q, Tressler R et al (2010) Telomerase inhibition targets clonogenic multiple myeloma cells through telomere length-dependent and independent mechanisms. PLoS One 5: e12487.

Brischwein K, Schlereth B, Guller B et al (2006) MT110: a novel bispecific single-chain antibody construct with high efficacy in eradicating established tumors. Mol Immunol 43:1129–43.

Bross PF, Beitz J, Chen G et al (2001) Approval summary: gemtuzumab ozogamicin in relapsed acute myeloid leukemia. Clin Cancer Res 7:1490–6.

Butler JM, Kobayashi H, Rafii S (2010) Instructive role of the vascular niche in promoting tumour growth and tissue repair by angiocrine factors. Nat Rev Cancer 10:138–46.

Cantley L, Carpenter CL (2008) Cell Signaling. In: Devita, Hellman & Rosenberg's Cancer: Principles & Practice of Oncology, 8th edn. Lippincott Williams & Wilkins, Philadelphia.

Castelo-Branco P, Zhang C, Lipman T et al (2011) Neural Tumor-Initiating Cells Have Distinct Telomere Maintenance and Can be Safely Targeted for Telomerase Inhibition. Clin Cancer Res 17:111–21

Charrad RS, Gadhoum Z, Qi J et al (2002) Effects of anti-CD44 monoclonal antibodies on differentiation and apoptosis of human myeloid leukemia cell lines. Blood 99:290–9.

Chen KH, Hsu CC, Song WS et al (2010) Celecoxib enhances radiosensitivity in medulloblastoma-derived CD133-positive cells. Childs Nerv Syst 26:1605–12.

Chen X, Deng Y (2009) Simulations of a specific inhibitor of the dishevelled PDZ domain. J Mol Model 15:91–6.

Clarke WT, Marks PW (2010) Gemtuzumab ozogamicin: is there room for salvage? Blood 116:2618–9.

Croom KF, Perry CM (2003) Imatinib mesylate: in the treatment of gastrointestinal stromal tumours. Drugs 63:513–22.

Deng L, Hu S, Baydoun AR et al (2009) Aspirin induces apoptosis in mesenchymal stem cells requiring Wnt/beta-catenin pathway. Cell Prolif 42:721–30.

Deng Y, Chan SS, Chang S (2008) Telomere dysfunction and tumour suppression: the senescence connection. Nat Rev Cancer 8:450–8.

Deonarain MP, Kousparou CA, Epenetos AA (2009) Antibodies targeting cancer stem cells: a new paradigm in immunotherapy? MAbs 1:12–25.

Diaz R, Nguewa PA, Parrondo R et al (2010) Antitumor and antiangiogenic effect of the dual EGFR and HER-2 tyrosine kinase inhibitor lapatinib in a lung cancer model. BMC Cancer 10:188.

Dick JE (2008) Stem cell concepts renew cancer research. Blood 112:4793–807.

Doggrell SA (2010) The hedgehog pathway inhibitor GDC-0449 shows potential in skin and other cancers. Expert Opin Investig Drugs 19:451–4.

Emami KH, Nguyen C, Ma H et al (2004) A small molecule inhibitor of beta-catenin/CREB-binding protein transcription. Proc Natl Acad Sci USA 101:12682–7.

Entimov VJ, Brown TJ (2010a) Evaluation of activated CD44 as a biological target in the eradication of breast cancer stem cells. Cancer Stem Cell Therapeutics, American Association of Cancer Research (AACR) 101st Annual Meeting in Washington, DC 2010.

Entimov VJ, BrownTJ (2010b) HA-Irinotecan targeting of activated CD44 is an effective therapy for the eradication of putative colon cancer stem cells. Cancer Stem Cell Therapeutics, American Association of Cancer Research (AACR) 101st Annual Meeting in Washington, DC 2010.

Fletcher JI, Haber M, Henderson MJ, Norris MD (2010) ABC transporters in cancer: more than just drug efflux pumps. Nat Rev Cancer 10:147–56.

Gadhoum Z, Delaunay J, Maquarre E et al (2004) The effect of anti-CD44 monoclonal antibodies on differentiation and proliferation of human acute myeloid leukemia cells. Leuk Lymphoma 45:1501–10.

Gires O, Klein CA, Baeuerle PA (2009) On the abundance of EpCAM on cancer stem cells. Nat Rev Cancer 9:143.

Griffero F, Daga A, Marubbi D et al (2009) Different response of human glioma tumor-initiating cells to epidermal growth factor receptor kinase inhibitors. J Biol Chem 284:7138–48.

Gupta PB, Chaffer CL, Weinberg RA (2009) Cancer stem cells: mirage or reality? Nat Med 15:1010–2.

Gupta PB, Onder TT, Jiang G et al (2009) Identification of selective inhibitors of cancer stem cells by high-throughput screening. Cell 138:645–59.

Halsen G, Krämer I (2010) Assessing the risk to health care staff from long-term exposure to anticancer drugs - the case of monoclonal antibodies. J Oncol Pharm Pract, Jul 28.

He B, Lee AY, Dadfarmay S et al (2005) Secreted frizzled-related protein 4 is silenced by hypermethylation and induces apoptosis in beta-catenin-deficient human mesothelioma cells. Cancer Res 65:743–8.

He B, You L, Uematsu K et al (2004) A monoclonal antibody against Wnt-1 induces apoptosis in human cancer cells. Neoplasia 6:7–14.

Hidalgo M, Maitra A (2009) The Hedgehog Pathway and Pancreatic Cancer. N Engl J Med 361:2094–6.

Hoey T, Yen WC, Axelrod F et al (2009) 1DLL4 Blockade Inhibits Tumor Growth and Reduces Tumor-Initiating Cell Frequency. Cell Stem Cell 5:168–177.

Jin L, Hope KJ, Zhai Q et al (2006) Targeting of CD44 eradicates human acute myeloid leukemic stem cells. Nat Med 2:1167–74.

Jin L, Lee EM, Ramshaw HS et al (2009) Monoclonal antibody-mediated targeting of CD123, IL-3 receptor alpha chain, eliminates human acute myeloid leukemic stem cells. Cell Stem Cell 5:31–42.

Jordan CT, Upchurch D, Szilvassy SJ et al (2000) The interleukin-3 receptor α chain is a unique marker for human acute myelogenous leukemia stem cells. Leukemia 14:1777–84.

Joseph I, Tressler R, Bassett E et al (2010) The telomerase inhibitor imetelstat depletes cancer stem cells in breast and pancreatic cancer cell lines. Cancer Res 70:9494–504.

Kang KB, Wang TT, Woon CT et al (2007) Enhancement of glioblastoma radioresponse by a selective COX-2 inhibitor celecoxib: inhibition of tumor angiogenesis with extensive tumor necrosis. Int J Radiat Oncol Biol Phys 67:888–96.

Katayama R, Koike S, Sato S et al (2009) Dofequidar fumarate sensitizes cancer stem-like side population cells to chemotherapeutic drugs by inhibiting ABCG2/BCRP-mediated drug export. Cancer Sci 100:2060–8.

Khanim FL, Hayden RE, Birtwistle J et al (2009) Combined bezafibrate and medroxyprogesterone acetate: potential novel therapy for acute myeloid leukaemia. PLoS One. 4: e8147.

Kim H, Won S, Hwang DY et al (2010) Downregulation of Wnt/beta-catenin signaling causes degeneration of hippocampal neurons in vivo. Neurobiol Aging doi:10.1016/j.neurobiolaging.2010.03.013|

King PJ, Guasti L, Laufer E (2008) Hedgehog signalling in endocrine development and disease. J Endocrinol 198:439–50.

Kitazaki T, Oka M, Nakamura Y et al (2005) Gefitinib, an EGFR tyrosine kinase inhibitor, directly inhibits the function of P-glycoprotein in multidrug resistant cancer cells. Lung Cancer 49:337–43.

Koch U, Radtke F (2010) Notch signaling in solid tumors. Curr Top Dev Biol 92:411–55.

Koppe M, Schaijk F, Roos J et al (2004) Safety, pharmacokinetics, immunogenicity, and biodistribution of (186)Re-labeled humanized monoclonal antibody BIWA 4 (Bivatuzumab) in patients with early-stage breast cancer. Cancer Biother Radiopharm 19:720–9.

LaBarge MA (2010) The difficulty of targeting cancer stem cell niches. Clin Cancer Res 16:3121–9.

Levitzki A (2002) Tyrosine kinases as targets for cancer therapy. Eur J Cancer 38 Suppl 5:S11–8.

LoRusso PM, Ryan AJ, Boerner SA (2008) Small Molecule Tyrosine Kinase Inhibitors. In Devita, Hellman & Rosenberg's Cancer: Principles & Practice of Oncology 8th Edn. Williams & Wilkins, Philadelphia.

Luistro L, He W, Smith M et al (2009) Preclinical profile of a potent gamma-secretase inhibitor targeting notch signaling with in vivo efficacy and pharmacodynamic properties. Cancer Res 69:7672–80.

Marangoni E, Lecomte N, Durand L et al (2009) CD44 targeting reduces tumour growth and prevents post-chemotherapy relapse of human breast cancers xenografts. Br J Cancer 100:918–22.

Marian CO, Cho SK, McEllin BM et al (2010) The telomerase antagonist, imetelstat, efficiently targets glioblastoma tumor-initiating cells leading to decreased proliferation and tumor growth. Clin Cancer Res 16:154–63.

Marks PA (2007) Discovery and development of SAHA as an anticancer agent. Oncogene 26:1351–6.

Martínez-Iglesias O, Ruiz-Llorente L, Sánchez-Martínez R et al (2008) Histone deacetylase inhibitors: mechanism of action and therapeutic use in cancer. Clin Transl Oncol 10:395–8.

Massard C, Deutsch E, Soria JC (2006) Tumour stem cell-targeted treatment: elimination or differentiation. Ann Oncol 17:1620–4.

Merchant AA, Matsui W (2010) Targeting Hedgehog--a cancer stem cell pathway. Clin Cancer Res 16:3130–40.

Mimeault M, Johansson SL, Henichart JP et al (2010) Cytotoxic effects induced by docetaxel, gefitinib, and cyclopamine on side population and non side population cell fractions from human invasive prostate cancer cells. Mol Cancer Ther 9:617–30.

Mittal S, Mifflin R, Powell DW (2009) Cancer stem cells: the other face of Janus. Am J Med Sci 338:107–12.

Munz M, Baeuerle PA, Gires O (2009) The emerging role of EpCAM in cancer and stem cell signaling. Cancer Res 69:5627–9.

Murphy CG, Fornier M (2010) HER2-positive breast cancer: beyond trastuzumab. Oncology (Williston Park) 24:410–5.

Murray JA, Khanim FL, Hayden RE et al (2010) Combined bezafibrate and medroxyprogesterone acetate have efficacy without haematological toxicity in elderly and relapsed acute myeloid leukaemia (AML). Br J Haematol 149:65–9.

Mustjoki S, Rohon P, Rapakko K et al (2010) Low or undetectable numbers of Philadelphia chromosome-positive leukemic stem cells (Ph(+)CD34(+)CD38(neg)) in chronic myeloid leukemia patients in complete cytogenetic remission after tyrosine kinase inhibitor therapy. Leukemia 24:219–22.

Naka K, Hoshii T, Hirao A (2010) Novel therapeutic approach to eradicate tyrosine kinase inhibitor resistant chronic myeloid leukemia stem cells. Cancer Sci 101:1577–81.

Neyns B, Sadones J, Chaskis C et al (2010) Phase II study of sunitinib malate in patients with recurrent high-grade glioma. J Neurooncol Sep 25.

Nowak D, Stewart D, Koeffler HP (2009) Differentiation therapy of leukemia: 3 decades of development. Blood 113:3655–65.

Osada T, Hsu D, Hammond S et al (2010) Metastatic colorectal cancer cells from patients previously treated with chemotherapy are sensitive to T-cell killing mediated by CEA/CD3-bispecific T-cell-engaging BiTE antibody. Br J Cancer 102:124–33.

O'Sullivan B, Thomas R (2004) Recent advances on the role of CD40 and dendritic cells in immunity and tolerance. Curr Opin Hematol 10:272–8.

Pannuti A, Foreman K, Rizzo P, Osipo C (2010) Targeting Notch to Target Cancer Stem Cells . Clin Cancer Res 16:3141–52.

Phay JE, Shah MH (2010) Targeting RET receptor tyrosine kinase activation in cancer. Clin Cancer Res 16:5936–41.

Ramalingam SS, Belani CP, Mack PC et al (2010) Phase II study of Cediranib (AZD 2171), an inhibitor of the vascular endothelial growth factor receptor, for second-line therapy of small cell lung cancer (National Cancer Institute #7097). J Thorac Oncol 5:1279–84.

Razavi R, Gehrke I, Gandhirajan RK et al (2011) Nitric oxide-donating acetylsalicylic acid induces apoptosis in chronic lymphocytic leukemia cells and shows strong anti-tumor efficacy in vivo. *Clin Cancer Res* 2011: published online 11 January, doi:10.1158/1078–0432.

Redova M, Chlapek P, Loja T et al (2010) Influence of LOX/COX inhibitors on cell differentiation induced by all-trans retinoic acid in neuroblastoma cell lines. Int J Mol Med 25:271–80.

Reya T, and Clevers H (2005) Wnt signalling in stem cells and cancer. Nature 434:843–850.

Riccioni R, Dupuis ML, Bernabei M et al (2010) The cancer stem cell selective inhibitor salinomycin is a p-glycoprotein inhibitor. Blood Cells Mol Dis 45:86–92.

Roccaro AM, Leleu X, Sacco A et al (2008) Resveratrol exerts antiproliferative activity and induces apoptosis in Waldenström's macroglobulinemia. Clin Cancer Res 14:1849–58.

Roesler R, Cornelio DB, Abujamra AL, Schwartsmann G (2010) HER2 as a cancer stem-cell target. Lancet Oncol 11:225–6.

Rosato RR, Grant S (2004) Histone deacetylase inhibitors in clinical development. Expert Opin Investig Drugs 13:21–38.

Rudin CM, Hann CL, Laterra J et al (2009) Low JA.Treatment of medulloblastoma with hedgehog pathway inhibitor GDC-0449. N Engl J Med 361:1173–8.

Rupp U, Schoendorf-Holland E, Eichbaum M et al (2007) Safety and pharmacokinetics of bivatuzumab mertansine in patients with CD44v6-positive metastatic breast cancer: final results of a phase I study. Anticancer Drugs 18:477–85.

Scatena R, Bottoni P, Giardina B (2008) Mitochondria, PPARs, and Cancer: Is Receptor-Independent Action of PPAR Agonists a Key? PPAR Res 2008: 256251.

Scatena R, Bottoni P, Giardina B (2008) Modulation of cancer cell line differentiation: A neglected proteomic analysis with potential implications in pathophysiology, diagnosis, prognosis, and therapy of cancer. Proteomics Clin Appl 2:229–37.

Scatena R, Bottoni P, Pontoglio A, Giardina B (2010) Revisiting the Warburg effect in cancer cells with proteomics. The emergence of new approaches to diagnosis, prognosis and therapy. Proteomics Clin Appl 4:143–58.

Scatena R, Bottoni P, Pontoglio A, Giardina B (2011). Cancer stem cells: the development of new cancer therapeutics. Expert Opin Biol Ther. Mar 30.

Schuler M et al (2008) First results from a phase Ib study of the anti-EpCAM antibody adecatumumab (MT201) in combination with docetaxel in patients with metastatic breast cancer. *Annual Meeting of ESMO*, Abstract No. 485p

Shackleton M, Quintana E, Fearon ER, Morrison SJ (2009) Heterogeneity in cancer: cancer stem cells versus clonal evolution. Cell 138:822–9.

Shojaei F, Lee JH, Simmons BH et al (2010) HGF/c-Met acts as an alternative angiogenic pathway in sunitinib-resistant tumors. Cancer Res 70:10090–100.

Singh B, Cook KR, Vincent L et al (2010) Role of COX-2 in Tumorospheres Derived from a Breast Cancer Cell Line. J Surg Res: published online 26 Mar 2010 doi:10.1016/j.jss.2010.03.003

So PL, Tang JY, Epstein EH (2010) Novel investigational drugs for basal cell carcinoma. Expert Opin Investig Drugs 19:1099–112.

Subramaniam V, Vincent IR, Gilakjan M, Jothy S (2007) Suppression of human colon cancer tumors in nude mice by siRNA CD44 gene therapy. Exp Mol Pathol 83:332–40.

Takahashi-Yanaga F, Kahn M (2010) Targeting Wnt signaling: can we safely eradicate cancer stem cells? Clin Cancer Res 16:3153–62.

Tang C, Ang BT, Pervaiz S (2007) Cancer stem cell: target for anti-cancer therapy. FASEB J 21: 3777–85.

Tao LY, Liang YJ, Wang F et al (2009) Cediranib (recentin, AZD2171) reverses ABCB1- and ABCC1-mediated multidrug resistance by inhibition of their transport function. Cancer Chemother Pharmacol 64:961–9.

Trumpp A, Wiestler OD (2008) Mechanisms of Disease: cancer stem cells-targeting the evil twin. Nat Clin Pract Oncol 5:337–47.

van der Heijden MS, Bernards R (2010) Inhibition of the PI3K pathway: hope we can believe in? Clin Cancer Res 16:3094–9.

Vanamala J, Reddivari L, Radhakrishnan S, Tarver C (2010) Resveratrol suppresses IGF-1 induced human colon cancer cell proliferation and elevates apoptosis via suppression of IGF-1R/Wnt and activation of p53 signaling pathways. BMC Cancer 10:238.

Von Hoff DD, LoRusso PM, Rudin CM et al (2009) Inhibition of the hedgehog pathway in advanced basal-cell carcinoma. N Engl J Med 361:1164–72.

Wang JCY, Dick JE (2008) Cancer Stem Cells. In: Devita, Hellman & Rosenberg's Cancer: Principles & Practice of Oncology 8th Edn. Lippincott Williams & Wilkins, Philadelphia.

Wang Y, Chen X, Zhu W et al (2006) Growth inhibition of mesenchymal stem cells by aspirin: involvement of the WNT/beta-catenin signal pathway. Clin Exp Pharmacol Physiol 33:696–701.

Wei P, Walls M, Qiu M et al (2010) Evaluation of selective gamma-secretase inhibitor PF-03084014 for its antitumor efficacy and gastrointestinal safety to guide optimal clinical trial design. Mol Cancer Ther 9:1618–28.

Wicha MS (2009) Targeting breast cancer stem cells. Breast 18 Suppl 3:S56–8.

Wu Y, Cain-Hom C, Choy L et al (2010) Therapeutic antibody targeting of individual Notch receptors. Nature 464:1052–1059.

Yauch RL, Dijkgraaf GJ, Alicke B et al (2009) Smoothened mutation confers resistance to a Hedgehog pathway inhibitor in medulloblastoma. Science 326:572–4.

Yin L, Velazquez OC, Liu ZJ (2010) Notch signaling: emerging molecular targets for cancer therapy. Biochem Pharmacol 80:690–701.

You L, He B, Xu Z et al (2004) An anti-Wnt-2 monoclonal antibody induces apoptosis in malignant melanoma cells and inhibits tumor growth. Cancer Res 64:5385–9.

Younus J, Verma S, Franek J, Coakley N (2010) Sunitinib malate for gastrointestinal stromal tumour in imatinib mesylate-resistant patients: recommendations and evidence. Curr Oncol 17: 4–10.

Zama IN, Hutson TE, Elson P et al (2010) Sunitinib rechallenge in metastatic renal cell carcinoma patients. Cancer 116: 5400–6.

Zheng LS, Wang F, Li YH et al (2009) Vandetanib (Zactima, ZD6474) antagonizes ABCC1- and ABCG2-mediated multidrug resistance by inhibition of their transport function. PLoS One 4: e5172.

Zhou BB, Zhang H, Damelin M et al (2009) Tumour-initiating cells: challenges and opportunities for anticancer drug discovery. Nat Rev Drug Discov 8:806–23.

Zibat A, Missiaglia E, Rosenberger A et al (2010) Activation of the hedgehog pathway confers a poor prognosis in embryonal and fusion gene-negative alveolar rhabdomyosarcoma. Oncogene 29:6323–30.

Chapter 16
Cancer Stem Cell and ATP-Binding Cassette: Which Role in Chemoresistance?

Andrea Silvestrini, Elisabetta Meucci, Giuseppe Ettore Martorana, Bruno Giardina, and Alvaro Mordente

Introduction

"Man spends the first half of his life to ruin his health and the second half in search of healing himself." This aphorism of Leonardo da Vinci is cited here to point out a significant feature of the strategy against cancer: the presence of a plethora of drugs with broad activity is intended at challenging neoplastic cells in the near future and introduce humans to the *second half* of chemotherapy era, i.e., the "personal targeted therapy" and/or the safe combination therapeutic treatment *in search of healing*.

Surgery and/or radiotherapy are often not sufficient to induce long-lasting tumor regression in patients with cancer. Chemotherapy is therefore also required for the successful treatment of several neoplasias. Patients, however, almost invariably experience a recurrence after therapy and exhibit a so-called multidrug-resistant phenotype, i.e., chemoresistance or resistance of a particular tumor to chemotherapy (Marin et al. 2010). Some possible reasons for this failure include the intrinsic drug resistance of cancer stem cells (CSCs) and/or the inadequacy of the treatment. The phenomenon of chemoresistance becomes a central problem when toxicity of a drug increases to reach the same dosage necessary to kill cancer cells which then becomes the rate-limiting dose.

Exposure of cancer cells to a single anticancer drug may induce the achievement of multidrug resistance (MDR) phenotype, thus resulting in concurrent resistance to structurally distinct anticancer drugs (Assaraf 2006).

A. Silvestrini • E. Meucci • G.E. Martorana • B. Giardina • A. Mordente (✉)
Institute of Biochemistry and Clinical Biochemistry, Catholic University,
School of Medicine, Largo F. Vito 1, 00168 Rome, Italy
e-mail: alvaro.mordente@rm.unicatt.it

Furthermore, antineoplastic drugs can fail to kill cancer cells for various reasons (Broxterman et al. 2009; Marin et al. 2010). First of all, activation of detoxifying proteins (e.g., cytochrome P450) can promote drug resistance by inactivation/modification of chemotherapeutics agents. Otherwise, disruptions in apoptotic signaling pathways (e.g., p53 mutations) allow cells to become resistant to drug-induced cell death via apoptosis. Moreover, tumor cells can also activate mechanisms that repair DNA damage (e.g., DNA methylation changes upon exposure to the drug). Finally, active pumping drugs out of cells thus decreasing intracellular concentration can result from enhanced activity of efflux pumps, e.g., ATP-binding cassette transporters (ABC transporters). For all the above said reasons antitumor drug chemoresistance continues to create major obstacles to drug treatment of various human neoplasias. Here we provide an overview of the last point (i.e., efflux transporters) inferred from the most significant papers in this field.

ABC transporters function as efflux pumps which can extrude an array of structurally and functionally distinct cytotoxic drugs and may lead to failure of chemotherapeutic regimens in different human cancers.

The majority of these transporters actively pumps out of cells a plethora of physiological compounds, including peptides, steroids, ions, and lipids. Eukaryotes have eight ABC subfamilies (A–H) with seven of these (A–G) present in the human genome (Dean et al. 2001). The proteins expressed in humans are present in 49 ABC genes and their distribution is on different chromosomes (Tirona and Kim 2002).

Classification of ABC Transporters

ABC transporters represent a large superfamily of membrane proteins which mediate the transport of a multitude of molecules across membranes in every living organism (Saurin et al. 1999).

Whereas the nucleotide-binding domains (NBDs) are responsible for the binding and hydrolysis of ATP and, consequently, for the generation of driving force, the transmembrane domains (TMDs) form the translocation pathway for transported substrates across the membrane. Due to their common substrate (i.e., ATP), NBDs exhibit a number of conserved sequence motifs, including Walker A, Walker B, and the ABC signature, which is the peculiarity of the ABC superfamily. In contrast, the TMDs are more heterogeneous in sequence and structure, reflecting the diversity of transported compounds.

Physiological substrates of ABC transporters include endogenous molecules or metabolites (e.g., leukotrienes, steroids, bile salts, organic anions), and/or xenobiotics. Noteworthy, it is also clear that the physiological functions of these proteins should be diverse and organ specific (Johnstone et al. 2000).

Structural domains and ABC pump organization are reviewed in Sarkadi et al. (2006). Briefly, the structural requirements for functionally active transporters consist of two sets of hydrophobic segments that span the membrane (TMDs) and are thought to confer all or most of the substrate specificity of the transporter, and a

16 Cancer Stem Cell and ATP-Binding Cassette: Which Role in Chemoresistance?

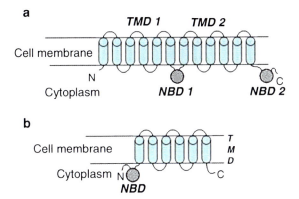

Fig. 16.1 Structural features of ABC transporters. Most of the transporters are membrane-associated with six membrane-spanning regions, and are characterized by the presence of the TMD region (ABC region). (**a**) ABCB1 typically is a full-length transporter of two identical halves as shown, with two NBDs that contain conserved sequences of the ABC. (**b**) ABCG2, on the other hand, is a half-transporter consisting of one NBD containing one TMD, composed by a six membrane-spanning domain

Table 16.1 Selected ABC transporters involved in MDR and class of antitumor drugs substrates. Overlapping substrate specificities of ABC transporters confer MDR to cancer cells (adapted from Szakács et al. 2006)

Name of ABC transporter	Drug class
ABCB1, ABCC1, ABCG2	Anthracyclines
ABCB1, ABCC1, ABCG2	Podophyllotoxins
ABCB1, ABCC1, ABCC2	Vinca alkaloids
ABCB1, ABCC2, ABCG2	Camptothecins
ABCB1, ABCC2, ABCG2	Kinase inhibitors

pair of NBDs. ABC genes either encode a full transporter encoding all four domains, or a half-transporter with a single TMD and a single NBD (Fig. 16.1). The so-called half-transporter proteins consisting of one TMD fused to one NBD (e.g., ABCG2) that can dimerize as either a homo- or heterodimer to form a biologically active and complete transporter complex. The classification of ABC transporters is based on the sequence analysis of the aminoacids in the ATP-binding domain. Thus, the ABC transporters are grouped into subfamilies based on the conservation of the NBD aminoacid sequence. Moreover, the ABC superfamily includes more than 300 proteins among which there are transporters of quite different compounds (Dean et al. 2001). The human genome encodes 49 ABC transporters that have been divided into seven groups (i.e., ABCA1-ABCA12, ABCB1-ABCB11, ABCC1-ABCC13, ABCD1-ABCD4, ABCE1, ABCF1-ABCF3, and ABCG1-ABCG5). Of these transporters, three are most often associated with MDR (see Table 16.1): the P-glycoprotein (P-gp), encoded by the *ABCB1* (or MDR-1) gene; the MDR-associated protein-1 (MRP-1) encoded by the *ABCC1* (or MRP-1) gene; and the breast cancer resistance protein (BCRP or ABCG2) encoded by the *ABCG2* gene.

ABC Transporters and MDR

It is particularly noteworthy that MDR tumors are a major barrier to effective tumor therapy and, along with metastasis, are estimated to be major contributors to death by cancer. Therefore, understanding the biochemical basis of MDR in order to develop clinical drugs or strategies to prevent the occurrence of resistance is a crucial goal for treating tumors nowadays. Reduction in cellular accumulation of drugs occurs via increased expression of ABC transporters. Considerably three transporters, belonging to the ABC family, have been implicated as major contributors to MDR in cancer. Discovered over 30 years ago, P-glycoprotein (P-gp; MDR1; ABCB1), MRP-1 (or ABCC1) and, more recently, ABCG2 (alias the BCRP) also appear to function as clinically relevant drug efflux pumps proteins. All these three proteins were discovered as factors overexpressed in MDR cell lines in cell culture and they have since been detected in patients with MDR tumors in vivo (Gottesman et al. 2002).

Moreover, these pumps are important for the absorption, distribution, and excretion of drugs, xenobiotics, and/or their modified metabolites. There is evidence that the intrinsic occurrence of ABC proteins modulates the resistance of tumors to a wide variety of structurally distinct chemotherapeutic drugs through their overexpression (Scotto and Johnson 2001). Two of the most widely studied transporters, P-gp/MDR-1 (ABCB1) and MRP-1 (ABCC1) have both been demonstrated to efflux a wide variety of the most commonly used anticancer drugs out of tumor cells (Table 16.1). Their overexpression correlates broadly with drug resistance in many different forms of neoplasias including pancreatic cancer (O'Driscoll et al. 2007), non-small cell lung cancer (NSCLC) (Roy et al. 2007), and breast cancer (Larkin et al. 2004), as well as in glioma (Calatozzolo et al. 2005). The P-glycoprotein, encoded by the *ABCB1* gene, was the first ABC transporter found to be overexpressed in MDR tumor cell lines (Riordan et al. 1985). Therefore, overcoming MDR phenotype is the major challenge to the successful chemotherapeutic treatment of many types of cancers in humans.

P-gp, MRP-1, and ABCG2 all exhibit an unusually broad range of substrate specificity, the so-called polyspecificity. These proteins have the potential to interact with several drugs as substrates (some in Fig. 16.2).

The upregulation of ABCB1 and ABCG2 transporters confers MDR to CSCs that may drive tumor progression and poor outcome of chemotherapy in anaplastic thyroid carcinoma (Zheng et al. 2010). Thus, treatment with doxorubicin, extruded by ABC transporters, conferred a growth advantage to CSCs which overgrew the culture. In fact inhibition of both ABCB1 and ABCG2 revealed that resistance of CSCs to doxorubicin may be mainly due to the overexpression of these ABC transporters (Zheng et al. 2010).

For these reasons, the missing piece of the puzzle is that of an inhibition of an ABC pump which can prevent MDR. The lack of response to this sentence implies that there are redundant mechanisms for resistance to drugs that are P-gp substrates, so that inhibition of this transporter alone may not sensitize cancer cells. In fact several clinical trials with inhibitors of P-gp fail to sensitize tumors to drugs.

Fig. 16.2 Chemical structure of some selected chemotherapeutic drug substrates of P-gp, MRP-1, and ABCG2

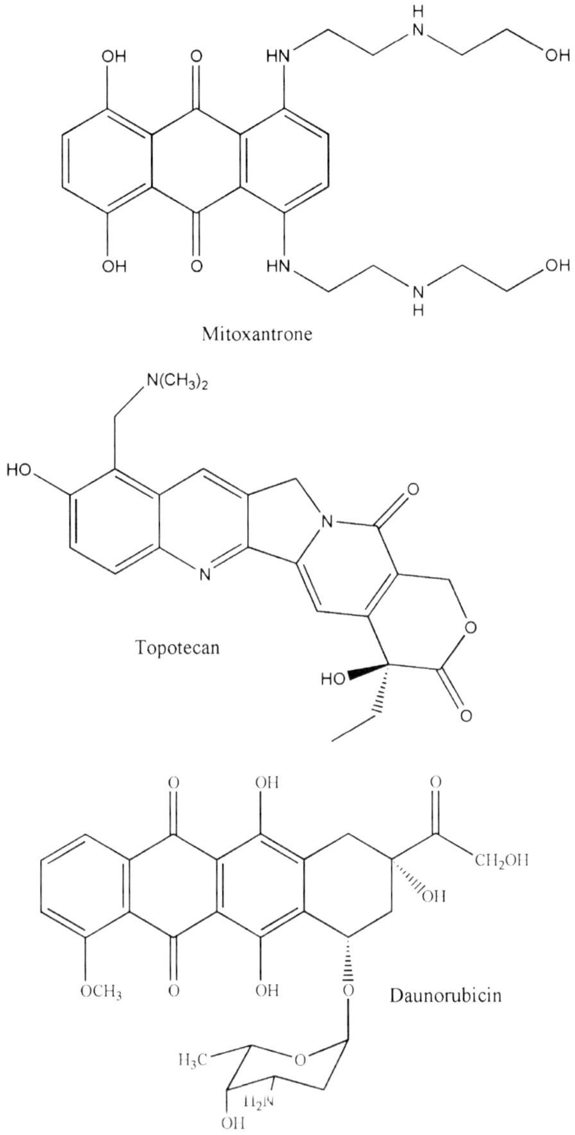

In this context, ABC proteins can, therefore, affect strongly drug therapy and resistance to treatment by multiple drugs has been associated with ABC protein expression in the target tissue. For instance, MDR to chemotherapeutic drugs is a serious barrier to successful treatment of many human cancers. To understand the importance of this phenomenon, all cancer-related deaths in the clinics are considered to be essentially a result of chemotherapy failure.

Table 16.2 Human ABC transporters classification with subfamily and indication of protein that confer MDR with organ or tissue localization

Subfamily	Members	Protein that confer MDR	Alias	Localization	References
ABCA	12	ABCA2	ABC2	B, K, L	Dean et al. (2001)
ABCB	11	ABCB1	P-gp/MDR1	MT, I, P, BBB, Lv, K	Ambudkar et al. (1999)
ABCC	13	ABCC1	MRP/MRP-1	MT, K, P, L, PBMC	Jedlitschky et al. (1996)
ABCD	4				
ABCE	1				
ABCF	3				
ABCG	6	ABCG2	BCRP/MXR	MT, P, Br, Lv, I	Doyle et al. (1998)

BBB blood–brain barrier, *B* brain, *Br* breast, *K* kidney, *L* lung, *P* placenta, *PBMC* peripheral blood mononuclear cells, *Lv* liver, *I* intestine, *MT* many tissues

In conclusion, MDR can have many causes but one important mechanism of drug resistance is the expression of active drug efflux pumps in the membranes of cancer cells and CSCs (Kakarala and Wicha 2008).

ABCB Subfamily: Characteristics and Tissue Distribution

Human ABCB subfamily consists of 11 members and includes both full transporters and half transporters. The most famous component of ABCB subfamily is ABCB1 (Fig. 16.1a) also known as P-gp discovered more than 30 years ago (Juliano and Ling 1976). The human *ABCB1* gene, containing 27 exons spans over 209 kb, is sited on chromosome 7q21–31 (Kolwankar et al. 2005). Structurally, the P-gp consists of 1,280 amino acids residues forming a full transporter configuration of 170 kDa. The amino acid sequence of P-gp is arranged as two repeating units of 610 residues that are joined by a linker region of about 60 amino acids (Chen et al. 1986). Each repeat has six TMD segments and a hydrophilic domain containing an ATP-binding site (NBD) (Fig. 16.1a).

Of the two human genes, encoding for P-gp (i.e., *MDR1* and *MDR2*), *MDR1* seems to confer most of drug resistance (Ambudkar et al. 2003).

It is particularly noteworthy that hydrophobicity, planar aromatic rings, and tertiary amino groups favor interaction with P-gp, but no highly conserved elements of recognition have been found. How a single protein can accommodate so many different structures is an unresolved mystery (Borst and Elferink 2002).

Substrates that bind to P-gp are generally organic molecules of amphipathic or lipid-soluble nature which frequently possess aromatic ring systems.

P-gp was found at the apical surface of cells in the kidney, liver, pancreas, the villous membrane of the small and large intestine, and the suprarenal glands (Thiebaut et al. 1987) (Table 16.2). Furthermore, it is highly expressed in bone marrow, at the blood–brain barrier (BBB), in placenta and the testes (Cascorbi 2006). In particular, the presence of P-gp in hematopoietic progenitor cells of the bone marrow protects these vital cells from drug toxicity during chemotherapy (van Tellingen et al. 2003). On the basis of tissue distribution, the physiological roles for P-gp have been speculated to be absorption, distribution, and excretion of xenobiotics, thus conferring one important function in the protection of tissues from toxic compounds. MDR has frequently been associated to the presence of P-gp, which is overexpressed in many drug-resistant cell lines and in a number of leukemias and solid tumors. Accordingly, P-gp seems to be a main player in clinical drug resistance in metastatic breast cancer (Fojo and Coley 2007). Drug-resistant cell lines treated with ABCB1 siRNA display increased intracellular drugs accumulation, leading to increased anticancer treatment sensitivity (Jonsson et al. 1999).

More recently, ABCB5 was found as a novel ABCB subfamily transporter encoded on chromosome 7p21–15.3 in human malignant melanoma (Frank et al. 2003). The human *ABCB5* gene consists of 16 exons and spans over 108 kb (Frank et al. 2003). ABCB5 is the third member of the human P-gp family next to its structural paralogs ABCB1 (2–5) and ABCB4. ABCB5, expressed on a subset of chemoresistant cells, functions as a rhodamine efflux transporter and regulates membrane potential and cell fusion (Frank et al. 2003). Moreover, ABCB5 has also been involved in doxorubicin efflux transport and it has been already exploited as therapeutic target by development of a specific antibody (Frank et al. 2005). The ABCB5-expressing cells accumulated significantly less drugs compared with melanoma cells that did not express ABCB5 (Frank et al. 2005). Furthermore, ABCB5 and ABCG2 positive cells were found expressed in a subpopulation of melanoma CSCs (Schatton et al. 2008) introducing a new perspective in therapeutic treatments.

ABCC Subfamily: Characteristics and Tissue Distribution

The human ABCC subfamily consists of ten members mostly implicated in MDR. This subfamily includes ABCC1 (MRP-1), ABCC2 (MRP-2), ABCC3 (MRP-3), ABCC4 (MRP-4), and other isoforms.

The most famous member is ABCC1 discovered by Cole et al. (1992) and originally called MRP-1, was found to mediate MDR in in vitro models of human lung cancer cell lines. Structurally, the human ABCC1 consists of 1531 aminoacid residues forming a full transporter with three transmembrane domains and two ATP-binding domains. Antitumor drug substrates of this transporter include epipodophyllotoxins, anthracyclines, camptothecins, and vinca alkaloids (Table 16.1).

Xenobiotics that enter in the body can be metabolized by oxidation (phase I metabolism) or made more hydrophilic by conjugation with glutathione (GSH), sulfate, or glucuronate (phase II metabolism). In physiological conditions, transported substrates of MRPs proteins appear in fact to be glucuronide- or glutathione- or sulfate-conjugated (Jedlitschky et al. 1996). As a result, transport by MRPs provides a link between drug efflux and the GSH system.

Single-nucleotide polymorphisms (SNPs) of ABC pump genes have been reported to play a key role in response to medication. Many SNPs in ABCC1 have been identified in human population and these SNPs are believed to result in differences in protein expression and/or function. The G1299T polymorphism resulted in increased doxorubicin resistance but decreased transport of some organic anions (Conrad et al. 2002).

In human beings, ABCC1 is ubiquitously expressed in the body (Table 16.2). The tissues showing the highest level of ABCC1 expression include the lung, testis, kidney, blood, and placenta (Sugawara et al. 1997). Moreover, it has been proposed that, in addition to extruding drugs through the plasma membrane, MRP-1 can confer drug-resistant phenotype to cells by sequestering the drugs into the intracellular compartments. This suggestion would resolve the contradiction of how a drug-resistant cell line expressing ABCC1 may exhibit the same level of intracellular drug accumulation as its drug-sensitive counterpart (Cole et al. 1992).

Increased levels of ABCC1 expression have been found in a wide range of hematological diseases [e.g., acute myeloblastic leukemia (AML), acute lymphoblastic leukemia (ALL), chronic lymphoblastic leukemia (CLL)] NSCLC and solid tumors (e.g., breast cancer, prostate cancer, gastric carcinoma, colorectal cancer, endometrial carcinoma, glioma, neuroblastoma, and retinoblastoma). Some of them, such as NSCLC or CLL, generally exhibit high level of ABCC1 expression and these tumors are therefore intrinsically multidrug resistant. Furthermore, ABCC1 can confer resistance to many commonly used neutral natural products, chemotherapeutic agents (i.e., vinca alkaloids, anthracyclines, podophyllotoxins) but also to various anionic compounds (i.e., methotrexate). Substrate specificity of ABCC1, and its distribution in tissues which are the major defense lines of the body, implies a physiological role for ABCC1 in protection against xenobiotics and toxins. Among the other ABCC members that appear to contribute to drug resistance, it must be remembered ABCC2 (MRP-2) that confers resistance to paclitaxel (Huisman et al. 2005). ABCC2 has a substrate selectivity analogous to that of ABCC1 but the tissue distribution is quite different from that of ABCC1. In fact, ABCC2 expression is restricted to the liver and kidney. Interestingly, ABCC1 and ABCC2 have been shown to act synergistically with several phase II conjugating enzymes including the GSH S-transferases (Leslie et al. 2004).

ABCC5, originally classified as an organic anion transporter, has been reported to confer resistance to several drugs (Wielinga et al. 2005).

Other ABCC isoforms (i.e., ABCC3-7, ABCC11, and ABCC12) exist, several of which are known to transport conjugated organic anions and could be involved in the protection of tissues from the toxic effects of arsenic (Leslie et al. 2004).

ABCG Subfamily: Characteristics and Tissue Distribution

ABCG subfamily consists of six members which have been shown to have mostly a role in transporting sterols across membranes. The most famous member of this subfamily, implicated in MDR, is ABCG2.

ABCG2, or BCRP (also named mitoxantrone resistance protein, MXR), is an ABC half-transporter (Fig. 16.1) that has been subjected to intense study since its discovery a decade ago (Miyake et al. 1999). *ABCG2* gene maps to chromosome 4q22, spans over 66 kb and consists of 16 exons and 15 introns. ABCG2 is a 72-kDa protein composed of 655 amino acids localized in plasma membrane (Bates et al. 2001). This transporter appears as a key drug extrusion pump in the context of anti-cancer multi drug resistance. It has an N-terminal ATP-binding domain (NBD) and a C-terminal transmembrane domain (TMD) (Fig. 16.1b), a structure half the size, and in reverse configuration, of most other ABC proteins which instead comprise two NBDs and two TMDs. Since ABCG2 is a half-transporter, it is believed to have to homodimerize, or possibly oligomerize, in order to function (Dean et al. 2001; Bates et al. 2001; Sharom 2008).

Variations at residue 482 of ABCG2 are found in many resistant cell lines, and the mutation of the wild-type arginine at this position to either threonine or glycine imparts the ability to transport rhodamine and changes the substrate specificity (Honjo et al. 2001) conferring MDR phenotype.

ABCG2 expression in tissues overlaps with P-gp, because the protein can be found in tissues such as the placenta, prostate, small intestine, brain, colon, liver, and ovary (Doyle et al. 1998) (Table 16.2). Moreover, the *ABCG2* gene is also expressed in the small intestine, thus its inhibition can also improve the systemic availability of the cancer drugs that have limited intestinal absorption due to active efflux by this transporter.

Notably, ABCG2 is often expressed in CSC populations, where it plays a crucial role in cellular protection, resulting in drug resistance and failure of cancer chemotherapy (Hirschmann-Jax et al. 2004; Ishikawa and Nakagawa 2009). ABCG2 is also found to be expressed in human hematopoietic stem cells (Scharenberg et al. 2002). Moreover, ABCG2 null hematopoietic cells were significantly more sensitive to mitoxantrone in vivo (Zhou et al. 2002). The suppression of ABCG2, by RNA interference, could significantly inhibit cancer cell proliferation (Chen et al. 2010). The overexpression of ABCG2 in various stem cells, makes this protein as a marker of the so-called SP (side population) cells (see below in section "Cancer Stem Cells' Chemoresistance"), representing pluripotent stem cells (Kim et al. 2002). The fact that ABCG2, which could reduce accumulation of chemotherapeutic agent, is especially highly expressed in stem cells makes it reasonable to assume that drug resistance is due to ABCG2 overexpressing in CSCs (Zhang et al. 2004).

Furthermore, ABCG2 is expressed not only in some cancer cells but also in a variety of normal tissues. For instance, ABCG2 is present in the apical membrane of placental syncytiotrophoblasts, in the endocrine cells of the pancreas, in the luminal membranes of villous epithelial cells in the small intestine and colon, in the bile canalicular membrane of hepatocytes, in ducts and lobules of the breast, and in venous and capillary endothelial cells of almost all tissues (Doyle et al. 1998; Sarkadi et al. 2004).

While ABCG2 is overexpressed in a variety of normal and malignant cells to efflux chemotherapeutic agents, endogenous ABCG2 expression in certain cancers is considered as a reflection of the differentiated phenotype of the cell of origin and likely contributes to intrinsic drug resistance.

Moreover, ABCG2 exhibits a broad range of substrate specificity (Table 16.1). Anticancer drug substrates of ABCG2 include, but are not limited to, the commonly used anticancer drugs like doxorubicin, mitoxantrone, and topotecan as well as the fluorescent dye Hoechst 33342.

The substrate specificity of ABCG2 is clearly distinct from other G-subfamily members, such as ABCG1, ABCG5, and ABCG8, which were all identified as cholesterol transporters (Schmitz et al. 2001), although cholesterol itself may affect ABCG2 activity (Storch et al. 2007).

Furthermore, ABCG2 transports a wide range of compounds, including large uncharged molecules or compounds with an amphiphilic character (Krishnamurthy and Schuetz 2006). A considerable overlap in anticancer drug substrate specificity between ABCG2 and P-gp should be noted, although there are also several differences in the substrate specificities of both transporters (Bates et al. 2001). Like P-gp, ABCG2 does not require glutathione (Krishnamurthy and Schuetz 2006), but, in contrast to P-gp, is able to transport phase two metabolites also conjugated with glucuronic acid and sulfates compounds (Ebert et al. 2005; Zamek-Gliszczynski et al. 2006).

In addition, ABCG2 expression appears to be sex-specific (Merino et al. 2005) and may be highly influenced by sexual steroids (Wang et al. 2008).

ABC Transporter Inhibitors

Since we have a better defined picture of the role of the ABC efflux pumps, the use of inhibitors have been obviously investigated in detail in studies on strategies to overcome MDR in cancer cell lines.

The ultimate goal is in fact to co-administer inhibitors with the anticancer compounds to make the treatment more effective and with minimal drug side-effects.

A variety of compounds have been discovered, known as modulators, inhibitors, or chemosensitizers that can reverse MDR mediated by the ABC multidrug efflux pumps. These molecules are able to reverse MDR in intact cells in vitro by interfering with the ability of the transporter to efflux drugs. Modulators generally do not kill MDR cells directly, but when they are co-administered with a cytotoxic drug, they restore cytotoxicity. Efflux of the drug is diminished or blocked, so that cancer cells are killed. Several inhibitors appear to interact with the substrate-binding pocket of the protein and compete with cytotoxic drugs for transport. This has led, initially, to the development of P-gp inhibitors. The concurrent presence of several ABC pump in tumors can, however, complicate the use of inhibitors.

First-generation P-gp inhibitors such as cyclosporin and verapamil (Fig. 16.3) are substrates of P-gp competing for the active binding site with drugs. It has been shown that these compounds inhibit drug pump function in MDR cell lines in vitro. Unfortunately, their use was limited by unacceptable toxicity and they failed in clinical settings, showing also an induction of P-gp activity on long-term administration (Lemma et al. 2006).

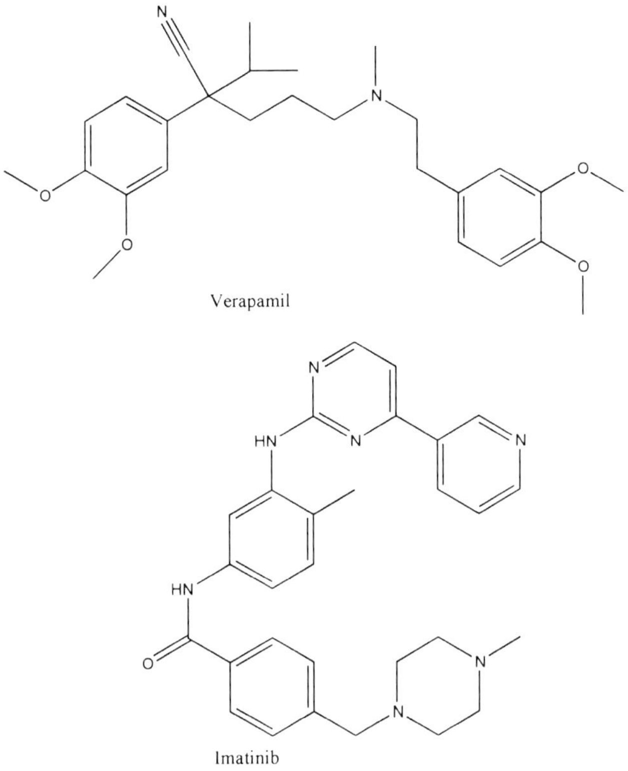

16 Cancer Stem Cell and ATP-Binding Cassette: Which Role in Chemoresistance?

Fig. 16.3 Chemical structure of representative ABC inhibitors; verapamil is a first-generation inhibitor and imatinib a tyrosine kinase inhibitor

The second generation agents, as the cyclosporine derivative valspodar (PSC-833), had unpredictable pharmacokinetic interactions targeting also other transporters. Moreover, this class of chemosensitizers acts as competitive substrates for the binding active site of the pump (Modok et al. 2006). The third-generation of P-gp inhibitors such as tariquidar, zosuquidar, and elacridar (Fig. 16.4), were developed to have a weak pharmacokinetic interaction. These drugs were designed in the first instance as ABC transporter inhibitors/competitors, in particular as P-gp inhibiting compounds (Stein and Walther 2006). These compounds have a high target affinity and specificity for P-gp and are being tested in phase III clinical trials in conjunction with chemotherapy agents to determine whether P-gp inhibition can restore, enhance or prolong drug sensitivity of cancer cells (Redmond et al. 2008).

The modulatory effects of plant flavonoids (Fig. 16.5) on cell MDR mediated by P-gp glycoprotein and related ABC transporters have been already reviewed by Di Pietro et al. (2002). Furthermore, natural products of relatively low toxicity, including curcumin, are reported to be inhibitors of ABC transporters (Anuchapreeda et al. 2002; Chearwae et al. 2004). Using curcumin as inhibitor has multiple advantages among which a low toxicity compared with most of third-generation inhibitors and a broad

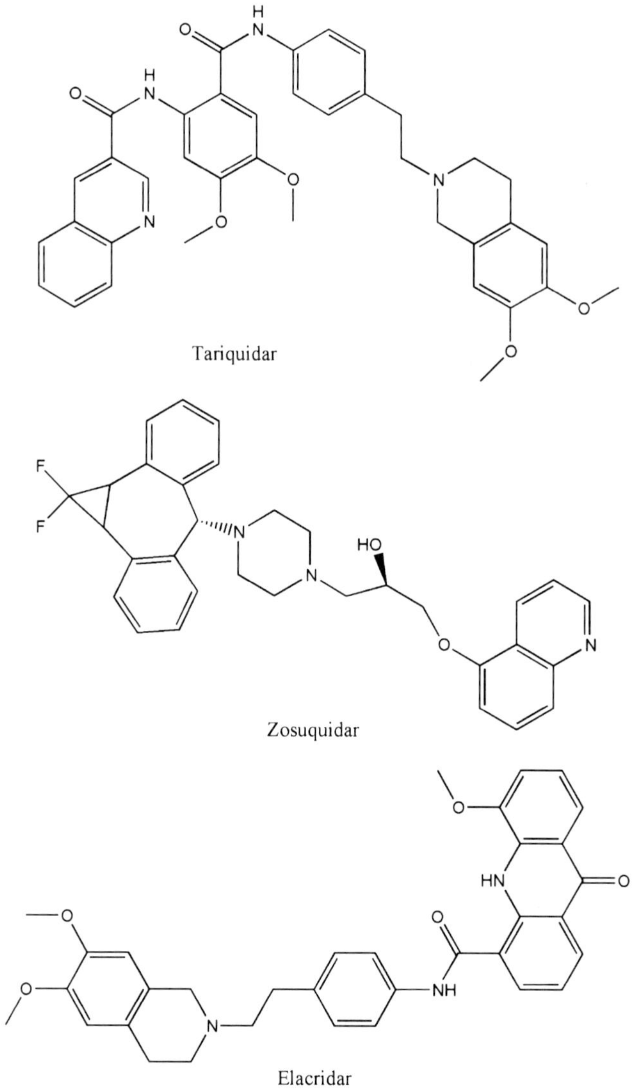

Fig. 16.4 Chemical structure of third-generation ABC inhibitors under clinical evaluation

spectrum of modulatory effects on ABC transporters. Limtrakul et al. (2007) have demonstrated that curcumin can inhibit the efflux function of ABCB1, ABCC1, and ABCG2 by direct binding to the ABC transporters.

In general, the protective action of flavonoids was attributed to their ability to bind to the active site of the transporters. A variety of flavonoid molecules have been shown to modulate ABC transporters activity in vitro and in cultured cells (Versantvoort et al. 1994; Ji and He 2007). Some of them have been also shown to have

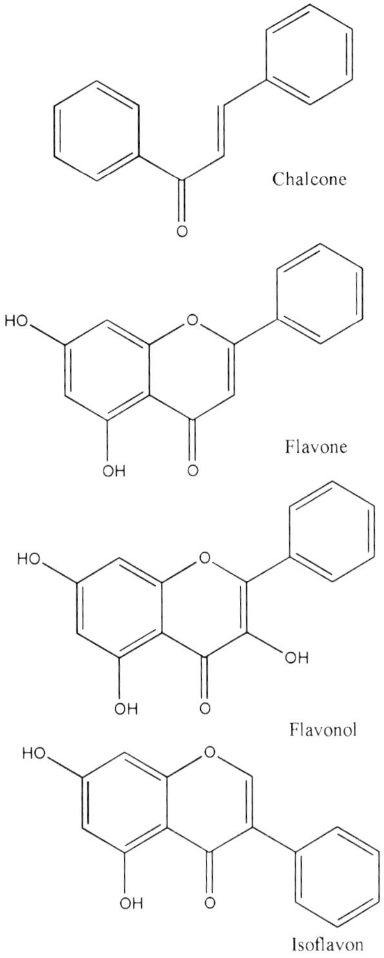

Fig. 16.5 Structure of the major classes of flavonoids

modulatory effects on both ABCC1 and ABCG2, vs. which specific new inhibitors have been identified (Zhang et al. 2004). Moreover, flavonoids can increase the oral bioavailability of paclitaxel in rats (Choi et al. 2004). The MDR efflux pump was inhibited by isoflavonoids (Fig. 16.5) such as genistein, daidzoin, sophoraisoflavone, licoisoflavone, and chrysin (Bobrowska-Hagerstrand et al. 2001). It has been suggested that isoflavones interact directly with the substrate-binding site of ABC transporters acting just like competitive inhibitors (Ji and He 2007).

Dualistic effects, i.e., P-gp modulation and antitumor activity, of flavonoids may synergistically act in cancer chemotherapy. The application of flavonoids as P-gp modulators to improve efficacy of drugs like taxanes, anthracyclines, epipodophyllotoxins, camptothecins and vinca alkaloids could be explored (Bansal et al. 2009). Thus the inhibition of ABC transporters by flavonoids may provide an innovative approach in reversing MDR in CSCs.

Clinical evidence indicates that the emergence of drug-resistant clones is through the acquisition of mutations and clonal evolution, such as the *BCR–ABL* mutations that arise in imatinib-resistant in chronic myeloid leukemia (Lee et al. 2008).

One of the most successful targeted therapies is represented by tyrosine kinase inhibitors (TKIs) such as imatinib (Gleevec) (Fig. 16.3) a drug-inhibiting activated ABL in patients with CML or with ALL associated with translocation t(9;22) (q34;q11). Imatinib is both an ABCG2 substrate and inhibitor, susceptible to efflux from stem cells that express this transporter. However, leukemia stem cells are not dependent on ABL for growth. Therefore, since imatinib successfully inhibits the non-stem cells and induces remission, the patient must remain on the drug. Alternative approaches using monoclonal antibodies have been used to mitigate or overcome MDR response of neoplastic cell. A monoclonal antibody anti-P-gp was shown to modulate the efflux of drugs in vitro (Mechetner and Roninson 1992).

Various interactions between cholesterol and P-gp have been suggested, including a role for the protein in transbilayer movement of cholesterol (Eckford and Sharom 2008). The ABC pumps appear also to require their substrates to be conjugated with a lipid. Statins are the widely used inhibitors of HMG-CoA reductase and they should also be able to mitigate MDR in cancer (Mehta and Mehta 2010). Moreover, it has been shown that statins enhance susceptibility to doxorubicin-induced apoptosis in human rhabdomyosarcoma and neuroblastoma cells and lead to higher drugs accumulation in tumor cells via inhibition of ABC transporters (Sieczkowski et al. 2010). Interestingly, the same authors found that full maturation of glycosylated ABCB1 is affected by statins. Glycosylation of ABCB1 is important for appropriate protein folding and plasma membrane export. The core-glycosylated in contrast to the fully glycosylated species of ABCB1 is inactive (Sieczkowski et al. 2010).

Cancer Stem Cells' Chemoresistance

During the past few years, various studies have suggested that tumors are composed of various cell populations having different properties, among which a population of cancer cells called CSCs that maintain tumor formation and growth. In CSCs, the pathway of self-renewal and differentiation are deregulated with consequent unlimited self-renewal and a buildup of excess CSCs. Moreover, CSCs have unusual differentiation programs that generate progenitor tumor cells, which then proliferate to form the bulk of the tumor (Zhou et al. 2009). Support on CSCs was first documented in leukemia and myeloma, and, so far, their existence has been validated in several solid tumors, such as colon, breast, liver, and pancreas (Ischenko et al. 2008). Investigators have thus suggested that the cell surface markers could be used to identify and purify CSCs from tumors (Li et al. 2007).

Furthermore, the CSC hypothesis offers an attractive model of carcinogenesis and, at the same time, also helps explain the mechanism(s) of drug resistance and tumor relapse. On the basis of CSC model, a tumor contains a heterogeneous population of adult cancer cells and a small number of CSCs (Dean et al. 2005; Zhou et al. 2009).

Therapies have been mainly developed to kill most of the tumor cells, but CSCs, which have intrinsic detoxifying mechanisms, can easily escape conventional treatments and result refractory. The CSC model thus explains why conventional chemotherapy may result in tumor cells reduction and, on the other hand, why most tumors relapse showing MDR.

In CML, a TKI dramatically depleted adult cells but failed to reduce CSCs, which then leaded to disease development. In mantle cell lymphoma CSC-targeted therapy is mandatory to overcome MDR and treat definitively tumor cells (Kahl 2009).

Furthermore, it has been described that several TKIs are able to interact with members of the ABC family transporters such as ABCG2 and ABCB1, increasing the accumulation of anticancer drugs in ABC transporter-overexpressing cells (Shi et al. 2007). These studies have been focused on the interaction between TKIs and ABCG2, while limited information is available for the interaction of ABCC1 or other members of the ABCC subfamily with these drugs.

Although already proposed some years ago (Lapidot et al. 1994; Goodell et al. 1996; Reya et al. 2001), only recently the CSC hypothesis has come into focus. CSCs have been defined as "a small subset of cancer cells within a cancer that constitute a reservoir of self-sustaining cells with the exclusive ability to self-renew and to cause the heterogeneous lineages of cancer cells that comprise the tumor" (Clarke et al. 2006).

Since the expression and activity of ABC transporters are elevated in normal stem cells, this led to testing whether these pumps were able to efflux lipophilic fluorescent DNA intercalating dyes. Thus cells that were able to efflux dyes have been termed the "side population" cells, since they are identified in the fluorescence-activated cell sorter as cells that do not retain the dye (Goodell et al. 1996).

"Side population" (SP), a subpopulation of cells that is thus distinguished from the main population on the basis of dye exclusion was initially used to identify the pluripotent hematopoietic stem cell compartment first discovered within the bone marrow (Tang et al. 2007). These cells have the potential to repopulate their own "self-renewing" pool and manage hematopoietic stores or differentiate into lineage-specific lymphoid and myeloid cells to replenish the turnover of cells within the immune system. One idea was that these isolated "side population" stem-like cells evolved mechanisms to avoid natural xenobiotic toxicity by expressing ATP-dependent cell surface pumps referred to as ABC transporters.

A loss of expression leads to cell differentiation, indicating that P-gp and ABCG2 might determine stem cell-induced tissue remodeling through their differential expression. In fact, SP cells have been implicated in the regeneration of various organs, such as liver (Lagasse et al. 2000), skeletal muscles (Jackson et al. 1999), and cardiac muscles (Jackson et al. 2001).

The identification of CSCs, or tumor-initiating cells, has focused renewed attention on the role of ABC transporters in drug resistance, and as cancer target therapy.

It assumes that the malignancy contains a small subpopulation of CSCs possessing the ability to generate tumors. These cells are intrinsically multidrug resistant through their ABC transporter expression as well as their capacity for DNA repair (Al-Hajj et al. 2003). Thus, drug treatment does not kill CSCs and these cells support relapse of the tumor. Most CSCs appear to evade cytotoxic therapies or irradiation through active mechanisms.

Another clinically relevant inherent property of stem cells is their ability to pump drugs out of the cell through the use of the ABC family of drug transporters. If these efflux pumps could be inhibited, CSCs could be more susceptible to current or newly designed chemotherapeutic agents used in conjunction.

An important milestone was that overexpression of ABC transporters is thought to be central to the acquisition of multidrug-resistant phenotype in CSCs in primary human brain tumors (Bredel 2001) in leukemia and lymphoma cells (Dean et al. 2005). Since this class of proteins were relatively recently discovered, there is an increasing body of evidence that their expression and activity correlate with cancer stem-like phenotypes (Wu and Alman 2008).

Interestingly, the fact that ABCG2 could reduce accumulation of chemotherapeutic agent, and is especially highly expressed in stem cells makes it reasonable to assume that intrinsic drug resistance of CSCs is due to ABCG2 overexpression (Wu and Alman 2008).

At last, CSCs seem to become resistant to anticancer drugs by several mechanisms. In this scenario, there are three major mechanisms of drug chemoresistance in CSC: (1) decreased uptake of water-soluble drugs which require transporters to enter cells; (2) various changes in cells that affect the capacity of cytotoxic drugs to kill cells (e.g., increased repair of DNA damage, reduced apoptosis); and (3) increased ATP-dependent efflux of drugs.

These concepts suggest the clinical relevance of CSCs and drive the study of a "future targeted therapy" to these cells in order to reduce the relapse of cancer.

Conclusions and Perspectives

The effective chemotherapy of cancer continues to be hindered by the resistance of tumor cells to chemotherapeutic agents.

At the moment of this writing, the model is that CSCs are resistant to chemotherapy through their relative quiescence, their capacity for DNA repair, decreased entry into apoptosis, and ABC transporter overexpression. All this provides mechanisms by which at least some tumor stem cells survive at chemotherapy and could relapse even several years after treatments. Thus, in order to treat cancer, it is essential to focus on the removal of CSCs. It is apparent that expression of critical ABC transporters remains on in certain adult tissues such as in the kidney. In fact, in renal cancer cells, ABCB1 is expressed in all cells and these tumors thus rarely respond to primary chemotherapy treatment. Therefore, a CSC model of drug resistance has been popularized.

A priori, it is unlikely that some tumors would not just use such a wonderful mechanism to defend themselves against drugs. As a result, overexpression of ABC transporters occurs in cancer cell lines and tumors that are multidrug resistant.

To date, more than 300 ABC transporters have been described, classified, localized, and functionally evaluated in diverse organisms from microbes to humans. The majority of these proteins actively transport an array of biological compounds. Several ABC transporters have been recognized as a source of drug resistance in the treatment of malignancies. In particular, ABCG2 is the latest of drug efflux ABC transporters discovered from a doxorubicin-resistant MCF-7 breast cancer cell line (Scheffer et al. 2000). Since then, the function of this transporter has been studied extensively in terms of MDR. So that ABCG2 has been considered as one of the major transporters causing drug resistance in CSCs.

Actually, the ability to predict response to chemotherapy and to prevent chemoresistance with the targeted therapy will permit selection of the best adjuvant therapy for human beings. Finally, administration of MDR inhibitors as adjuvant therapy is shown to improve the remission rate of patients with acute myeloid leukemia (Chauncey et al. 2000). Thus, in the next future the advances in our understanding of multidrug ABC transporters can provide clinical solution. Understanding the basis of CSC behavior will allow for the design of new strategies, including combination therapies to counteract MDR. Encouragingly, limiting chemoresistance induced by ABC transporters could be important for ameliorating cancer patients; this may be achieved by combining standard cytotoxic chemotherapy with targeted approaches in a "personal" combination therapy with inhibitors/modulators of ABC transporters. Thus, the design of a personally tailored therapy and a precocious diagnosis has a crucial role to accompany our knowledge on the *second half* of the chemotherapy era.

References

Al-Hajj, M, Wicha, MS, Benito-Hernandez, A, Morrison, SJ, Clarke, MF. (2003) Prospective identification of tumorigenic breast cancer cells. Proc Natl Acad Sci USA. 100(7):3983–8.

Ambudkar, SV, Dey, S, Hrycyna, CA, Ramachandra, M, Pastan,I, Gottesman, MM. (1999) Biochemical, cellular, and pharmacological aspects of the multidrug transporter. Annu Rev Pharmacol Toxicol. 39: 361–98.

Ambudkar, SV, Kimchi-Sarfaty, C, Sauna, ZE, Gottesman, MM (2003) P-glycoprotein: from genomics to mechanism. Oncogene 22(47): 7468–85.

Anuchapreeda, S, Leechanachai, P, Smith, M M, Ambudkar, S V, and Limtrakul, P N (2002) Modulation of P-glycoprotein expression and function by curcumin in multidrug-resistant human KB cells. Biochem Pharmacol 64: 573–582.

Assaraf, Y G (2006) The role of multidrug resistance efflux transporters in antifolate resistance and folate homeostasis. Drug Resist. Updat. 9: 227–246.

Bansal, T, Jaggi, M, Khar, RK, Talegaonkar, S (2009) Emerging significance of flavonoids as P-glycoprotein inhibitors in cancer chemotherapy. J Pharm Pharm Sci. 12(1):46–78.

Bates, SE, Robey, R, Miyake, K, Rao, K, Ross, DD, Litman, T (2001) The role of half-transporters in multidrug resistance. J. Bioenerg. Biomembr. 33: 503–11.

Bobrowska-Hagerstrand, M, Wrobel, A, Rychlik, B, Bartosz, G, Soderstrom, T, Shirataki, Y, Motohashi, N, Molnar, J, Michalak, K, Hagerstrand, H (2001) Monitoring of MRP-like activity in human erythrocytes: inhibitory effect of isoflavones. Blood Cells Mol Dis 27: 894–900.

Borst, P, Elferink, RO (2002) Mammalian ABC transporters in health and disease. Annu Rev Biochem. 71:537–92.

Bredel M (2001) Anticancer drug resistance in primary human brain tumors. Brain Res Brain Res Rev 35: 161–204.

Broxterman, HJ, Gotink, KJ, Verheul, HM (2009) Understanding the causes of multidrug resistance in cancer: a comparison of doxorubicin and sunitinib. Drug Resist Updat. 12(4-5):114–26.

Calatozzolo, C, Gelati, M, Ciusani, E, Sciacca, FL, Pollo, B, Cajola, L, Marras, C, Silvani, A, Vitellaro-Zuccarello, L, Croci, D, Boiardi, A, Salmaggi, A (2005). Expression of drug resistance proteins P-gp, MRP1, MRP3, MRP5 and GST-pi in human glioma. J Neurooncol. 74(2):113–21.

Cascorbi I (2006) Role of pharmacogenetics of ATP-binding cassette transporters in the pharmacokinetics of drugs. Pharmacol Ther. 112(2):457–73.

Chauncey, TR, Rankin, C, Anderson,JE, Chen, I, Kopecky, KJ, Godwin, JE, Kalaycio, ME, Moore, DF, Shurafa, MS, Petersdorf, SH, Kraut, EH, Leith, CP, Head, DR, Luthardt, FW, Willman, CL, Appelbaum, FR (2000) A phase I study of induction chemotherapy for older patients with newly diagnosed acute myeloid leukemia (AML) using mitoxantrone, etoposide, and the MDR modulator PSC 833: a southwest oncology group study 9617. Leuk Res 24(7): 567–74.

Chearwae, W, Anuchapreeda, S, Nandigama, K, Ambudkar, SV, Limtrakul, P (2004) Biochemical mechanism of modulation of human P-glycoprotein (ABCB1) by curcumin I, II, and III purified from Turmeric powder. Biochem Pharmacol. 68(10): 2043–2052.

Chen, CJ, Chin, JE, Ueda, K, Clark,DP, Pastan, I, Gottesman, MM, Roninson, IB (1986) Internal duplication and homology with bacterial transport proteins in the mdr1 (P-glycoprotein) gene from multidrug-resistant human cells. Cell. 47(3): 381–9.

Chen, Z, Liu, F, Ren, Q, Zhao, Q, Ren, H, Lu, S, Zhang, L, Han, Z (2010) Suppression of ABCG2 inhibits cancer cell proliferation. International Journal of Cancer 126 (4): 841–851.

Choi, J S, Jo, B W, Kim, Y C (2004) Enhanced paclitaxel bioavailability after oral administration of paclitaxel or prodrug to rats pretreated with quercetin. Eur J Pharm Biopharm, 57: 313–318.

Clarke, M F, Dick, J E, Dirks, P B, Eaves, C J, Jamieson, Catriona HM, Jones, D L, Visvader, J, Weissman, I L, Wahl, G M (2006) Cancer Stem Cells-Perspectives on Current Status and Future Directions: AACR Workshop on Cancer Stem Cells. Cancer Res 66: 9339–9344.

Cole, S P, Bhardwaj, G, Gerlach, J H, Mackie, J E, Grant, C E, Almquist, K C, Stewart, A J, Kurz, E U, Duncan, A M and Deeley, R G (1992) Overexpression of a transporter gene in a multidrug-resistant human lung cancer cell line. Science 258, 1650–1654.

Conrad, S, Kauffmann, HM, Ito, K, Leslie, EM, Deeley, RG, Schrenk, D, Cole, SP (2002). A naturally occurring mutation in *MRP1* results in a selective decrease in organic anion transport and in increased doxorubicin resistance. Pharmacogenetics 12: 321–330.

Dean, M, Fojo, T, Bates, S (2005) Tumour stem cells and drug resistance. Nat Rev Cancer 5: 275-284.

Dean, M, Rzhetsky, A, Allikmets, R (2001) The human ATP-binding cassette (ABC) transporter superfamily. Genome Res. 11(7):1156–66.

Di Pietro, A, Conseil, G, Perez-Victoria, JM, Dayan, G, Baubichon-Cortay, H, Trompier, D, Steinfels, E, Jault, J M, deWet, H, Maitrejean, M, Comte, G, Boumendjel, A, Mariotte, A M, Dumontet, C, McIntosh, D B, Goffeau, A, Castanys, S, Gamarro, F, Barron, D (2002) Modulation by flavonoids of cell multidrug resistance mediated by P-glycoprotein and related ABC transporters. Cell Mol Life Sci 59: 307–322.

Doyle, LA, Yang, W, Abruzzo, LV, Krogmann, T, Gao, Y, Rishi, AK, and Ross, DD (1998) A multidrug resistance transporter from human MCF-7 breast cancer cells. Proc Natl Acad Sci 95: 15665–15670.

Ebert, B, Seidel, A, Lampen A (2005) Identification of BCRP as transporter of benzo[a]pyrene conjugates metabolically formed in Caco-2 cells and its induction by Ah-receptor agonists. Carcinogenesis 26(10):1754–63.

Eckford, P D W, and Sharom, F J (2008) Interaction of the P-Glycoprotein Multidrug Efflux Pump with Cholesterol: Effects on ATPase Activity, Drug Binding and Transport. Biochemistry 47(51): 13686–13698.

Fojo, T, Coley, H M (2007) The role of efflux pumps in drug-resistant metastatic breast cancer: new insights and treatment strategies. Clin. Breast Cancer 7: 749–756.

Frank, NY, Margaryan, A, Huang, Y, Schatton, T, Waaga-Gasser, AM, Gasser, M, Sayegh, MH, Sadee, W, Frank, MH (2005) ABCB5-mediated doxorubicin transport and chemoresistance in human malignant melanoma. Cancer Res. 65(10):4320–33.

Frank, NY, Pendse, SS, Lapchak, PH, Margaryan, A, Shlain, D, Doeing, C, Sayegh, MH, Frank, MH. (2003) Regulation of progenitor cell fusion by ABCB5 P-glycoprotein, a novel human ATP-binding cassette transporter. J Biol Chem 278: 47156–65.

Goodell, MA, Brose, K, Paradis, G, Conner, AS, Mulligan, RC (1996) Isolation and functional properties of murine hematopoietic stem cells that are replicating in vivo. J Exp Med. 183(4):1797–806.

Gottesman, MM, Fojo, T, Bates, SE (2002) Multidrug resistance in cancer: role of ATP-dependent transporters. Nat Rev Cancer. 2(1): 48–58.

Hirschmann-Jax, C, Foster, AE, Wulf, GG, Nuchtern, JG, Jax, TW, Gobel, U, Goodell, MA, Brenner, MK (2004) A distinct "side population" of cells with high drug efflux capacity in human tumor cells. Proc Natl Acad Sci USA. 101: 14228–14233.

Honjo, Y, Hrycyna, C A, Yan, Q W, Medina-Perez, W Y, Robey, R W, van de Laar, A, Litman, T, Dean, M, Bates, S E (2001) Acquired mutations in the MXR/BCRP/ABCP gene alter substrate specificity in MXR/BCRP/ABCP-overexpressing cells. Cancer Res. 61: 6635–9.

Huisman, M T, Chhatta, A A, van Tellingen, O, Beijnen, J H, Schinkel, A H (2005) MRP2 (ABCC2) transports taxanes and confers paclitaxel resistance and both processes are stimulated by probenecid. Int. J. Cancer 116: 824–9.

Ischenko, I, Seeliger, H, Schaffer, M, Jauch, KW, Bruns, CJ (2008) Cancer stem cells: how can we target them? Curr Med Chem. 15(30): 3171–84.

Ishikawa, T, Nakagawa, H (2009) Human ABC transporter ABCG2 in cancer chemotherapy and pharmacogenomics. J Exp Ther Oncol. 8(1):5–24.

Jackson, KA, Majka, SM, Wang, H, Pocius, J, Hartley, CJ, Majesky, MW, Entman, ML, Michael, LH, Hirschi, KK, Goodell, MA (2001) Regeneration of ischemic cardiac muscle and vascular endothelium by adult stem cells. J Clin Invest. 107(11):1395–402.

Jackson, KA, Mi, T, Goodell, MA (1999) Hematopoietic potential of stem cells isolated from murine skeletal muscle. Proc Natl Acad Sci USA. 96(25):14482–6.

Jedlitschky, G, Leier, I, Buchholz, U, Barnouin, K, Kurz, G, Keppler, D (1996) Transport of glutathione, glucuronate, and sulfate conjugates by the MRP gene-encoded conjugate export pump. Cancer Res. 56(5): 988–94.

Ji, BS, He, L (2007) CJY, an isoflavone, reverses P-glycoprotein-mediated multidrug-resistance in doxorubicin-resistant human myelogenous leukaemia (K562/DOX) cells. J Pharm Pharmacol. 59(7):1011–5.

Johnstone, RW, Ruefli, AA, Smyth, MJ. (2000) Multiple physiological functions for multidrug transporter P-glycoprotein? Trends Biochem Sci 25:1–6.

Jonsson, O, Behnam-Motlagh, P, Persson, M, Henriksson, R, Grankvist, K. (1999) Increase in doxorubicin cytotoxicity by carvedilol inhibition of P-glycoprotein activity. Biochem. Pharmacol. 58(11) 1801–1806.

Juliano, R L, Ling, V (1976) A surface glycoprotein modulating drug permeability in Chinese hamster ovary cell mutants. Biochim. Biophys. Acta 455: 152–162.

Kahl, BS (2009) Frontline therapy in mantle cell lymphoma: the role of high-dose therapy and integration of new agents. Curr Hematol Malig Rep. 4(4):213–7.

Kakarala, M, Wicha, M S (2008) Implications of the cancer stem-cell hypothesis for breast cancer prevention and therapy. J Clin Oncol 26:2813–20.

Kim, M, Turnquist,H, Jackson, J, Sgagias, M, Yan, Y, Gong, M, Dean, M, Sharp, J G, Cowan, K (2002) The multidrug resistance transporter ABCG2 (breast cancer resistance protein 1) effluxes Hoechst 33342 and is overexpressed in hematopoietic stem cells. Clin. Cancer Res. 8: 22–28.

Kolwankar, D, Glover, DD, Ware, JA, Tracy, TS (2005) Expression and function of ABCB1 and ABCG2 in human placental tissue. Drug Metab. Dispos. 33(4) 524–529.

Krishnamurthy, P, Schuetz, JD (2006) Role of ABCG2/BCRP in biology and medicine. Annu Rev Pharmacol Toxicol. 46: 381–410.

Lagasse, E, Connors, H, Al-Dhalimy, M, Reitsma, M, Dohse, M, Osborne, L, Wang, X, Finegold, M, Weissman, IL, Grompe, M (2000) Purified hematopoietic stem cells can differentiate into hepatocytes in vivo. Nat Med. 6(11):1229–34.

Lapidot, T, Sirard, C, Vormoor, J, Murdoch, B, Hoang, T, Caceres-Cortes, J, Minden, M, Paterson, B, Caligiuri, MA, Dick, JE (1994) A cell initiating human acute myeloid leukaemia after transplantation into SCID mice. Nature 367(6464):645–8.

Larkin, A, O'Driscoll, L, Kennedy, S, Purcell, R, Moran, E, Crown, J, Parkinson, M, Clynes, M (2004) Investigation of MRP-1 protein and MDR-1 P-glycoprotein expression in invasive breast cancer: a prognostic study. Int J Cancer. 112(2): 286–94.

Lee, F, Fandi, A, Voi, M (2008) Overcoming kinase resistance in chronic myeloid leukemia. Int J Biochem Cell Biol. 40(3):334–43.

Lemma, GL, Wang, Z, Hamman, MA, Zaheer, NA, Gorski, JC, Hall, SD (2006) The effect of short- and long-term administration of verapamil on the disposition of cytochrome P450 3A and P-glycoprotein substrates. Clin Pharmacol Ther. 79(3):218–30.

Leslie, E M, Haimeur, A, Waalkes, MP (2004) Arsenic transport by the human multidrug resistance protein 1 (MRP1/ABCC1): Evidence that a tri-glutathione conjugate is required. J. Biol. Chem. 279: 32700–32708.

Li, C, Heidt, DG, Dalerba, P, Burant, CF, Zhang, L, Adsay, V, Wicha, M, Clarke, MF, Simeone, DM (2007) Identification of pancreatic cancer stem cells. Cancer Res 67: 1030–7.

Limtrakul, P, Chearwae, W, Shukla, S, Phisalphong, C, Ambudkar, SV (2007) Modulation of function of three ABC drug transporters, P-glycoprotein (ABCB1), mitoxantrone resistance protein (ABCG2) and multidrug resistance protein 1 (ABCC1) by tetrahydrocurcumin, a major metabolite of curcumin. Mol Cell Biochem. 296(1-2): 85–95.

Marin, JJ, Romero, MR, Briz, O (2010) Molecular bases of liver cancer refractoriness to pharmacological treatment. Curr Med Chem. 17(8): 709–40.

Mechetner, EB, Roninson, IB (1992) Efficient inhibition of P-glycoprotein-mediated multidrug resistance with a monoclonal antibody. Proc Natl Acad Sci USA. 89(13): 5824–5828.

Mehta, NG, Mehta, M (2010) Overcoming multidrug-resistance in cancer: Statins offer a logical candidate. Med Hypotheses 74(2):237–9.

Merino, G, van Herwaarden, AE, Wagenaar, E, Jonker, JW, Schinkel, AH (2005) Sex-dependent expression and activity of the ATP-binding cassette transporter breast cancer resistance protein (BCRP/ABCG2) in liver. Mol Pharmacol. 67(5): 1765–1771.

Miyake, K, Mickley, L, Litman, T, Zhan, Z, Robey, R, Cristensen, B, Brangi, M, Greenberger, L, Dean, M, Fojo, T, Bates, SE (1999) Molecular cloning of cDNAs which are – highly overexpressed in mitoxantrone-resistant cells: demonstration of homology to ABC transport genes. Cancer Res. 59: 8–13.

Modok, S, Mellor, HR, Callaghan, R (2006) Modulation of multidrug resistance efflux pump activity to overcome chemoresistance in cancer. Curr Opin Pharmacol. 6(4):350–4.

O'Driscoll, L, Walsh, N, Larkin, A, Ballot, J, Ooi, WS, Gullo, G, O'Connor, R, Clynes, M, Crown, J, Kennedy, S (2007) MDR1/P-glycoprotein and MRP-1 drug efflux pumps in pancreatic carcinoma. Anticancer Res. 27: 2115–20.

Redmond, KM, Wilson, TR, Johnston, PG, Longley, DB (2008) Resistance mechanisms to cancer chemotherapy. Front Biosci. 13:5138–54.

Reya, T, Morrison, SJ, Clarke, MF, Weissman, IL (2001) Stem cells, cancer, and cancer stem cells. Nature. 414(6859):105–11.

Riordan, JR, Deuchars, K, Kartner, N, Alon, N, Trent, J, Ling, V (1985) Amplification of P-glycoprotein genes in multidrug-resistant mammalian cell lines. Nature 316(6031):817–9.

Roy, S, Kenny, E, Kennedy, S, Larkin, A, Ballot, J, Perez, De Villarrea,l M, Crown, J, O'Driscoll, L (2007) MDR1/P-glycoprotein and MRP-1 mRNA and protein expression in non-small cell lung cancer. Anticancer Res. 27: 1325–30.

Sarkadi, B, Homolya, L, Szakács, G, Váradi, A (2006) Human multidrug resistance ABCB and ABCG transporters: participation in a chemoimmunity defense system. Physiol Rev. 86(4):1179–236.

Sarkadi, B, Ozvegy-Laczka, C, Német, K, Váradi, A (2004) ABCG2 – a transporter for all seasons. FEBS Lett. 567(1):116–20.

Saurin, W, Hofnung, M, Dassa, E (1999) Getting in or out: early segregation between importers and exporters in the evolution of ATP-binding cassette (ABC) transporters, J. Mol. Evol. 48: 22–41.

Scharenberg, CW, Harkey, MA, Torok-Storb, B (2002) The ABCG2 transporter is an efficient Hoechst 33342 efflux pump and is preferentially expressed by immature human hematopoietic progenitors. Blood 99(2): 507–512.

Schatton, T, Murphy, G F, Frank, N Y, Yamaura, K, Waaga-Gasser, A M, Gasser, M, Zhan, Q, Jordan, S, Duncan, L M, Weishaupt, C, Fuhlbrigge, R C, Kupper, T S, Sayegh, M H, Frank, M H (2008) Identification of cells initiating human melanomas. Nature 451: 345–349.

Scheffer, GL, Maliepaard, M, Pijnenborg, AC, van Gastelen, MA, de Jong, MC, Schroeijers, AB, van der Kolk, DM, Allen, JD, Ross, DD, van der Valk, P, Dalton, WS, Schellens, JH, Scheper, RJ (2000) Breast cancer resistance protein is localized at the plasma membrane in mitoxantrone- and topotecan-resistant cell lines. Cancer Res. 60(10):2589–93.

Schmitz, G, Langmann, T, Heimerl, S (2001) Role of ABCG1 and other ABCG family members in lipid metabolism. J Lipid Res. 42: 1513–1520.

Scotto, KW, Johnson, RA (2001) Transcription of the multidrug resistance gene MDR1: a therapeutic target. Mol Interv. 1(2):117–25.

Sharom, FJ (2008) ABC multidrug transporters: structure, function and role in chemoresistance. Pharmacogenomics. 9(1):105–127.

Shi, Z, Peng, XX, Kim, IW, Shukla, S, Si, QS, Robey, RW, Bates, SE, Shen, T, Ashby, CR Jr, Fu, LW, Ambudkar, SV, Chen, ZS (2007) Erlotinib (Tarceva, OSI-774) antagonizes ATP-binding cassette subfamily B member 1 and ATP-binding cassette subfamily G member 2-mediated drug resistance. Cancer Res. 67(22):11012–20.

Sieczkowski, E, Lehner, C, Ambros, PF, Hohenegger, M (2010) Double impact on p-glycoprotein by statins enhances doxorubicin cytotoxicity in human neuroblastoma cells. Int J Cancer. 126(9): 2025–35.

Stein, U, Walther, W (2006) Reversal of ABC transporter-dependent multidrug resistance in cancer, a realistic option? Am. J. Cancer 5: 285–297.

Storch, CH, Ehehalt, R, Haefeli, WE, Weiss, J (2007) Localization of the human breast cancer resistance protein (BCRP/ABCG2) in lipid rafts/caveolae and modulation of its activity by cholesterol in vitro. J Pharmacol Exp Ther. 323(1): 257–64.

Sugawara, I, Akiyama, S, Scheper, RJ, Itoyama, S (1997) Lung resistance protein (LRP) expression in human normal tissues in comparison with that of MDR1 and MRP. Cancer Lett. 15;112(1): 23–31.

Szakács, G, Paterson, JK, Ludwig, JA, Booth-Genthe, C, Gottesman, MM (2006) Targeting multidrug resistance in cancer. Nat Rev Drug Discov. 5(3):219–34.

Tang, C, Ang, BT, Pervaiz, S (2007) Cancer stem cell: target for anti-cancer therapy. FASEB J. 21: 3777–3785.

Thiebaut, F, Tsuruo, T, Hamada, H, Gottesman, M M, Pastan, I, Willingham, M C (1987) Cellular localization of the multidrug-resistance gene product P-glycoprotein in normal human tissues. PNAS 84: 7735–7738.

Tirona, RG, Kim, RB (2002) Pharmacogenomics of organic anion-transporting polypeptides (OATP). Adv Drug Deliv Rev 54:1343–1352.

van Tellingen, O, Buckle, T, Jonker, JW, van der Valk, MA, Beijnen, JH (2003) P-glycoprotein and Mrp1 collectively protect the bone marrow from vincristine-induced toxicity in vivo. Br J Cancer. 89(9): 1776–82.

Versantvoort, CHM, Broxterman, HJ, Lankelma, J, Feller, N, Pinedo, HM (1994) Saturation and inhibition of the ATP-dependent daunorubicin transport in an MRP overexpressing multidrug resistant human small cell lung cancer cell line. Biochem Pharmacol 48:1129–1136.

Wang, H, Unadkat, JD, Mao, Q (2008) Hormonal regulation of BCRP expression in human placental BeWo cells. Pharm Res. 25(2): 444–452.

Wielinga, P, Hooijberg, JH, Gunnarsdottir, S, Kathmann, I, Reid, G, Zelcer, N, van der Born, K, de Haas, M, van der Heijden, I, Kaspers, G, Wijnholds, J, Jansen, G, Peters, G, Borst, P (2005) The human multidrug resistance protein MRP5 transports folates and can mediate cellular resistance against antifolates. Cancer Res. 65(10): 4425–4430.

Wu, C, Alman, BA (2008) Side population cells in human cancers. Cancer Lett. 268(1): 1–9.

Zamek-Gliszczynski, MJ, Hoffmaster, KA, Nezasa, K, Tallman, MN, Brouwer, KL (2006) Integration of hepatic drug transporters and phase II metabolizing enzymes: mechanisms of hepatic excretion of sulfate, glucuronide, and glutathione metabolites. Eur J Pharm Sci. 27(5):447–86.

Zhang, S, Yang, X, Morris, ME (2004) Flavonoids are inhibitors of breast cancer resistance protein (ABCG2)-mediated transport. Mol Pharmacol. 65(5):1208–16.

Zheng, X, Cui, D, Xu, S, Brabant, G, Derwahl, M (2010) Doxorubicin fails to eradicate cancer stem cells derived from anaplastic thyroid carcinoma cells: characterization of resistant cells. Int J Oncol. 37(2): 307–15.

Zhou, S, Morris, JJ, Barnes, YX, Lan, L, Schuetz, JD, Sorrentino, BP (2002) Bcrp1 gene expression is required for normal numbers of side population stem cells in mice, and confers relative protection to mitoxantrone in hematopoietic cells in vivo. Proceedings of the National Academy of Sciences of the United States of America 99(19):12339–12344.

Zhou, BB, Zhang, H, Damelin, M, Geles, KG, Grindley, JC, Dirks, PB (2009) Tumour-initiating cells: challenges and opportunities for anticancer drug discovery. Nat Rev Drug Discov. 8(10): 806–23.

Chapter 17
Stem Cells and Cancer Stem Cells: Biological and Clinical Interrelationships

Cinzia Bagalà and Carlo Barone

Introduction

Stem cells are virtually present in all adult tissues and play a fundamental role in tissue development, replacement, and repair. They have been characterized as having low proliferative rates, existing as minority populations within tissues in defined niches, and having responses to extracellular stimuli that are distinct from those of the more differentiated cells within the organ. They also exhibit a peculiar ability to undergo self-renewal as well as multi-lineage differentiation; in fact they are able to divide symmetrically, thus producing two daughter stem cells, or asymmetrically producing a daughter stem cell and a cell that leaves the stem cell niche to differentiate.

Stem cells were also isolated in acute myeloid leukemia in 1994 by Lapidot et al., whose findings were confirmed by other authors in the following years; finally in 2003, Al-Hajj et al. identified a subpopulation of breast cancer cells which was phenotypically different from other breast cancer cells and highly tumorigenic in vivo. Since then cancer stem subpopulations have been identified in the majority of human cancers thanks to the technique of sorting cells based on cell surface antigens and to tumor initiation assay. Cancer stem cells express peculiar surface antigen such as CD44, a cell adhesion molecule involved in cellular binding to hyaluronic acid, and exhibit low level of CD24, a negative regulator of the chemokine receptor CXCR4 involved in cancer metastasis (phenotype $CD44^+/CD24^{low}$). Tumoral stem cells are able to form tumors after injection in NOD/SCID mice with a greater efficiency that unsorted tumoral cells; in fact, as few as 100 cells with this phenotype were able to induce tumors whereas tens of thousands of cells with alternative phenotype failed to do so, thus explaining why an increased number of cancer stem cells in a tumor may be correlated with a poor clinical outcome and may be responsible of recurrence.

C. Bagalà • C. Barone (✉)
Division of Medical Oncology, Department of Internal Medicine,
Catholic University, Largo A. Gemelli 8, 00168 Rome, Italy
e-mail: carlobarone@rm.unicatt.it

Origin and Regulation of Tumoral Stem Cell

One major question which remains to be answered regards the possibility that tumoral stem cell may derive from normal stem cells. The cancer stem-cell hypothesis proposes that cancer arises in stem and/or progenitors cells through dysregulation of the normally tightly regulated processes of self-renewal and differentiation, alternatively CSCs may arise by genetic reprogramming of differentiated somatic cells during transformation that endows them with stem cell properties (Passegue et al. 2003). Cancer and normal stem cells share many gene expression profiles and signaling pathways such as *Hedgehog, Notch,* and *Wnt* which need to be tightly regulated in order to drive a correct development of organs and tissues (Table 17.1 and Fig. 17.1, reproduced from Batra and Ponnusamy 2008 with permission from J Ovarian Res).

One example is provided by the Hedgehog–Gli pathway in which the secreted glycoproteins of the Hedgehog family (*Sonic, Desert,* and *Indian* Hedgehog) bind to a membrane receptor complex formed by Patched (PTCH1) and Smoothened (SMOH) thus modulating the transcriptional activity of Gli 1, 2 and 3 proteins (Ruiz i Altaba et al. 2002). This pathway must be off most of the time and only active at the precise points and locations at which the Hedgehog signal is necessary, while it results abnormally activated in precursor cells and some sporadic cancer including basal cell carcinomas, medulloblastomas and some gliomas. Hedgehog signals induce cellular proliferation through upregulation of n-Myc, Cyclin-D and E and FOXM1, and also upregulate Jag2 and Wnt proteins such as Wnt2b and Wnt5a (Katoh and Katoh 2009); it also induces BCL2 and CFLAR to promote cell survival and it upregulates key transcription factors such as Snail, Slug, ZEB1, ZEB2, Twist2 and FOXC2 promoting epithelial-to-mesenchymal transition, a process which converts epithelial cells into mesenchymal cells through profound disruption of cell–cell junctions and extensive reorganization of the actin cytoskeleton (Katoh and Katoh 2009). These events are presumed to be required for tumor invasion and metastasis of carcinoma cells by promoting loss of contact inhibition, increased cell motility and enhanced invasiveness, and there are increasing evidences that the induction of epithelial-to-mesenchymal transition in epithelial tumor cells can result in the generation of cells with stem cell properties (Battula et al. 2010). Hedgehog signaling induces stem cell markers such as CD44, CD133, BMI1, and LGR5; Bar et al. (2007) observed that cyclopamine, a plant alkaloid that inhibits the action of Smoothened in the membrane receptor complex thus blocking the Hedgehog

Table 17.1 Major self-renewal pathways in CSCs

Molecular pathway	Mechanism
Hedgehog-Gli	Timely activation of transcriptional activity of Gli proteins. Promotion of epithelial-to-mesenchymal transition
Notch	Trascriptional control of genes involved in stem cell self-renewal and differentiation. Linking of angiogenesis to CSCs self-renewal
Wnt	Regulation of cytoplasmic β-catenin

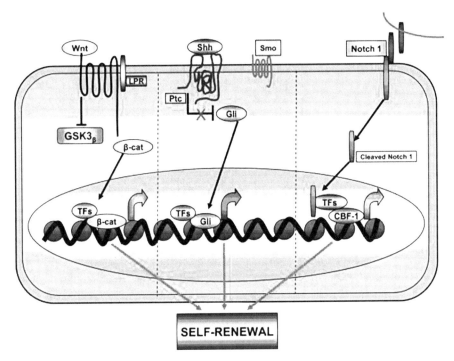

Fig. 17.1 Schematic diagram of signaling pathways that are involved in normal and cancer stem cell biology. Wnt, Shh and Notch1 pathways have been shown to contribute to the self-renewal of stem cells and/or progenitors in a variety of organs; when deregulated, these pathways can contribute to oncogenesis (reproduced from Batra and Ponnusamy 2008 with permission from Journal of Ovarian Research)

signaling, is able to significantly reduce the stem-like fraction in gliomas to the extent that viable glioblastoma cells treated with cyclopamine were no longer able to form *neurosphere* (floating spherical colonies allowing propagation of stem and progenitor cells in an undifferentiated state) "in vitro" and to induce tumors in athymic mice after intracranial injection. The same authors found that radiation treatment increased the percentage of stem-like cells in glioblastoma cell populations suggesting that this standard therapy preferentially targets differentiated neoplastic cells.

Similar results were obtained blocking the Notch signaling pathway in glioblastoma and breast tumor models. Notch encodes a trans-membrane receptor that upon binding with specific ligands (Jagged 1 and 2, Delta 1, 3 and 4) is cleaved by gamma-secretase, releasing an intracellular domain (NICD) that is directly involved in transcriptional control of multiple genes (Fortini 2009). The Notch pathway plays a major role in the maintenance of the stem cell state in the nervous system, in the breast and the intestinal tract promoting self-renewal and repressing differentiation. Aberrant activation of Notch signaling is an early event in breast cancer and high expression of NICD in ductal carcinoma in situ (DCIS) predicts a reduced time to recurrence 5 years after surgery. Farnie and Clarke (2007) observed that a gamma-secretase inhibitor and a Notch4 neutralizing antibody impaired the self-renewal capacity of primary DCIS tissue reducing *mammosphere* formation in vitro. Similarly, Fan et al. (2010) observed that gamma-secretase inhibitors deplete the stem cancer cell population in glioblastoma in vitro culture through reduced proliferation and increased apoptosis; these events were associated with decreased AKT and STAT3 phosphorylation. Therefore, there are growing evidences that Notch is involved in normal and cancer stem cell self-renewal. This pathway may be also involved in controlling stem cell differentiation through members of the basic helix-loop-helix family Hes and Hey. In particular Hes1, a trascriptional repressor activated by Notch and also Hedgehog signaling pathways is rapidly upregulated by each of the three quiescence signals (loss of adhesion, contact inhibition, and mitogen withdrawal) and is one of the genes that might protect quiescent cells from differentiation (Park et al. 2004). Hes1 level is often high in tumors such as rhabdomyosarcomas, as a consequence of Notch and also Hedgehog activation and this may protect cancer cells against differentiation; in fact it has been shown that expressing a dominant-negative form of Hes1 in rhabdomyosarcoma cell lines induces myogenic differentiation and decreases proliferation.

Hovinga et al. (2010) demonstrated that in a three-dimensional explant of glioblastoma Notch signaling targets cancer stem cells also indirectly through controlling endothelial cell survival. In fact they observed that Notch inhibition results in a decreased number of endothelial cells within the tumor explants thus disrupting the perivascular niche harboring stem cells; this results in a decreased self-renewal of tumor stem cells which are dependent on factors created by the vasculature itself like normal stem cells. The authors conclude that Notch pathway plays a critical role in linking angiogensis and cancer stem cell self-renewal.

Wnt signaling has also been showed to be involved in regulating the self-renewal and differentiation of a variety of stem cells (Katoh and Katoh 2007). Activation of the canonical Wnt pathway begins with the binding of Wnt proteins to cell surface receptor of the Frizzled family and to the low-density lipoprotein receptor-related proteins LRP5 and LRP6. This signaling reduces the activity of glycogen synthase 3β (GSK3β), a serine/threonine kinase which phosphorylates β-catenin, and directs it to the proteosomal degradation pathway; the activation of Wnt pathway increases cytoplasmic β-catenin which translocates to the nucleus where it binds to transcription factors in the LEF1/TCF family activating the transcription of target genes such as FGF20, DKK1, WISP1, MYC and CCND1 thus inducing proliferation of precursors cells. Shimizu et al. (2008) also demonstrated that the nuclear accumulation of β-catenin may be induced by FGF2 through activation of phosphatidylinositol-3-kinase and inhibition of GSK3β; the authors also observed that nuclear accumulated β-catenin forms a molecular complex with Notch1 which binds to the Hes1 promoter region, thus inducing Hes1 gene expression which inhibits progenitor cells differentiation.

More recently, it has been suggest that pluripotency is a reprogrammable state depending on a transcriptional circuit involving key stem cell transcription factors and microRNAs (Table 17.2). In fact the introduction of defined transcription factors into mouse and human somatic cells has recently been shown to reprogram the developmental state of mature cells into that of pluripotent embryonic cells, generating

Table 17.2 Factors involved in reprogrammation of pluripotency

Yamanaka factors	Oct4, Sox2, c-Myc, Klf4
Thomson factors	Oct4, Sox2, Nanog, LIN28
miRNAs	miR-290, miR-295, miR-302, let-7
Others	Bmi1, SUZ12, EZH1/2, Cyclins, FGFs, ZFP42/Rex1, Wnt/β-catenin, TGFβ, ras, LOGs

so-called induced pluripotent stem (iPS) cells (Kashyap et al. 2009). Transcription factors associated with pluripotency and self-renewal are Oct4, Sox2, KLF4, C-Myc, Nanog, and LIN28; in particular it seems that greatest reprogramming efficiency is achieved when a combination of four factors such as Oct4, Sox2, KLF4 and c-Myc (so-called *Yamanaka factors*) or a combination of Oct4, Sox2, Nanog and LIN28 (known as *Thomson factors*) is introduced in differentiated cells (Kashyap et al. 2009).

Oct4 and Sox2 are critical factors required for maintaining self-renewal and pluripotency of mouse and human stem cells; they act synergistically to regulate their own transcription as well the expression of other key stem cell genes including Nanog, FGF4, Zfp42/Rex1 (a zinc finger protein belonging to the YY1 family of transcription factors), Wnt/β-catenin, and TGFβ family members. They occupy collectively about 10% of the promoters in the human genome, and they also bind to gene regions associated with loci encoding microRNAs, small (19–22 nucleotide long) noncoding RNAs that inhibit gene expression by binding primarily to target mRNA at specific sequence motifs within the 3′UTR of the transcript. Given the frequency with which mRNA target motifs are conserved within 3′UTR, it is estimated that 20–30% of all human genes are targets of miRNAs. A subset of miRNAs is preferentially expressed in embryonic stem (ES) cells such as miR-290, -295 and -302 which are found to be induced by Oct4, Nanog and Sox2 and also target these genes in a incoherent feed-forward loop. Recently miR-302 was demonstrated to convert human skin cancer cells into pluripotent ES-like cells. Also LIN-28, one of the pluripotency factors, is a RNA-binding protein which binds and represses the processing of let-7 (*lethal-7*) miRNA, a regulator of cell cycle exit which inhibits self-renewal in both normal and cancer stem cells and promotes terminal differentiation thus behaving as a tumor suppressor. In *C. elegans*, Let-7 mutants fail to exit the cell cycle at the correct time and instead undergo an extra round of division and terminally differentiate one stage later than normal (Nimmo and Slack 2009). In human cancer cell lines, Let-7 represses cell cycle regulators such as Cyclin D2, CDC251 and CDK6, promoters of growth including ras and c-Myc, and 12 *Let-7 regulated Oncofetal Genes* (LOGs) (Gunaratne 2009). The top three LOGs in cancer and stem cells include: HMGA2, IMP-1, and LIN28b. HMGA2 (LOG1) promotes self-renewal of young stem cells by repressing the cell cycle regulators $p16^{Ink4a}$ and $p19^{Arf}$. HMGA2 expression declines in aging stem cells partly in consequence of Let7b upregulation. IMP-1(LOG2), which is a member of an RNA binding proteins family including IMP-2 (LOG6), behaves as a classical oncofetal protein expressed only early during fetal life and re-expressed in many human cancers. It acts stabilizing target RNAs such as IGFII and c-Myc by shielding them from degradation.

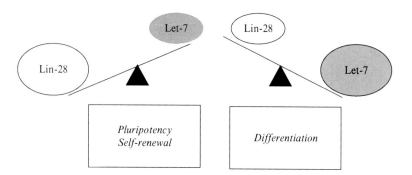

Fig. 17.2 The Lin-28/Let-7 switch. Bistable switches may regulate stem cell differentiation via double-negative feedback loops between *let-7* and its targets, *lin-28* and *lin-41*. The roles of *lin-28* and *let-7* as an oncogene and tumor suppressor suggests that stem cells and cancer cells share a common strategy for regulating the balance between self-renewal and differentiation (reproduced from Nimmo and Slack 2009 with permission from Chromosoma)

LIN28b (LOG3) is a structural and functional homolog of LIN28; recently, it was found by two groups of researchers that LIN28/LIN28b acts as a selective inhibitor of Let7 and it has been proposed that LIN28/Let-7 pair may act as a switch that balances the decision to maintain pluripotency versus differentiation (Fig. 17.2, reproduced from Nimmo and Slack 2009, with permission from Chromosoma).

c-Myc is also recognized as a pluripotency factor which activates the expression of miRNA 17–92 cluster through its interaction with the putative promoter region; miRNAs from this cluster target tumor suppressor genes such as E2F1, PTEN and TGFβRII thus controlling the G1 to S transition which is fundamental for ES self-renewal and cell proliferation. Activation of miR-17-92 and downregulation of Let-7 is frequently found in multiple cancers, suggesting that any perturbations in key ES cell transcription factors–miRNAs network may generate cancer stem cells (Gunaratne 2009).

This is particularly evident in some type of cancer such as a subset of sarcomas and hematopoietic malignancies which, at least in their early developmental event phases, display only a single detectable oncogenic event usually consequent to a nonrandom reciprocal chromosomal translocation. This generates a functional fusion gene believed to initiate tumor development through generation of a CSC population. This has been observed in Ewing sarcoma which is associated with a unique chromosomal translocation that generates the EWS-FLI-1 fusion protein composed of EWS and a member of *ets* transcription factor family, behaving as an aberrant transcription factor. Riggi et al. (2010) very recently observed that the expression of EWS-FLI-1 in human pediatric mesenchymal stem cells, under appropriate culture conditions, generated a subpopulation of cells displaying Ewing Sarcoma cancer stem cell features; this subset of cells showed a genetic reprogramming including the induction of the embryonic stem cell genes Oct4, Nanog and Sox2 in part as a consequence of the micro-RNA 145 repression. Therefore, it seems that regulation

17 Stem Cells and Cancer Stem Cells: Biological and Clinical Interrelationships

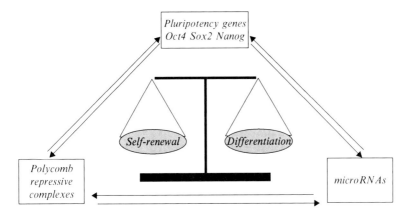

Fig. 17.3 The reciprocal regulatory circuit composed of Oct4–Sox2–Nanog; polycomb repressive complexes and microRNAs. Regulation of stem cell pluripotency and differentiation involves a mutual regulatory circuit of the NANOG, OCT4, and SOX2 pluripotency transcription factors with polycomb transcription repressors and stem cell microRNAs (reproduced from Kashyap et al. 2009 with permission from Stem Cells Dev)

of stem cell self-renewal and differentiation involves a mutual regulatory circuit comprising of the Nanog, Oct4 and Sox2 transcription factors with stem cell microRNAs and also polycomb repressive complexes 1 and 2 (including Bmi1 and EZH1/2 methyltransferase) which contribute to epigenetic regulation of key gene expression via dynamic regulation of chromatin/histone modifications (Fig. 17.3, reproduced from Kashyap et al. 2009, with permission from Stem Cell Dev). Bmi-1, a member of the *Polycomb* group (PcG) of transcription repressors, is required for the maintenance of tissue-specific stem cells and is involved in carcinogenesis within the same tissues. Bmi-1 promotes self-renewal of stem cells largely by interfering with two central cellular tumor suppressor pathways, $p16^{Ink4a}$/retinoblastoma protein (Rb) and $p19^{Arf}$/p53, whose disruption is a hallmark of cancer (Sang et al. 2010). In normal stem cells, p16 is repressed in a Bmi-1-dependent manner and cyclin D/Cdk4/6 complex can phosphorylate pRB allowing the E2F-dependent transcription that leads to cell cycle progression and DNA synthesis. In addition, Bmi 1 also represses p19 thus inducing MDM-mediated p53 degradation which prevents cell cycle arrest and apoptosis (Fig. 17.4, reproduced from Park et al. 2004 with permission from J Clin Invest). The oncogenic role of Bmi-1 is confirmed by its amplification in some lymphomas and breast cancer cell lines. Among PcG proteins SUZ12 is overexpressed in breast and colon cancer while EZH2 is upregulated in lymphomas as well in breast and prostate cancer. Moreover, Bmi-1 and SUZ12 are downstream target of Sonic hedgehog (Shh) and Wnt signaling, respectively, providing for a connection between epigenetic change regulators (PcG) and developmental-signaling pathways.

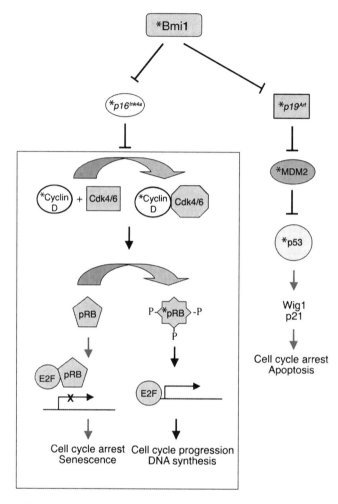

Fig. 17.4 Regulation of cell cycle, apoptosis, and senescence by Bmi-1. In normal stem cells, *p16Ink4a* and *p19Arf* genes are repressed in a Bmi1-dependent manner. In the absence of *p16Ink4a*, the cyclin D/Cdk4/6 complex can phosphorylate pRB, allowing the E2F-dependent transcription that leads to cell cycle progression and DNA synthesis. In addition, MDM2-mediated p53 degradation causes low p53 levels in the absence of *p19Arf*, thus preventing cell cycle arrest and apoptosis. Proteins affected by high and low levels of *Bmi1* are shown by *black* and *red arrows*, respectively. Sites of frequent mutations associated with cancer are shown by *asterisks* (reproduced from Park et al. 2004 with permission from J Clin Invest)

Cancer Stem Cell and Cancer Therapy

The cancer stem cell hypothesis has important clinical implications since cancer stem cells show low sensitivity to conventional chemotherapy, thus becoming responsible for cancer recurrence (Table 17.3). This is due to different mechanisms: first of all, they are slowly proliferating and in the G0 phase of the cell cycle for

Table 17.3 CSCs as cause of cancer recurrence

Slowly proliferating mainly G0 cells
Increased expression of ABC proteins and ALDH
Increased expression of anti-apoptotic proteins
Higher levels of phosphorylated checkpoint kinases making DNA-repair feasible

extended periods of time, thus being resistant to cell-cycle active chemotherapeutic agents; also they express increased adenosine triphosphate-binding cassette (ABC) proteins known to efflux chemotherapeutic drugs and they show elevated expression of enzymes such as ALDH able to metabolize cytotoxic agents such as cyclophosphamide; finally, they express increased levels of anti-apoptotic proteins such as survivin and bcl-2 proteins (Eyler and Rich 2008). Also, stem cells are radioresistant since they repair the DNA damage induced by radiation more rapidly than non-CSC; this is due to higher basal levels of phosphorylated checkpoint kinases, *Chk1* and *Chk2*, which cause cell cycle arrest until lethal DNA damage can be repaired. This suggests that in addition to their primary drug resistance, cancer stem cell subpopulation are primed to respond to genomic insults. Also aberrant activation of Notch and Wnt signaling seems to contribute to cancer stem cell radioresistance in human tumors such as gliomas and breast cancers; in fact, the expression of the constitutively active intracellular domains of Notch1 and Notch2 protects glioma stem cells against radiation while inhibition with gamma-secretase inhibitors or knockdown of Notch1 and 2 renders the glioma stem cells more sensitive to radiations at clinically relevant doses by reducing Akt activity and Mcl-1 levels (Eyler and Rich 2008).

The relative resistance of cancer stem cells to radiation and cytotoxic therapy highlights the need to develop agents able to target this cell population. One of the more significant advances in breast cancer therapy has been the development of HER2-targeted therapies for the treatment of HER2-overexpressing breast cancers. Recent neoadjuvant studies demonstrated a significant increase in the percentage of C44$^+$/CD24^{low} breast cancer stem cells in core biopsies after 12 weeks of conventional neoadjuvant chemotherapy with adriamicin and cyclophosphamide or docetaxel and cyclophosphamide, while in tumor biopsies from patients treated with lapatinib, a small molecule dual tyrosine kinase inhibitor of epidermal growth factor receptor (EGFR) and human-epidermal growth factor receptor type 2 (HER2), there was a nonstatistically significant reduction in the number of C44$^+$/CD24^{low} cells and in the *mammosphere*-formation efficiency after 6 weeks of treatment (Li et al. 2008). In a randomized second-line phase III trial comparing capecitabine alone or combined with lapatinib for women with relapsing HER-2 positive locally advanced or metastastic breast cancer, time to disease progression and progression-free survival improved in the lapatinib arm (Geyer et al. 2006). The beneficial effect of lapatinib in breast cancer may be due to selective inhibition of breast cancer stem cells. This hypothesis is also supported by Korkaya et al. (2008) who observed that transfection of HER2 into breast cancer cell lines increased the cancer stem-cell fraction and that trastuzumab was able to inhibit the growth of this subpopulation. Taken together, these studies suggest that the effectiveness of HER-2 inhibitors such as trastuzumab and lapatinib may be related directly to the ability of these agents to target the cancer stem-cell population. These agents may be much more effective when administered in adjuvant rather than in the metastatic setting because an agent that only target cancer stem cells and not bulk tumor cells would be predicted to have only modest effects on tumor size but it could have dramatic effects in preventing tumor recurrence in the adjuvant setting (Liu and Wicha 2010). If this is the case, cancer stem-cell models may have important implications for the development of adjuvant therapies. Almost three large randomized breast cancer adjuvant studies, in fact, have shown that the addition of trastuzumab to chemotherapy reduces the 3-year risk of recurrence by half, showing a trend toward an overall survival benefit (Baselga et al. 2006). On the contrary, the failure of EGFR-targeting agents in the adjuvant treatment of colon cancer has been ascribed to an epithelial–mesenchymal transition of circulating CSC driven by the lack of stromal interaction resulting into changes of cell membrane arrangement (Goldberg et al. 2010).

Inhibitors of Wnt, Hedgehog, and Notch signaling pathways should also be considered for CSCs therapy. Recently in phase I clinical trials in patients with advanced basal cell carcinomas (BCC) and medulloblastoma (MB), *Vismodegib* (GDC-0449), a small, orally administrable molecule inhibiting the Hedgehog pathway demonstrated antitumor activity (Von Hoff et al. 2009) and is currently undergoing phase II clinical trials for the treatment of advanced basal cell carcinoma, medulloblastoma, metastatic colorectal cancer, ovarian cancer, and other solid tumors (De Smaele et al. 2010). Though cyclopamine also showed an anti-tumoral effect in many "in vitro" and "in vivo" tumor models, its potential toxicity in nontumoral cells has driven the research for semi-synthetic analogues with improved pharmacological properties and a more favorable pharmacokinetic profile; IPI-926, one of these analogues, induced complete tumor regression in a Hedgehog-dependent medulloblastoma allograft model after daily oral administration and it is a drug candidate for clinical trials (Tremblay et al. 2009). Gamma-secretase inhibitors (GSIs), preventing the final cleavage step of the Notch receptors, showed anti-tumoral activity in preclinical studies; their clinical use, however, might still be limited due to their side-effects such as gastrointestinal toxicity which could be minimized by lowering the dose of GSIs when used in combination with other chemotherapeutic agents. This approach was demonstrated to be effective in "in vitro" studies enhancing the cytotoxic effect of traditional antineoplastic agents (Meng et al. 2009). Elucidation of other pathways that regulate self-renewal and differentiation of cancer stem cells may provide new targets for a more effective treatment of human malignancies.

Finally, a word should be said about the current use of autologous and allogeneic hematopoietic stem cell transplantation (HSCT) after myeloablative doses of chemotherapy. The identification of the bone marrow as a source of hematopoietic stem cells allows to administer cytotoxic therapy at high doses resulting in the permanent loss of bone marrow function; this approach requires the rescue with hematopoietic stem cells which are administered as an intravenous infusion and produces increased killing of tumoral cells allowing to cure patients who would otherwise relapse or progress after conventional treatment (Jeng and Van den Brink 2010). Allogeneic HSCT is reserved for high-risk patients with leukemia (Wayne et al. 2010), while autologous HSCT plays an important role in the therapeutic approach of relapsed non-Hodgkin's lymphoma (Nademanee et al. 2000), platinum-refractory nonseminomatous germ-cell tumors (Einhorn et al. 2007) and some pediatric tumors such as Ewing Sarcoma and neuroblastoma (Barrett et al. 2010).

References

Al-Hajj M, Wicha MS, Benito-Hernandez A, et al. (2003) Prospective identification of tumorigenic breast cancer cells. Proc Natl Acad Sci U S A 100(7):3983–8.

Bar EE, Chaudhry A, Lin A, et al (2007) Cyclopamine-mediated hedgehog pathway inhibition depletes stem-like cancer cells in glioblastoma. Stem Cells 25(10):2524–33.

Barrett D, Fish JD, Grupp SA (2010) Autologous and allogeneic cellular therapies for high-risk pediatric solid tumors. Pediatr Clin North Am 57(1):47–66

Baselga J, Perez EA, Pienkowski T, et al (2006) Adjuvant trastuzumab: a milestone in the treatment of HER-2-positive early breast cancer. Oncologist 11 Suppl 1:4–12

Batra SK and Ponnusamy MP (2008) Ovarian cancer: emerging concept on cancer stem cells. J Ovarian Res 1(1):4

Battula VL, Evans KW, Hollier BG, et al (2010) Epithelial-Mesenchymal Transition-Derived Cells Exhibit Multi-Lineage Differentiation Potential Similar to Mesenchymal Stem Cells. Stem Cells 28(8): 1435–45

De Smaele E, Ferretti E, Gulino A (2010) Vismodegib, a small-molecule inhibitor of the hedgehog pathway for the treatment of advanced cancers. Curr Opin Investig Drugs 11(6):707–18

Einhorn LH, Williams SD, Chamness A, et al (2007) High-dose chemotherapy and stem-cell rescue for metastatic germ-cell tumors. N Engl J Med 357(4):340–8

Eyler CE, Rich JN (2008) Survival of the fittest: cancer stem cells in therapeutic resistance and angiogenesis. J Clin Oncol 26(17):2839–45

Fan X, Khaki L, Zhu TS, et al (2010) NOTCH pathway blockade depletes CD133-positive glioblastoma cells and inhibits growth of tumor neurospheres and xenografts. Stem Cells 28(1):5–16

Farnie G, Clarke RB (2007) Mammary stem cells and breast cancer--role of Notch signalling. Stem Cell Rev (2):169–75

Fortini ME (2009) Notch signaling: the core pathway and its posttranslational regulation. Dev Cell. 16(5):633–47. Review

Geyer CE, Forster J, Lindquist D, e al (2006) Lapatinib plus capecitabine for HER2-positive advanced breast cancer. N. Engl J Med 355(26):2733–43

Goldberg RM, Sargent DJ, Thibodeau SN, et al (2010) Adjuvant mFOLFOX6 plus or minus cetuximab (Cmab) in patients (pts) with KRAS mutant (m) resected stage III colon cancer (CC): NCCTG Intergroup Phase III Trial N0147. J Clin Oncol 28:15s, (suppl; abstr 3508)

Gunaratne PH (2009) Embryonic stem cell microRNAs: defining factors in induced pluripotent (iPS) and cancer (CSC) stem cells? Curr Stem Cell Res Ther 4(3):168 77

Hovinga KE, Shimizu F, Wang R, et al (2010) Inhibition of notch signaling in glioblastoma targets cancer stem cells via an endothelial cell intermediate. Stem Cells 28(6):1019–29

Jeng RR, Van den Brink MRM (2010) Allogeneic heamatopoietic stem cell transplantation: individualized stem cell and immune therapy of cancer. Nat Rev Cancer 10(3):213–21

Kashyap V, Rezende NC, Scotland KB, et al (2009) Regulation of stem cell pluripotency and differentiation involves a mutual regulatory circuit of the NANOG, OCT4, and SOX2 pluripotency transcription factors with polycomb repressive complexes and stem cell microRNAs. Stem Cells Dev 18(7):1093–108. Review

Katoh Y, Katoh M (2009) Hedgehog target genes: mechanisms of carcinogenesis induced by aberrant hedgehog signaling activation. Curr Mol Med 9(7):873–86

Katoh M, Katoh M (2007) WNT signaling pathway and stem cell signaling network. Clin Cancer Res 13(14):4042–5

Korkaya H, Paulson A, Iovino F, et al (2008) HER2 regulates the mammary stem/progenitor cell population driving tumorigenesis and invasion. Oncogene 27(47):6120–30. Epub 2008 Jun 30.;13(14):4042–5

Lapidot T, Sirard C, Vormoor J, et al (1994) A cell initiating human acute myeloid leukaemia after transplantation into SCID mice. Nature 367(6464):645–8

Li X, Lewis MT, Huang J,et al (2008) Intrinsic resistance of tumorigenic breast cancer cells to chemotherapy. J Natl Cancer Inst.100(9):672–9

Liu S, Wicha MS (2010) Targeting Breast Cancer Stem Cells. J Clin Oncol 28(25):4006–12

Meng RD, Shelton CC, Li YM,et al (2009) Gamma-Secretase inhibitors abrogate oxaliplatin-induced activation of the Notch-1 signaling pathway in colon cancer cells resulting in enhanced chemosensitivity. Cancer Res 69(2):573–82

Nademanee A, Molina A, Dagis A, et al (2000) Autologous stem-cell transplantation for poor-risk and relapsed intermediate- and high-grade non-Hodgkin's lymphoma. Clin Lymphoma 1(1):46–54

Nimmo RA, Slack FJ (2009) An elegant miRror: microRNAs in stem cells, developmental timing and cancer. Chromosoma 118(4):405–18

Park IK, Morrison SJ, Clarke MF (2004) Bmi1, stem cells, and senescence regulation. J Clin Invest 113(2):175–9

Passegue E, Jamieson CH, Ailles LE, et al. (2003) Normal and leukemic hematopoiesis: are leukemias a stem cell disorder or a reacquisition of stem cell characteristics? *Proc Natl Acad Sci USA* 100 (Suppl 1):11842–11849

Riggi N, Suvà ML, De Vito C, et al (2010) EWS-FLI-1 modulates miRNA145 and SOX2 expression to initiate mesenchymal stem cell reprogramming toward Ewing sarcoma cancer stem cells. Genes Dev 24(9):916–32

Ruiz i Altaba A, Sánchez P, Dahmane N (2002) Gli and hedgehog in cancer: tumours, embryos and stem cells. Nat Rev Cancer 2(5):361–72. Review

Sang L, Roberts JM, Coller HA (2010) Hijacking HES1: how tumors co-opt the anti-differentiation strategies of quiescent cells. Trends Mol Med 16(1):17–26

Shimizu T, Kagawa T, Inoue T, et al (2008) Stabilized beta-catenin functions through TCF/LEF proteins and the Notch/RBP-Jkappa complex to promote proliferation and suppress differentiation of neural precursor cells. Mol Cell Biol 28(24):7427–41

Tremblay MR, Lescarbeau A, Grogan MJ (2009) Discovery of a potent and orally active hedgehog pathway antagonist (IPI-926). J Med Chem 52(14):4400–18

Von Hoff DD, LoRusso PM, Rudin CM, et al (2009) Inhibition of the hedgehog pathway in advanced basal-cell carcinoma. N Engl J Med 361(12):1164–72

Wayne AS, Baird K, Egeler RM (2010) Hematopoietic stem cell transplantation for leukemia. Pediatr Clin North Am 57(1):1–25

Chapter 18
Immunomodulatory Functions of Cancer Stem Cells

Tobias Schatton, Jennifer Y. Lin, and Markus H. Frank

Introduction

The concept that tumors and stem cells may share common biological characteristics is not novel (Bruce and Van Der Gaag 1963; Hamburger and Salmon 1977; Park et al. 1971). In fact, the defining stem cell characteristics of (1) self-renewal, (2) generation of differentiated progeny, and (3) potential for unlimited proliferation are commonly observed during tumor development (Gupta et al. 2009a; Schatton et al. 2009). Furthermore, many of the same signaling cascades and interactions with stromal elements that orchestrate physiologic stem cell behavior, and consequently development, are also found to play important roles in the initiation and propagation of tumors (Reya et al. 2001). For example, physiologic stem cells exhibit immunomodulatory properties (Le Blanc and Ringden 2007; Uccelli et al. 2008) that also apply to tumor evasion of host immunity and, as a result, neoplastic progression (Dunn et al. 2002; Mapara and Sykes 2004). The emerging literature on cancer stem cells (CSCs) and their interaction with the host immune system (Schatton and Frank 2009) will be the focus of this chapter. The CSC concept

T. Schatton (✉)
Transplantation Research Center, Children's Hospital Boston and Brigham and Women's Hospital, Harvard Medical School, 300 Longwood Avenue, Boston, MA 02115, USA
e-mail: tobias.schatton@tch.harvard.edu

J.Y. Lin
Department of Dermatology, Brigham and Women's Hospital,
Harvard Medical School, 77 Avenue Louis Pasteur, Boston, MA 02115, USA

M.H. Frank
Transplantation Research Center, Children's Hospital Boston and Brigham and Women's Hospital, Harvard Medical School, 300 Longwood Avenue, Boston, MA 02115, USA

Department of Dermatology, Brigham and Women's Hospital,
Harvard Medical School, 77 Avenue Louis Pasteur, Boston, MA 02115, USA

provides a rationale for the development of novel treatment modalities that specifically target CSCs and their biological functions, of which modulation of the immune response will be a critical one.

Cancer Stem Cells: Defining Characteristics and Roles in the Tumorigenic Process

Cancer is not a homogeneous disease. In fact, heterogeneity – both at the genetic and cellular levels – is a fundamental property of cancer biology (Hanahan and Weinberg 2000). Several theories have been postulated to account for the generation and maintenance of heterogeneity in tumors. According to the classic view of tumorigenesis, tumor heterogeneity can be explained by both intrinsic factors (i.e., progressive accumulations of genetic alterations over time) and extrinsic stimuli (e.g., distinct cues from the tumor microenvironment) (Hanahan and Weinberg 2000). This so-called stochastic theory of tumor initiation postulates that all cells within a cancer have biologically equivalent capacities to proliferate, form new tumors, and cause relapse (Nowell 1976). The cancer stem cell (CSC) hypothesis, provides an alternative explanation for tumor heterogeneity (Reya et al. 2001): It posits that cancers, like physiologic tissues, are organized as developmentally defined hierarchies of cells with divergent differentiation features and disparate capabilities for self-renewal and neoplastic proliferation. The CSC paradigm thus proposes that only a subpopulation of tumor cells within a cancer – namely CSCs – bears the competence to fuel tumor growth by continuously undergoing self-renewal and differentiation, whereas the bulk of differentiated cancer components lacks the capacity for tumor initiation and unlimited proliferation (Schatton et al. 2009).

According to a consensus definition (Clarke et al. 2006), a CSC is a cell within a tumor that possesses the capacity to undergo both self-renewing cell divisions that expand the CSC pool and cell divisions that result in more differentiated cancer cell progeny. Therefore, CSCs can only be defined experimentally by their ability to recapitulate the generation of a continuously growing tumor (Clarke et al. 2006). Accordingly, the experimental characterization of a putative CSC population relies on the use of an in vivo model system that allows for a rigorous confirmation of the traits used to define CSCs. The gold standard assay that fulfills this criterion is serial xenotransplantation at limiting dilution of marker-defined clinical cancer subpopulations into an orthotopic site of immunocompromised mice (typically NOD/SCID), which, although imperfect, is regarded as the best experimental system to evaluate CSC activity (Clarke et al. 2006). Using this approach, CSCs capable of sustained self-renewal and tumor propagation were first described in cancers of the hematopoietic lineage (Bonnet and Dick 1997). These initial studies demonstrated that it is possible to isolate from a single tumor sample two distinct cancer subpopulations that differ in their cell surface antigen profile and their tumor-seeding properties: (1) a CSC-enriched subset, as defined by its exclusive ability to self-renew as well as differentiate into nontumorigenic cancer cell progeny and its competence to seed

Table 18.1 Cell surface phenotype of CSCs in human malignancies[a]

Tumor type	Cell surface marker(s)	Reference
AML	CD34⁺CD38⁻	Bonnet and Dick (1997)
	CD34⁺CD38⁻	Ishikawa et al. (2007)
B-ALL	CD34⁺CD10⁻/CD34⁺CD19⁻	Cox et al. (2004)
	CD34⁺CD38⁻CD19⁻	Castor et al. (2005)
Bladder	CD44⁺CK5⁺CK20⁻Lineage⁻	Chan et al. (2009)
Breast	CD44⁺CD24⁻/low ESA⁺Lineage⁻	Al-Hajj et al. (2003)
CNS	CD133⁺	Singh et al. (2004)
Colon	CD133⁺	O'Brien et al. (2007)
	CD133⁺	Ricci-Vitiani et al. (2007)
	CD44⁺ESA^high Lineage⁻(CD166⁺)	Dalerba et al. 2007
Ewing	CD133⁺	Suva et al. (2009)
Head and Neck	CD44⁺Lineage⁻	Prince et al. (2007)
Liver	CD90⁺CD45⁻(CD44⁺)	Yang et al. (2008)
Melanoma	ABCB5⁺	Schatton et al. (2008)
Ovarian	CD44⁺CD117⁺	Zhang et al. (2008)
Pancreas	CD44⁺CD24⁺ESA⁺	Li et al. (2007)
	CD133⁺	Hermann et al. (2007)
T-ALL	CD34⁺CD4⁻/CD34⁺CD7⁻	Cox et al. (2007)

ABCB5 ATP-binding cassette, subfamily B, member 5, *ALL* acute lymphoblastic leukemia, *AML* acute myeloid leukemia, *CD* cluster of differentiation, *CK* cytokeratin, *CNS* central nervous system, *ESA* epithelial specific antigen

[a] Only studies that demonstrated sustained CSC self-renewal through serial xenotransplantation are listed in this table

new tumors upon serial xenotransplantation, and (2) the bulk of tumor cells that lack the capacity to generate tumors in animal hosts (Bonnet and Dick 1997). Subsequent studies extended these findings to a variety of additional hematological malignancies and solid tumor entities (Al-Hajj et al. 2003; Castor et al. 2005; Chan et al. 2009; Cox et al. 2004, 2007; Dalerba et al. 2007; Hermann et al. 2007; Ishikawa et al. 2007; Li et al. 2007; O'Brien et al. 2007; Prince et al. 2007; Ricci-Vitiani et al. 2007; Schatton et al. 2008; Singh et al. 2004; Suva et al. 2009; Yang et al. 2008; Zhang et al. 2008) (the markers used for the prospective characterization of CSCs in these various cancers are listed in Table 18.1). Hierarchical tumor organization was recently also confirmed in syngeneic mouse models, in which only fractions of murine tumor cells possessed the fundamental CSC features of extensive self renewal, differentiation, and enhanced tumorigenic capacity (Cho et al. 2008; Deshpande et al. 2006; Held et al. 2010; Wu et al. 2008).

Despite these seminal advances in our understanding of functional tumor heterogeneity, the CSC model remains a topic of considerable controversy (Gupta et al. 2009a). Some of this controversy seems to arise from confusion regarding the term "CSC." For instance, many interpret the term CSC to mean that the cellular precursors of such tumorigenic subpopulations were originally physiologic stem cells, which accumulated genetic alterations resulting in cancerous transformation. While this may be the case in some malignancies (Barker et al. 2009; Zhu et al. 2009), CSCs in other cancers may originate from more differentiated cells that reacquired stem-like properties through a series of mutagenic events (Huntly et al. 2004; Jamieson et al. 2004; Krivtsov et al. 2006). Additionally, differentiation in the context of CSC biology does not refer to oligo- or multipotent differentiation plasticity as it occurs during organogenesis or physiologic tissue regeneration, but rather to the ability of CSCs to give rise to cancer cells that lack tumor-initiating capacity (Clarke et al. 2006). Furthermore, in contrast to physiologic stem cells, which represent only a small cellular fraction of a particular tissue, CSCs may represent larger relative proportions of a total cancer cell population, depending on tumor type, variance of genetic alterations, and stage of disease progression (Gupta et al. 2009a). The number of cells needed to initiate a tumor is not part of the CSC definition (Reya et al. 2001; Schatton et al. 2009). In support of this notion, the frequency of leukemic CSCs varied more than 100-fold between patient specimens (Bonnet and Dick 1997). Given the potential confusion associated with the term "CSC," many investigators in the field refer to them as tumor-initiating or tumor-propagating cells (Clarke et al. 2006).

The determination of the relative frequency of CSCs may further be complicated by the experimental model system used to assess cancer "stemness" (Bonnet and Dick 1997; Lapidot et al. 1994; Quintana et al. 2008; Schatton et al. 2008). In this regard, it has been established for some time that biological aspects of the tumor microenvironment, including growth factor availability, extracellular matrix (ECM) constitution, or the degree of vascularization, as well as host immunocompetence can govern self-renewal capacity and tumorigenic potential (Scadden 2006). Given this dependence of defining CSC features on microenvironmental factors and the immune status of the host, it is not surprising that animal models that offer a more hospitable microenvironment for tumor growth – that is through the exogenous addition of ECM factors (e.g., Matrigel) (Quintana et al. 2008) and/or the use of more severely immunocompromised mice (Bonnet and Dick 1997; Quintana et al. 2008) – yielded higher relative CSC representation compared to CSC frequencies assessed in the absence of cografted stromal factors in more immunocompetent mouse models (Lapidot et al. 1994; Quintana et al. 2008; Schatton et al. 2008). The complexity of CSC biology and its implications for the type of animal model utilized for their characterization is further highlighted by the identification of novel CSC functions (Frank et al. 2010), including their intrinsic property to evade or actively modulate antitumor immune responses (Chan et al. 2009; Majeti et al. 2009; Di Tomaso et al. 2010; Schatton and Frank 2009; Schatton et al. 2010; Todaro et al. 2009; Wei et al. 2010a, b). Such mechanisms, which may confer selective growth advantages to the CSC pool, need to be taken into consideration when designing biologically relevant assays for their characterization. These findings highlight the importance of establishing translationally relevant assays for the study of CSCs, which accurately mimic the environmental factors found in clinical cancers (e.g., low-nutrient levels, necrosis, hypoxia, and relatively intact antitumor immunity) rather than further deviating from them. In addition to their pertinence for the design of clinically relevant CSC model systems, findings of CSC-driven immunomodulation may have far reaching implications, as they are likely to (1) advance our knowledge of the biological mechanisms by which CSCs may drive neoplastic growth and progression, and (2) help identify novel immunological interactions through which tumors may develop resistance to current immunotherapies (Schatton and Frank 2009).

This chapter focuses on immunomodulatory functions of CSCs. We discuss these recent findings both in the context of known immunomodulatory properties of physiologic stem cells (Le Blanc and Ringden 2007; Uccelli et al. 2008) and in relation to mechanisms responsible for the downregulation of immune responses against cancers (Dunn et al. 2002; Mapara and Sykes 2004). We propose that this novel CSC-specific capability may promote tumorigenic growth and resistance to current immunotherapeutic regimens. Accordingly, CSC-driven tumor escape from immune-mediated clearance has important implications for the design of more effective cancer immunotherapies.

Immunity and Cancer: The Concepts of Tumor Immunosurveillance and Immunological Tolerance

In 1957, Sir Frank Macfarlane Burnet and Lewis Thomas advanced the concept of "tumor surveillance" (Burnet 1957a, b), which posits that precancerous and cancerous cells might display "altered-self" antigens that enable the immune system to recognize and eliminate them during the early phases of tumorigenesis. While this hypothesis remains the topic of active controversy (Dunn et al. 2002), both clinical findings and experimental results generated over the past decades support its potential importance for the tumorigenic process (Mapara and Sykes 2004). For instance, mice with deficiencies in genes essential for the regulation of innate and adaptive immune responses, including NOD/SCID (nonobese diabetic severely combined immunodeficiency), RAG2$^{-/-}$ (recombination activation gene 2 knockout), IFN$\gamma^{-/-}$ (interferon-gamma knockout), and Pfp$^{-/-}$ (perforin knockout) mice, display increased incidences of spontaneous and carcinogen-induced sarcomas, lymphomas, and/or epithelial carcinomas (Dunn et al. 2002; Mapara and Sykes 2004; Shankaran et al. 2001). In addition, recent tumor xenotransplantation experiments demonstrated that the degree of host immunocompetence correlates with cancer cell numbers required for efficient tumor formation in immunocompromised mice (Bonnet and Dick 1997; Lapidot et al. 1994; Quintana et al. 2008; Schatton et al. 2008). For example, a minimum of 2×10^5 CD34$^+$CD38$^-$ patient-derived acute myeloid leukemia (AML) cells were required for efficient tumor formation in SCID recipients (Lapidot et al. 1994) compared to 5×10^3 AML cells of equal phenotype in more severely immunocompromised NOD/SCID mice (Bonnet and Dick 1997). Similarly, fewer human melanoma cells were required to cause tumor formation in IL-2R$\gamma^{-/-}$ (interleukin-2 receptor gamma chain null) NOD/SCID (also known as NOD/SCID gamma (NSG)) recipients (Quintana et al. 2008) compared with more immunocompetent NOD/SCID mice (Quintana et al. 2008; Schatton et al. 2008). Additional support for the notion that a functional immune system may prevent tumor initiation and growth comes from epidemiological studies of tumor incidence rates in immunocompromised patients (Dunn et al. 2002; Mapara and Sykes 2004). For example, HIV patients and transplant recipients on immunosuppressive medications have a markedly increased risk for developing a wide range of cancers (Grulich et al. 2007).

Importantly, numerous antigens have been identified that show selective expression and/or elevated expression levels in cancer cells compared to normal tissue cells (Parmiani et al. 2007; Rosenberg 1999), enabling the adaptive immune system to recognize tumors as foreign (Lee et al. 1999; Stockert et al. 1998). Such tumor antigens can be categorized into two distinct types (Rosenberg 1999): (1) tumor-specific antigens (TSAs), which are aberrant gene products resulting from mutations and/or chromosomal rearrangements, such as the leukemia-specific BCR-ABL fusion transcripts (Ben-Neriah et al. 1986), and (2) tumor-associated antigens (TAAs), which are encoded by cell lineage-specific genes that are transcriptionally and translationally activated in tumors compared to physiologic tissues. Common TAAs include the differentiation antigens MART-1 (melanoma antigen recognized by T cells), TRP-2 (tyrosinase-related protein 2), gp100 (glycoprotein 100), and the NY-ESO-1 or MAGE cancer testis antigens (CTAs) (Jager et al. 2000; Kawakami et al. 2000; Saikali et al. 2007). However, while TAA-specific immune effector cell responses are detectable in cancer patients, they are often incapable of rejecting the tumor (Khong et al. 2004; Lee et al. 1999).

One potential explanation for this observation is that tumors may contain highly aggressive, rapidly dividing cancer cell fractions that might simply outgrow the capacity of antitumor immune responses (Mapara and Sykes 2004). Consistent with this hypothesis, TAAs are nonuniformly expressed, allowing for the possibility that TAA-negative cancer cells may drive tumor growth in the presence of robust antitumor immunity (Schatton and Frank 2009; Schatton et al. 2010). An alternative explanation for the limited efficacy of the host immune system to fully eradicate tumors arises from the fact that neoplastic cells originate from the organism's own tissues and therefore predominantly express self-antigens to which host immune effector cells have been "tolerized" (Mapara and Sykes 2004). "Immunogenic tolerance" is the process by which an immune response does not attack a particular set of antigens (Hogquist et al. 2005; Ramsdell and Fowlkes 1990). Tolerance to self-antigens can be achieved by processes that result in either physical elimination of autoreactive immunocytes through apoptotic cell death (clonal deletion) (Kappler et al. 1987) or functional nonresponsiveness (clonal anergy) of antigen-reactive cells (Ramsdell et al. 1989). Self-tolerance refers to the ability of the body's immune system to recognize and protect self major histocompatibility complex (MHC)/*self* peptide complex-bearing cells from immune-mediated rejection while at the same time retaining its capacity to launch an immune response against cells expressing MHC/*foreign* peptide complexes (Hogquist et al. 2005; Ramsdell and Fowlkes 1990). Thus, the induction of immunological tolerance via positive and negative selection mechanisms prevents the emergence of autoimmune disorders under physiological conditions (Hogquist et al. 2005). In the cancer context, however, immune tolerance toward a tumor may facilitate tumorigenesis and neoplastic progression by preventing the host immune system from eliminating transformed cells (Mapara and Sykes 2004). This predicament has been demonstrated, for example, for the tumor suppressor protein and TAA, p53 (Theobald et al. 1997), which is aberrantly expressed by a variety of cancers (Kim and Deppert 2004). However, because of its low-level expression in normal tissues, p53-reactive cytotoxic T lymphocytes (CTLs) might be eliminated by clonal deletion and/or rendered anergic thereby impeding a potential antitumor immune response against p53-expressing cancer cells. Indeed, the functional avidity of p53-reactive CTLs was found to be approximately tenfold lower in syngeneic $p53^{+/+}$ compared to $p53^{-/-}$ transgenic mice (Theobald et al. 1997).

Taken together, findings of increased tumor incidence in immunocompromised individuals and animal models and the detection of TAA-directed immune responses in tumor patients support the possibility that the immune system can recognize and destroy nascent transformed cells, thereby promoting protection against tumor development (Dunn et al. 2002). However, this potential tumor suppressor role of the immune response could also facilitate the selection of cancer cells with the ability to escape from immune destruction (Dunn et al. 2002; Mapara and Sykes 2004). Emerging evidence now supports the possibility that the cells responsible for tumor initiation and growth, i.e., CSCs (Frank et al. 2010; Reya et al. 2001), could play pivotal roles in tumor immune evasion (Chan et al. 2009; Majeti et al. 2009; Di Tomaso et al. 2010; Schatton and Frank 2009; Schatton et al. 2010; Todaro et al. 2009; Wei et al. 2010a, b). Accordingly, such a CSC-associated function might importantly contribute to neoplastic development and progression (Schatton and Frank 2008, 2009). Here, we discuss recent findings of CSC-mediated immunomodulation in the context of established mechanisms responsible for the downregulation of immune responses against tumors and in relation to established immunomodulatory functions of physiologic stem cells.

Immunomodulatory Functions of Cancer Stem Cells: Mechanistic Insights

The CSC hypothesis predicts that (1) the CSC pool is required for tumor initiation and disease progression and (2) that targeted ablation of CSCs could eradicate cancers currently resistant to systemic therapy (Frank et al. 2010). Consequently, researchers have embarked on the quest of prospectively identifying CSC populations in a growing number of tumor entities (Schatton et al. 2009). Importantly, critical links between CSCs, neoplastic progression, and therapy resistance have emerged (Bao et al. 2006a; Li et al. 2008; Yu et al. 2007; Diehn et al. 2009; Dylla et al. 2008; Schatton et al. 2008), and proof-of-principle has now been established that selective eradication of CSCs can inhibit experimental tumor growth (Bao et al. 2008; Chan et al. 2009; Gupta et al. 2009b; Lathia et al. 2010; Li et al. 2009b; Majeti et al. 2009; Schatton et al. 2008; Yang et al. 2008). Despite these seminal advances, the precise mechanisms and pathways by which CSCs drive tumorigenicity and disease progression remain incompletely understood (Frank et al. 2010). Based on the demonstrated ability of cancer cell fractions to thwart the antitumor immune response in order to promote robust tumor growth (Dunn et al. 2002; Mapara and Sykes 2004) and the established capacity of physiologic stem cells to modulate allo- and autoimmunity (Le Blanc and Ringden 2007; Uccelli et al. 2008), we previously hypothesized that one important mechanism by which CSCs may drive the tumorigenic process might be their competence to preferentially evade an adequate antitumor response (Schatton and Frank 2008, 2009).

Indeed, several recent reports now demonstrate a specific relationship of CSCs to the evasion of host antitumor immunity (Chan et al. 2009; Majeti et al. 2009; Di Tomaso et al. 2010; Schatton and Frank 2009; Schatton et al. 2010; Todaro et al. 2009; Wei et al. 2010a, b). For example, in human malignant melanoma, the CSC or malignant melanoma-initiating cell (MMIC) fraction, which is marked by the chemoresistance determinant ABCB5 (Schatton et al. 2008), inhibited mitogen-activated peripheral blood mononuclear cell (PBMC) proliferation more efficiently than melanoma bulk populations (Schatton et al. 2010). Consistently, MMICs also preferentially inhibited production of the proliferative cytokine IL-2 by cocultured mitogen-activated PBMCs, and did not induce an IL-2 release by cocultured patient-identical PBMCs in the absence of mitogenic stimulation, whereas significant levels of IL-2 were detected in cocultures of melanoma bulk components with PBMCs (Schatton et al. 2010). Moreover, ABCB5$^+$ MMICs compared to bulk populations preferentially induced secretion of the immunosuppressive cytokine IL-10 by cocultured autologous PBMCs (Schatton et al. 2010). Similarly, glioblastoma stem-like cancer cells were found in three separate studies to suppress both mitogen and anti-CD3/CD28 stimulation-dependent T-cell proliferation (Di Tomaso et al. 2010; Wei et al. 2010a, b) and IL-2 and IFN-γ effector cytokine production (Wei et al. 2010a, b). Furthermore, Todaro et al. (2009) demonstrated increased resistance of colorectal cancer stem-like subsets vs. differentiated colon cancer cell lines to cytotoxic lysis by $\gamma\delta$ T cells. It should be noted that dissociated cancer cell populations isolated from tumor spheroid bodies grown in stem cell-permissive medium as opposed to prospectively purified, marker-defined CSCs were used in immune activation assays in these and other immunological CSC studies (Brown et al. 2009; Di Tomaso et al. 2010; Todaro et al. 2009; Wei et al. 2010a, b). Given the fact that tumor spheroids contain heterogeneous cell populations the composition of which may widely vary based on culture conditions (Jensen and Parmar 2006), it is difficult to draw definitive conclusions regarding an association between the immunomodulatory mechanisms described with CSC-specific behavior (Brown et al. 2009; Di Tomaso et al. 2010; Todaro et al. 2009; Wei et al. 2010a, b). For instance, while the glioma spheroid bodies reported by two independent groups (Brown et al. 2009; Wei et al. 2010a, b) were largely positive for the brain tumor CSC marker (Singh et al. 2004) CD133, Di Tomaso et al. (2010) immunologically characterized glioblastoma neurospheres that completely lacked CD133 expression. Marked differences were also reported with regard to expression levels of immune molecules, including, for example, class I and class II MHC molecules, in the distinct glioma spheroids characterized by different research laboratories (Brown et al. 2009; Di Tomaso et al. 2010; Wei et al. 2010a, b). Nonetheless, this research considerably strengthens the existing evidence of relative immune privilege of primitive cancer subpopulations and supports the hypothesis that evasion of immune-mediated elimination might be one important mechanism by which CSCs may sustain the tumorigenic process.

Several immunological mechanisms by which CSCs might modulate the antitumor immune response are now beginning to be unraveled (Chan et al. 2009; Majeti et al. 2009; Di Tomaso et al. 2010; Schatton and Frank 2009; Schatton et al. 2010; Todaro et al. 2009; Wei et al. 2010a, b). Moreover, additional CSC-associated immunoevasive strategies may be anticipated based on known tumor escape mechanisms and in light of established immunomodulatory properties of physiologic stem cells (Schatton and Frank 2009). For example, one important mechanism by which tumors can escape destruction by the anticancer immune response is by downregulating the expression of TAAs (Khong et al. 2004). In consideration of the CSC hypothesis, it seems plausible that the more undifferentiated cancer subpopulations responsible for tumor initiation and growth, i.e., CSCs, may not express common TAAs (Schatton and Frank 2009) (Fig. 18.1a). Indeed, MMICs demonstrated low to absent expression of the TAAs MART-1 (Schatton and Frank 2009; Schatton et al. 2010), NY-ESO-1, MAGE-A, and ML-IAP (melanoma inhibitor of apoptosis protein, also named livin) compared to tumor bulk populations (Schatton et al. 2010). Comparably, stem-like glioma cells were found to lack expression of several TAAs, including gp100, NY-ESO-1, MAGE, and IL-13Rα2 (IL-13 receptor alpha 2) (Di Tomaso et al. 2010). Consequently, CSCs might not be recognized by the anticancer immune response, which may render them resistant to rejection by immune effector populations. Taken together, these findings might thus provide for a novel explanation for the relative ineffectiveness of CD8$^+$ tumor-reactive T cells to fully eradicate cancers (Khong et al. 2004).

Another potential mechanism through which CSCs could evade rejection by T effector cells might be through downmodulation or absence of MHC class I antigen expression (Schatton and Frank 2009) (Fig. 18.1a). MHC class I molecules play critical roles in the recognition of malignant cells by CD8$^+$ cytotoxic T lymphocytes (CTLs) and, to a lesser degree, by CD4$^+$ T cells (Nishimura et al. 1999; Ruiter et al. 1991). Accordingly, partial or complete loss of MHC class I molecules may render class I-restricted CTLs or CD4$^+$ T cells unable to lyse tumor target cells (Aptsiauri et al. 2007; Bubenik 2003; Khong et al. 2004). Importantly, MHC class I expression was significantly reduced both in ABCB5$^+$ MMICs vis-à-vis melanoma bulk components (Schatton et al. 2010) and in glioma spheroid bodies compared to cancer cells cultured in the presence of fetal bovine serum (FBS) (Di Tomaso et al. 2010). Of note, decreased MHC class I expression has been associated with neoplastic progression, therapeutic unresponsiveness, and adverse clinical outcome in human patients (Aptsiauri et al. 2007; Cabrera et al. 2007; Carretero et al. 2008; van Houdt et al. 2008), which may at least in part relate to the inability of the antitumor immune response to eliminate the MHC class I$^-$ CSC pool.

It is important to recognize that low MHC class I levels may increase the susceptibility of tumor cells to natural killer (NK)-mediated cell lysis (Bubenik 2003). Owing to their cytolytic activity, NK cells are important effector cells of the innate immune system that form the first line of defense against pathogens and transformed cells (Moretta 2002). The function of NK cells is closely regulated by distinct cell

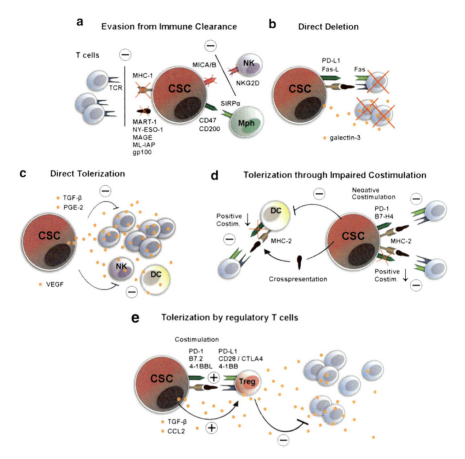

Fig. 18.1 Mechanisms of cancer stem cell (CSC)-mediated immunomodulation. (a) CSCs may evade rejection by CD8[+] T cells through absent or decreased expression of tumor-associated antigens (TAAs), such as MART-1, NY-ESO-1, MAGE, ML-IAP, or gp100, or through reduced MHC class I expression (TCR: T-cell receptor). To evade natural killer (NK)-mediated lysis, CSCs could either downmodulate their expression of activating NK receptor ligands (e.g., MICA or MICB) or induce decreased expression of activating surface receptors (e.g., NKG2D) on NK cells. In addition, CSCs may block the phagocytic activity of macrophages (Mph) through surface expression of the inhibitory SIRPα ligand CD47. Similarly, CD200 expression might enable CSCs to inhibit macrophage activation. (b) Direct deletion through the induction of immune effector cell apoptosis (e.g., via PD-L1-, Fas/Fas-L-, and/or galectin-3) might represent an additional mechanism of CSC-driven immune evasion. (c) CSCs might also directly tolerize immune effector populations, including T cells, NK cells, and dendritic cells (DCs), by secreting immunosuppressive factors, such as, for example, TGF-β, PGE-2, or VEGF. (d) Specifically, with regard to DCs, CSC-secreted molecules could inhibit their maturation. Cross-presentation of TAAs or CSC-specific antigens by such immature or functionally impaired DCs incapable of adequate costimulation might render tumor-reactive T cells anergic. Alternatively, MHC class II-expressing CSCs could function as antigen-presenting cells (APCs) that might tolerize tumor-specific T effector cells through absent positive costimulation or by delivering a negative costimulatory signal (e.g., PD-1 or B7-H4). (e) Finally, CSCs might actively induce and/or recruit regulatory T (Treg) cells to mitigate the antitumor immune response. Costimulatory signaling networks (i.e., PD-1/PD-L1, B7.2/CTLA4, or 4-1BBL/4-1BB) and/or soluble mediators (e.g., TGF-β or CCL2) could thereby facilitate functional interactions between CSCs and Treg cells

surface receptors, such as, for example, NKG2D (natural killer group 2, member D), that can trigger activating or inhibitory signals upon engagement with target cell ligands (Bauer et al. 1999; Diefenbach et al. 2001). Interestingly, mesenchymal stem cells, which, like CSCs (Di Tomaso et al. 2010; Schatton et al. 2010), may express reduced levels of MHC class I (Le Blanc et al. 2003), have been described to inhibit NK cell-mediated cytotoxicity by downregulating the expression of activating surface receptors, particularly on resting NK cells (Spaggiari et al. 2008). Similarly, malignant tumors, including CSCs, could develop means to control the expression of activating vs. inhibitory receptors on NK cells (Zhang et al. 2005) (Fig. 18.1a). Alternatively, CSCs might downregulate the expression of activating NK cell ligands and/or could express inhibitory ligands on their cell surface (Fig. 18.1a). Initial experimental support for this possibility is given by findings of little to no expression of the activating NKG2D ligands MICA and MICB (MHC class I-related proteins A and B) and the UL16-binding proteins 1–4 (ULBP1–4) on both glioma (Di Tomaso et al. 2010) and colorectal cancer spheroid cells (Todaro et al. 2009).

Additional mediators of the innate immune response involved in the recognition and clearance of foreign or malignant cells include macrophages (Jaiswal et al. 2010). While macrophages have predominantly been described to support protumorigenic activities such as tumor angiogenesis and metastasis formation, particularly under hypoxic conditions (Du et al. 2008), they can also act as phagocytes that remove foreign or transformed cells, for example, via Fc or complement receptor-dependent mechanisms (Fadok et al. 2001). CD200 surface receptor (CD200R) signaling can negatively regulate macrophage activation and inflammatory status (Nathan and Muller 2001). Notably, expression of the CD200R ligand, CD200, by cancer cells augments their ability to metastasize (Stumpfova et al. 2010). Intriguingly, CD200 was found preferentially expressed by CSC phenotype-expressing tumor subsets in breast, brain, and colon cancer (Kawasaki et al. 2007), allowing for the possibility that CSCs might modulate macrophage function to promote neoplastic progression (Fig. 18.1a). Signaling through the SIRPα (signal-regulatory protein alpha) receptor on macrophages can negatively regulate their phagocytic activity (Barclay and Brown 2006). For instance, upregulation of the anti-phagocytic SIRPα ligand CD47 (also known as integrin-associated protein, IAP) by circulating hematopoietic stem cells (HSCs) enables them to evade macrophage killing (Jaiswal et al. 2009). Importantly, AML CSCs were found to express elevated CD47 levels compared to their normal counterparts and increased CD47 expression predicted worse overall survival in AML patients (Majeti et al. 2009). Furthermore, monoclonal antibody-mediated CD47 blockade on AML CSCs inhibited their in vivo engraftment and anti-CD47 antibody treatment of human AML-bearing mice resulted in marked inhibition of disease propagation (Majeti et al. 2009). Similarly, CSC-directed CD47 blockade resulted in macrophage engulfment of bladder cancer cells in vitro (Chan et al. 2009). Together, these findings establish CD47 as an important CSC-associated immune evasion mechanism (Fig. 18.1a) and identify the SIRPα-CD47 pathway as a potential therapeutic target for tumor therapy.

In addition to their preferential evasion of CTL-, NK-, or macrophage-mediated lysis, CSCs might also engage in active tolerance induction in order to modulate the host antitumor immune response in favor of inexorable tumor growth. In support of this hypothesis, tumor-reactive T cells are often unable to eliminate TAA-bearing cancer populations upon continuous antigen exposure despite the initial occurrence of transient CD4$^+$ clonal expansions (Staveley-O'Carroll et al. 1998). One major mechanism of tolerance induction involves clonal deletion of antigen-reactive T cells through apoptotic cell death (Ramsdell and Fowlkes 1990). The secreted beta-galactoside-binding protein galectin-3 represents one important immune regulator of apoptosis, particularly of tumor-reactive CD8$^+$ T cells (Peng et al. 2008). Consequently, galectin-3 administration to tumor-bearing mice promoted neoplastic progression (Peng et al. 2008). Galectin-3 has also been implicated in mesenchymal stem cell-mediated immunomodulation (Sioud et al. 2010). Specifically, knockdown of galectin-3 using small-interfering RNA (siRNA) reduced the immunosuppressive effect of mesenchymal stem cells on mixed lymphocyte cultures (Sioud et al. 2010). Similarly, CD133$^+$ pulmonary adenocarcinoma cells induced CD8$^+$ T-cell apoptosis in a galectin-3 dependent manner (Li et al. 2010). Markedly increased galectin-3 levels were also detected in supernatants of glioma spheroid cultures compared to glioma cells cultured in the presence of differentiation factors (Wei et al. 2010b). Consistently, exogenous addition of galectin-3 to glioma stem-like cell/PBMC cocultures induced T-cell apoptosis (Wei et al. 2010b). This galectin-3-mediated apoptosis induction could be reversed by genetic knockdown of the STAT3 (signal transducer and activator of transcription 3) transcription factor (Wei et al. 2010b), which was recently also implicated in glioma CSC survival and tumor growth (Wang et al. 2009). An alternative mechanism by which glioma stem-like cells may induce T-cell apoptosis could involve the programmed death ligand 1 (PD-L1, also named B7-H1) (Wei et al. 2010b). PD-L1 is widely expressed by several cancers and can provide a molecular shield to a growing neoplasm by promoting apoptosis of tumor-infiltrating, cancer-reactive T cells (Dong et al. 2002; Hirano et al. 2005). Consistently, Wei et al. (2010b) reported that PD-L1 blockade on glioma stem-like cells could reverse apoptosis induction in cocultured T cells. Conversely, PD-L1 was not found differentially expressed in spheroid vs. adherent glioma cultures in a separate study (Di Tomaso et al. 2010) and was expressed at lower levels in CSCs compared to tumor bulk populations in human malignant melanoma (Schatton et al. 2010). Another important mediator of T-cell deletion is the Fas/Fas-L system (Strand et al. 1996). Tumors can actively destroy T cells by enhanced secretion of soluble Fas-L (Andreola et al. 2002; Hahne et al. 1996; Hallermalm et al. 2004; Neuber and Eidam 2006). Consistently, absence of Fas-L expression in tumor metastases correlated with better overall patient survival (Neuber and Eidam 2006). While a specific relationship between CSC-driven immune evasion and the Fas/Fas-L signaling axis, galectin-3-, or PD-L1-mediated apoptosis has not been established to date, the currently available scientific evidence, however, supports the possibility that CSCs might actively downregulate the antitumor immune response through apoptotic deletion of cancer-reactive T-cell clones (Fig. 18.1b).

Immunological tolerance can also be induced through functional inactivation of antigen-reactive lymphocytes (Ramsdell et al. 1989). Tolerance induction through nondeletional mechanisms is also referred to as clonal anergy (Ramsdell et al. 1989). One immunological process that has been implicated in the induction of anergy is direct inhibition of antigen-reactive cells via the secretion of immunosuppressive factors, including, for example, TGF-β (transforming growth factor beta) or PGE-2 (prostaglandin E2) (Mannie et al. 1995; Wahl et al. 2004). Notably, both TGF-β and PGE-2 are constitutively produced by mesenchymal stem cells and have been found to prominently contribute to their immunosuppressive effects on T cell, dendritic cell (DC), and NK cell activation (Aggarwal and Pittenger 2005; Djouad et al. 2007; Liu et al. 2004; Spaggiari et al. 2008). These soluble factors can also be produced by tumors to dampen the anticancer immune response (Gorelik and Flavell 2001; Herfs et al. 2009; Inge et al. 1992). Markedly elevated PGE-2 and TGF-β levels were also detected in spheroid glioma cultures compared to glioblastoma cells cultured in differentiation medium (Wei et al. 2010a) (Fig. 18.1c). Moreover, additional immunoregulatory members of the TGF-β axis are specifically activated in the CSC fraction of breast cancers (Shipitsin et al. 2007) and melanomas (Schatton et al. 2010), suggesting a potentially important role for TGF-β signaling in CSC-driven immunomodulation (Fig. 18.1c). Vascular endothelial growth factor (VEGF) represents an additional soluble molecule constitutively produced by mesenchymal stem cells (Aggarwal and Pittenger 2005), which, in addition to its angiogenesis-promoting effects (Risau 1997), can mediate immunosuppression by blocking the differentiation of bone marrow-resident lymphoid progenitor cells (Ohm et al. 2003). This surrogate VEGF activity might potentially also contribute to tumorigenesis. Interestingly, glioma spheroid cultures (Wei et al. 2010a) and CD133$^+$ glioma CSCs (Bao et al. 2006b) demonstrated enhanced VEGF production compared to more differentiated tumor cells, and in vivo VEGF blockade suppressed growth of glioblastoma CSC-derived xenografts (Bao et al. 2006b). However, whether immunomodulatory effects may contribute to CSC-mediated, VEGF-induced tumor growth requires further investigation. In sum, secretion of immunosuppressive cytokines and growth factors could represent one mechanism by which CSCs might render antigen-reactive lymphocytes anergic to fuel immune evasion and ultimately tumorigenic growth (Fig. 18.1c).

Induction of anergy can further result from impaired stimulation of antigen-specific immune cells (Li et al. 2009a). According to the "two-signal" paradigm, antigen-dependent T-cell activation requires two distinct but complimentary signals: naïve T cells receive signal 1 through T-cell receptor (TCR) engagement with the MHC/antigenic peptide complex presented by an APC (antigen-presenting cell) (Li et al. 2009a). Signal 2 is an antigen-nonspecific stimulus triggered through ligation of an APC-expressed positive costimulatory ligand to its respective receptor expressed on the T cell (Li et al. 2009a). Positive costimulatory signaling is required for full T-cell activation leading to IL-2 production, clonal expansion, and the acquisition of an effector/memory phenotype (Jenkins et al. 1991). Importantly, TCR signaling in the absence of positive costimulation may induce T-cell anergy and/or apoptosis (Schwartz 1990). Additionally, negative or inhibitory costimulatory signals may function to downregulate immune responses (Freeman et al. 2000; Li et al. 2009a). Costimulatory molecules can be grouped broadly into three distinct superfamilies based on structural homology: (1) the immunoglobulin (Ig) superfamily, which includes CD28, CTLA-4 (cytotoxic T lymphocyte antigen-4), and PD-1, (2) the tumor necrosis factor (TNF)/TNF receptor (TNFR) superfamily, in which the CD40/CD40L pathway is dominant, and (3) the emerging T-cell Ig domain and mucin domain family (TIM) (Li et al. 2009a). Of note, costimulatory signaling events are not restricted to T cell–APC interactions, but may also encompass interactions between T cells and nonlymphoid cells, including mesenchymal stem cells and cancer cells (Kroczek et al. 2004). It thus seems plausible that CSCs could interfere with costimulatory signaling events to mitigate the antitumor immune response in favor of neoplastic progression. For example, CSCs could inhibit T-cell-dependent tumor immunity by actively modulating the positive costimulatory molecule repertoire and hence the activation state of APCs (Fig. 18.1d). In support of this possibility, mesenchymal stem cells suppressed APC differentiation and function leading to T-cell unresponsiveness (Beyth et al. 2005; Jiang et al. 2005). In the cancer context, tolerance to a particular tumor epitope was induced through cross-presentation of the TAA by APCs incapable of providing adequate positive costimulation (Sotomayor et al. 2001). Consistently, stimulation of such dysfunctional APCs with activating antibodies against CD40 resulted in T-cell priming and subsequent regression of experimental tumors (Sotomayor et al. 1999).

It is also possible that CSCs themselves may serve as functional APCs (Fig. 18.1d). In fact, MMICs displayed aberrant positivity for MHC class II (Schatton et al. 2010). Similarly, glioma stem-like cells expressed MHC class II (Brown et al. 2009; Di Tomaso et al. 2010; Wei et al. 2010a, b). Importantly, continuous exposure to a particular antigen is required for the maintenance of T-cell anergy (Ramsdell and Fowlkes 1992). Presentation of a TAA by MHC class II-expressing CSCs, especially in the absence of concurrent positive costimulation, could thus potentially foster tumor escape from immunosurveillance by maintaining T-cell unresponsiveness. While direct evidence for this possibility in the context of CSCs has not been established to date, MHC class II$^+$ tumor cells were found to instigate T-cell anergy in MHC class II-restricted T-cell clones ex vivo (Becker et al. 1993). In human patients, MHC class II expression by tumor cells correlated with disease progression and adverse clinical outcome (Brocker et al. 1984; Ruiter et al. 1991). T-cell homing to lymph nodes is required for APC-mediated tolerance induction to alloantigens (Bai et al. 2002). Strikingly, compared to primary melanomas and visceral metastasis, melanoma metastasis to lymph nodes comprised an enhanced relative frequency of ABCB5$^+$ MMICs (Schatton et al. 2008), which also demonstrated selective expression of MHC class II compared to tumor bulk populations in a separate study (Schatton et al. 2010). Furthermore, both ABCB5$^+$ MMICs (Schatton et al. 2010) and glioma spheroid cultures (Di Tomaso et al. 2010; Wei et al. 2010a, b) showed absent to low expression of several prominent positive costimulatory molecules, including members of the CD28/B7 and CD40/CD40L signaling pathways. Taken together, these findings lend initial experimental support to the possibility that CSCs might actively present common TAAs or CSC-specific antigens, such as ABCB5 (Schatton et al. 2008), in the absence of positive costimulation to inactivate tumor-reactive T cells (Fig. 18.1d).

Alternatively, CSCs could also disrupt the antitumor response via the expression of negative costimulatory molecules (Fig. 18.1d). Indeed, tumorigenic MMIC fractions displayed selective expression for the negative costimulator PD-1 (Schatton et al. 2010). Similarly, glioma spheroids showed homogeneous positivity for both PD-1 (Di Tomaso et al. 2010) and its ligand PD-L1 (Di Tomaso et al. 2010; Wei et al. 2010a, b), suggesting a potentially important role for the PD-1-PD-L1/PD-L2 signaling axis in CSC-driven tumor immune evasion. In support of this hypothesis, tumor cell-expressed PD-L1 conferred resistance to CTL killing (Hirano et al. 2005). In addition to its role in negative costimulation, PD-L1 can also induce T-cell apoptosis in a PD-1 signaling-independent manner (discussed above) (Dong et al. 2002). While the involvement of PD-L1 on cancer cells in the escape of host antitumor immunity and neoplastic progression is now well established (Dong et al. 2002; Gao et al. 2009; Hamanishi et al. 2007; Hirano et al. 2005; Nomi et al. 2007), findings of PD-1 receptor expression on tumorigenic cancer cell subsets are novel (Schatton et al. 2010). In this regard, it is important to recognize that PD-1 receptor ligation may not only confer changes to the PD-1-expressing cell but can also lead to reverse signaling into ligand-positive immune cell populations (Kuipers et al. 2006; Dong et al. 2003). For example, soluble PD-1 inhibited DC activation (Kuipers et al. 2006) and induced production of the immunosuppressive cytokine IL-10 by CD4$^+$ T cells (Dong et al. 2003). In addition, blockade of the PD-1 ligand, PD-L2, on DCs prevented experimental tumor growth (Radhakrishnan et al. 2004). It is thus possible that CSCs might modulate antitumor immunity via reverse PD-1 signaling. Importantly, a monoclonal antibody directed at PD-1 (MDX-1106), which is thought to primarily act through PD-1 inhibition on T cells, is currently in phase I testing for various cancers, with partial and complete responses observed (Brahmer et al. 2010). Findings of unaltered primary tumor growth in pd-1$^{-/-}$ vs. wild-type mice (Iwai et al. 2005) could support the possibility that the therapeutic efficacy of MDX-1106 may not solely rely on the alteration of PD-1 signaling in T cells but also on the inhibition of PD-1-mediated evasion of antitumor immunity by CSCs. An additional costimulatory molecule with important roles in the modulation of both innate and adaptive immune responses (Yi and Chen 2009), which was found preferentially expressed by slow-cycling CD133$^+$ brain tumor cells (Yao et al. 2008), is the emerging negative costimulatory ligand B7-H4. Of note, tumor-specific B7-H4 expression correlated with cancer progression, decreased numbers of tumor-infiltrating lymphocytes, and adverse clinical outcome in various tumor entities (Krambeck et al. 2006; Miyatake et al. 2007; Mugler et al. 2007). Together these findings highlight the potential importance of negative costimulatory signaling for CSC-driven evasion of immune-mediated tumor rejection (Fig. 18.1d). However, the functional relevance of negative costimulatory molecule expression by stem-like cancer cells is yet to be elucidated.

Finally, the induction and/or active recruitment of regulatory T (Treg) cells might represent an additional mechanism by which CSCs may thwart the antitumor immune response (Fig. 18.1e). Treg cells can potently inhibit the activation and cytokine production of other immune cells and are thus essential for the maintenance of immunological self-tolerance and immune homeostasis (Hori et al. 2003;

Nishizuka and Sakakura 1969; Sakaguchi et al. 1995). Phenotypically, Treg cells are typically distinguished among CD4+ T cells by their high expression of the IL-2 receptor (also known as CD25) and positivity for the transcription factor FOXP3 (forkhead box P3) (Hori et al. 2003). Yet, alternative phenotypes, including CD8+ Treg cells have been described (Smith and Kumar 2008). Importantly, the generation and/or recruitment of Treg cells to inflammatory sites is one mechanism by which mesenchymal stem cells can induce tolerance to alloantigens (Aggarwal and Pittenger 2005; Casiraghi et al. 2008; Di Ianni et al. 2008). The induction of Treg cells has also been implicated in enhanced experimental tumor growth (Djouad et al. 2003). Accumulating evidence further suggests that Treg cells might also be important mediators of tumor immune evasion in oncology patients (Ahmadzadeh et al. 2008; Clark et al. 2008; Curiel et al. 2004; Liyanage et al. 2002; Woo et al. 2002). Specifically, Treg cells isolated from lung cancer specimens inhibited proliferation of autologous T cells (Woo et al. 2002). Moreover, increased Treg cell frequencies were detected in tumor lesions and peripheral blood of cancer patients compared to the respective physiologic tissues and blood of healthy individuals (Clark et al. 2008; Liyanage et al. 2002). Furthermore, elevated Treg cell numbers predicted reduced overall survival of ovarian carcinoma patients (Curiel et al. 2004). Importantly, both MMICs (Schatton et al. 2010) and glioma stem-like cells (Wei et al. 2010a, b) were found to induce Treg cells among cocultured PBMCs, supporting the possibility that CSC-mediated regulation of Treg cell behavior might foster tumor immune privilege.

Mechanistically, signaling through negative costimulatory molecules expressed by Treg cells, such as PD-L1 or CTLA-4, may control their tolerogenic effects (Wang et al. 2008; Wing et al. 2008) (Fig. 18.1e). Accordingly, PD-1 or B7.2 expression (Di Tomaso et al. 2010; Schatton et al. 2010) by CSCs might function to enable their interaction with Treg cells. To exert their immunosuppressive effects, Treg cells may further depend on strong positive costimulatory signaling, for example, through the CD28 or 4-1BB receptors (Hombach et al. 2007; Tsukahara et al. 2005; Zheng et al. 2004) (Fig. 18.1e). Strikingly, ABCB5+ MMICs showed preferential expression for both the CD28 ligand B7.2 and 4-1BBL, and MMIC-specific blockade of B7.2 decreased the abundance of Treg cells along with IL-10 production among cocultured mitogen-activated PBMCs (Schatton et al. 2010). These findings establish a functional link between B7.2 signaling and CSC-mediated Treg cell maintenance, with important implications for tumor immune evasion and cancer immunotherapy (Fig. 18.1e).

In addition to costimulatory signaling, paracrine production of immunosuppressive factors, including TGF-β, may govern the generation and function of Treg cells (Ostroukhova et al. 2006; Du et al. 2006) (Fig. 18.1e). Intriguingly, MMICs compared to tumor bulk populations expressed higher transcript levels of TGF-β2 and TGF-β3 (Schatton et al. 2010), both of which have been implicated in the induction of Treg cells (Namba et al. 2002; Shah and Qiao 2008) and in melanoma progression (Van Belle et al. 1996). Also, supernatants of cancer stem-like glioma cells contained increased TGF-β levels vs. supernatants from glioma cells cultured in differentiation medium (Wei et al. 2010a). An additional soluble mediator recently suggested as a CSC-secreted factor in glioma is the inflammatory chemokine CCL2 (Wei et al. 2010a). CCL2 can serve as a chemoattractant for Treg cells (Hasegawa et al. 2007) and has been associated with malignant transformation and tumor development (Soria and Ben-Baruch 2008). Taken together, these findings support the possibility that CSCs might modulate Treg cell behavior, including their homing patterns and immunosuppressive functions, to promote tumor immune evasion (Fig. 18.1e).

In summary, several recent reports (Chan et al. 2009; Majeti et al. 2009; Di Tomaso et al. 2010; Schatton and Frank 2009; Schatton et al. 2010; Todaro et al. 2009; Wei et al. 2010a, b) suggest that the CSC component within a tumor may possess a preferential ability to thwart the antitumor immune response. The mechanisms of CSC-mediated modulation of antitumor immunity are, however, only beginning to be unraveled. Interestingly, CSC-specific immunomodulatory functions parallel tolerogenic properties of physiological stem cells (Le Blanc and Ringden 2007; Uccelli et al. 2008) and mechanisms of cancer immunotherapy resistance (Dunn et al. 2002; Mapara and Sykes 2004). As such, insights generated in these related research areas may help furthering the scientific progress in the very exciting and highly promising CSC immunity field. In particular, CSC-mediated tumor immune escape from immune-mediated rejection has important implications for current immunotherapeutic strategies for various cancers.

Translational Relevance of Cancer Stem Cells to Tumor Immunotherapy

Tumor immunotherapy has emerged as a promising treatment option for patients with metastatic disease, with sometimes remarkable but nevertheless often limited success (Rosenberg et al. 2008). This particularly applies to two of the most chemoresistant and immunogenic cancers – that is malignant melanoma and renal cell carcinoma (Rosenberg et al. 2008). One major obstacle has been to develop strategies that efficiently antagonize mechanisms of tumor immune escape and resistance to immunotherapy (Dunn et al. 2002; Mapara and Sykes 2004). Cancer immunotherapeutic strategies can be broadly categorized into (1) immunomodulatory methods aimed at reinforcing host antitumor immunity, (2) active immunization protocols that involve whole cells, peptides, or immunizing vectors to sensitize the host immune system against the cancer, and (3) adoptive cell transfer (ACT) of ex vivo expanded autologous or allogeneic immunocytes reactive against TAAs (Rosenberg et al. 2008).

Immune activators approved for the treatment of tumor patients with refractory malignancy include IL-2 and IFN-α (Atkins et al. 1993, 1999; Flaherty et al. 2001; Schuchter 2004). Yet, many cancer patients do not benefit from monotherapies with these nonspecific immune enhancers, as evident by complete response rates of only about 5–15% (Atkins et al. 1993, 1999; Flaherty et al. 2001; Schuchter 2004). One explanation for the observed refractoriness of cancers to IL-2 immunotherapy is given by the importance of the cytokine not only for the activation of T effector populations but also for the induction of Treg cells (Ting et al. 1984). Indeed, IL-2 treatment was found to increase Treg cell frequencies in cancer patients (Ahmadzadeh and Rosenberg 2006). Accordingly, Treg cell depletion could represent a promising strategy to enhance cancer immunotherapeutic efficacy, as indicated by findings of enhanced antitumor immunity upon Treg cell reduction in experimental animal models (Jones et al. 2002) and human patients (Dannull et al. 2005). However, an inability of current Treg cell-depleting regimens to sustain a prolonged decrease of Treg cell numbers was observed by others (Attia et al. 2005; Powell et al. 2007). In light of the CSC concept, it seems plausible that adequate Treg cell depletion and thus IL-2 therapeutic efficiency might require the concurrent blockade of CSC-associated mechanisms responsible for Treg cell induction (Schatton et al. 2010; Wei et al. 2010a). Irrespective of an IL-2 effect on Treg cell maintenance, CSC-driven immunotherapy resistance is also suggested by findings of preferentially inhibited IL-2 cytokine production by autologous or mitogen-activated PBMCs cocultured in the presence of MMICs vs. melanoma bulk populations (Schatton et al. 2010). Similarly, glioma spheroid cells suppressed IL-2 production by cocultured autologous T cells (Wei et al. 2010b). These findings may ultimately provide novel insights into the mechanisms underlying immunotherapy resistance of human cancers. Moreover, they have profound implications for the design of experimental model systems aimed at the identification of CSCs. Specifically, tumorigenicity experiments performed in the absence of functional IL-2 signaling, as is the case, for example, in NSG mice (Quintana et al. 2008), might represent inadequate xenotransplantation assays for the characterization of CSCs. This possibility is further supported by the established negative correlation between IL-2 cytokine levels with tumorigenic growth in experimental animal models, including in syngeneic settings (Abdel-Wahab et al. 1994; Zatloukal et al. 1995). Given the potential importance of immunomodulation for CSC-mediated tumor initiation and growth (Chan et al. 2009; Majeti et al. 2009; Di Tomaso et al. 2010; Schatton and Frank 2009; Schatton et al. 2010; Todaro et al. 2009; Wei et al. 2010a, b), an ideal mouse model for the study of CSC biology would be one that allows CSC-immune cell interactions to take place in a manner closely resembling the clinical patient scenario, for example, by reconstituting immunocompromised mice with isogenic patient leukocytes (Melkus et al. 2006) prior to the transplantation of autologous tumor subpopulations.

More recently, additional immunotherapeutics aimed at modulating critical regulatory elements of patient immune cells to enhance their antitumor reactivity have entered clinical trials (Kirkwood et al. 2008). These include inhibitors of costimulatory molecules or paracrine immunosuppressive cytokines, including CTLA-4, PD-1, 4-1BB, and TGF-β (Fong and Small 2008; Kirkwood et al. 2008; Lahn et al. 2005; Lynch 2008). In contrast to current regimens involving traditional immune activators, these novel immunotherapeutic agents exert inhibitory effects not only on immune effector cells but also on Treg cells (Kirkwood et al. 2008). They might thus prove more efficient in inducing durable responses in cancer patients. Indeed, a recent phase 3 study, treatment of patients with therapy-resistant, unresectable stage III or IV melanoma with the anti-CTLA-4 antibody Ipilimumab resulted in improved overall survival compared to patients treated with a gp100 peptide vaccine (Hodi et al. 2010).

A potential additional explanation for this encouraging antimelanoma effect of CTLA-4 blockade arises from the recent demonstration that tumorigenic MMICs (1) selectively expressed the CTLA-4 ligand B7.2 and (2) induced Treg cells in a B7.2 signaling-dependent manner (Schatton et al. 2010). Inhibition of CSC-specific, B7.2-dependent immune escape mechanisms might thus at least in part contribute to the antitumor efficiency of Ipilimumab. Given the preferential expression of PD-1 (Schatton et al. 2010; Di Tomaso et al. 2010), 4-1BBL (Schatton et al. 2010), and TGF-β (Wei et al. 2010b) by cancer stem-like cells, partial and complete responses observed in tumor patients treated with the anti-PD-1 antibody MDX-1106 (Brahmer et al. 2010), or therapeutic agents directed at 4-1BB (Lynch 2008) or TGF-β (Kirkwood et al. 2008), could potentially also relate to the ability of these immunotherapeutics to block CSC-driven evasion of immune-mediated rejection. Together, these findings highlight the possibility that immunotherapeutic strategies aimed at enhancing the endogenous immune responses to cancer might prove most efficient if CSC-specific immune escape mechanisms are concurrently impaired. In light of this intriguing possibility, it might be relevant to analyze the clinical effectiveness of novel agents, including Ipilimumab and MDX-1106, not only with regard to the pattern and duration of immune responses (Reuben et al. 2006) but also in the context of their impact on the CSC subset and its immunomodulatory functions (Schatton and Frank 2009).

Another avenue of potentiating the antitumor immune response in the clinic is through active immunization regimens using peptides, whole cells, or antigen-pulsed DCs (Rosenberg et al. 2004). Such active immunization approaches often target known TAAs, which include MART-1, gp100, or CTAs (Rosenberg et al. 2004). Despite the frequently achieved induction of TAA-reactive lymphocytes in response to such cancer vaccines (van der Bruggen et al. 1991), only rare and highly sporadic regressions are observed in tumor patients (Rosenberg et al. 2004). The demonstration that MMICs display low to absent expression of MART-1 and the CTAs NY-ESO-1 and MAGE-A among other TAAs (Schatton and Frank 2009; Schatton et al. 2010) could provide a novel explanation for the failure of current active immunization therapies. Glioma spheroids were also found to express only low levels of certain TAAs, including gp100, NY-ESO-1, and MAGE (Di Tomaso et al. 2010), lending further support to the hypothesis that active immunization directed at common TAAs may spare the CSC fraction. A promising approach for enhancing the efficacy of cancer vaccines in light of the CSC concept might be the concurrent use of epigenetic and/or alternative sensitizing protocols that drive CSCs into differentiation. In this regard, Wei et al. (2010b) showed that immunosuppressive properties of glioma stem-like cells diminished upon altering their differentiation state. Comparably, Todaro et al. (2009) demonstrated that treatment of colorectal cancer spheroid cells with the aminobisphosphonate zoledronate, which causes intracellular accumulation of immunogenic phosphoantigens (Bonneville and Scotet 2006), sensitizes them to γδ T-cell-mediated target cell killing (Todaro et al. 2009). An alternative avenue that could potentially improve the therapeutic efficiency of vaccination strategies in light of the CSC theory would be to identify and target antigens that are specific to the CSC compartment. For instance, the ABCB5 antigen might represent a promising target for CSC-directed immunization protocols in human melanoma, where the molecule is principally expressed (Frank et al. 2005), with enhanced expression levels detected in more advanced disease stages (Schatton et al. 2008). For instance, in glioblastoma, stem-like cells could be used as antigen sources for DC vaccinations (Xu et al. 2009). A separate study demonstrated enhanced expression of the human epidermal growth factor receptor 2 (HER2) on CD133$^+$ glioblastoma cells compared to cancer bulk populations (Ahmed et al. 2010). In this study, T cells transduced with a retroviral vector encoding a HER2-specific chimeric antigen receptor killed autologous HER2$^+$ tumor cells both in vitro and in vivo, resulting in sustained regression of glioblastoma xenografts (Ahmed et al. 2010). Findings in a human breast cancer cell line, further described expression of the immunogenic Notch-1 and Numb-1 peptides on CD44^{hi}CD24^{lo} subsets (Mine et al. 2009). Whether these findings are relevant to clinical breast cancer, however, requires further investigation. Di Tomaso et al. (2010) found that T lymphocytes could elicit both Th1 and Th2 effector responses following stimulation with autologous glioma spheroid cells. Based on these findings the authors suggested that the CSC compartment in glioblastoma could express TAAs recognized by T cells. For instance, Sox2 was detectable in the majority of tumor spheroid cells in this study (Di Tomaso et al. 2010). Whether this TAA is specific for CSCs or was expressed by more differentiated cells present within glioblastoma spheres was, however, not examined in this study. Similarly, Brown et al. (2009) described efficient cell killing of brain tumor stem-like cells by CTLs and, as a result, inhibition of tumor xenograft growth. However, the patient-derived glioblastoma cells used in this study were transduced with the pp65 antigen (Brown et al. 2009). It is thus not surprising that pp65$^+$ glioma CSCs were cleared by human cytomegalovirus pp65-specific CTLs (Brown et al. 2009), precluding the general applicability of these findings to CSC immunotargeting. Clinically relevant findings supporting the potential importance of targeting antigens specific to the CSC compartment for effective immunotherapy, come from data generated in CML patients undergoing donor lymphocyte infusion (Biernacki et al. 2010). In this study, those CML patients who demonstrated apparent graft vs. leukemia effects typically showed reactivity to antigens expressed on CD34$^+$ CML progenitor cells as opposed to differentiated bulk components (Biernacki et al. 2010). Taken together, these findings highlight a putative advantage of targeting CSC-associated antigens over inducing antitumor immune responses to common TAAs, which might not be expressed by the CSC compartment (Di Tomaso et al. 2010; Schatton and Frank 2009; Schatton et al. 2010). CSC-specific immunization strategies might prove particularly effective when pursued in the context of concurrent differentiation regimens and/or if they are directed at antigens required for CSC function.

Finally, similar considerations might apply to ACT approaches. Comparable to cancer vaccines, infusion of cancer patients with ex vivo expanded, tumor-reactive lymphocyte clones can yield significant antitumor responses (Rosenberg et al. 2008). However, such immune responses may be limited due to restricted in vivo homing properties and limited life spans of tumor-specific T cells (Dudley et al. 2001). Current strategies aimed at improving ACT treatment efficacy involve concurrent inhibition of negative costimulatory receptors on tumor-reactive T cells (Phan et al. 2003), transduction of CTL clones with growth factors or positive costimulatory molecules (Liu and Rosenberg 2001), or prior depletion of host Treg cells (Antony et al. 2005). Because the CSC concept applies to tumor development and neoplastic progression (Frank et al. 2010), ACT of lymphocytes reactive against CSC-specific antigens might further enhance tumor eradication in patients with advanced disease. In view of the ability of CSCs to modulate antitumor immunity (Chan et al. 2009; Majeti et al. 2009; Di Tomaso et al. 2010; Schatton and Frank 2009; Schatton et al. 2010; Todaro et al. 2009; Wei et al. 2010a, b), future ACT regimens might also generate more durable anticancer effects if they concurrently inhibit the mechanisms of CSC-driven immune evasion.

Concluding Remarks

CSCs have been prospectively isolated from several human cancers, and some of the molecular and cellular apparatuses underlying CSC-driven tumorigenicity are currently being deciphered. Importantly, critical links between CSCs, neoplastic progression, and tumor therapy resistance have been established, emphasizing the necessity to target CSC-specific functions in order to efficiently eradicate malignant tumors in cancer patients. Robust scientific evidence has now been generated that one such CSC-associated mechanism is their unique ability to escape and/or modulate the antitumor immune response. The immunomodulatory repertoire of CSC subsets includes evasion from immune clearance, induction of clonal anergy or deletion, and activation of Treg cells. Strikingly, all of these CSC-associated functions have previously been linked to the failure of current cancer immunotherapies. As such, countering these newly unveiled CSC immunoevasive properties will be critical to developing more effective immunotherapeutic protocols with the promise to further reduce cancer morbidity and mortality in human patients.

Acknowledgments Our research is supported by the U.S. National Institutes of Health/National Cancer Institute (grants 1RO1CA113796, 1RO1CA138231, and 2P50CA093683-06A20006 to M. H. Frank). T. Schatton is the recipient of a Postdoctoral Fellowship Award from the American Heart Association Founders Affiliate.

References

Abdel-Wahab, Z., Li, W. P., Osanto, S., Darrow, T. L., Hessling, J., Vervaert, C. E., Burrascano, M., Barber, J. & Seigler, H. F. (1994), Transduction of human melanoma cells with interleukin-2 gene reduces tumorigenicity and enhances host antitumor immunity: a nude mouse model. Cell Immunol 159:26–39.

Aggarwal S & Pittenger MF (2005), Human mesenchymal stem cells modulate allogeneic immune cell responses. Blood 105:1815–22.

Ahmadzadeh M, Felipe-Silva A, Heemskerk B, Powell DJ Jr, Wunderlich JR, Merino MJ & Rosenberg SA (2008), FOXP3 expression accurately defines the population of intratumoral regulatory T cells that selectively accumulate in metastatic melanoma lesions. Blood 112:4953–60.

Ahmadzadeh M & Rosenberg SA (2006), IL-2 administration increases CD4+ CD25(hi) Foxp3+ regulatory T cells in cancer patients. Blood 107:2409–14.

Ahmed N, Salsman VS, Kew Y, Shaffer D, Powell S, Zhang YJ, Grossman RG, Heslop HE & Gottschalk S (2010), HER2-specific T cells target primary glioblastoma stem cells and induce regression of autologous experimental tumors. Clin Cancer Res 16:474–85.

Al-Hajj M, Wicha MS, Benito-Hernandez A, Morrison SJ & Clarke MF (2003), Prospective identification of tumorigenic breast cancer cells. Proc Natl Acad Sci USA 100:3983–8.

Andreola G, Rivoltini L, Castelli C, Huber V, Perego P, Deho P, Squarcina P, Accornero P, Lozupone F, Lugini L, et al. (2002), Induction of lymphocyte apoptosis by tumor cell secretion of FasL-bearing microvesicles. J Exp Med 195:1303–16.

Antony PA, Piccirillo CA, Akpinarli A, Finkelstein SE, Speiss PJ, Surman DR, Palmer DC, Chan CC, Klebanoff CA, Overwijk WW, et al. (2005), CD8+ T cell immunity against a tumor/self-antigen is augmented by CD4+ T helper cells and hindered by naturally occurring T regulatory cells. J Immunol 174:2591–601.

Aptsiauri N, Cabrera T, Mendez R, Garcia-Lora A, Ruiz-Cabello F & Garrido F (2007), Role of altered expression of HLA class I molecules in cancer progression. Adv Exp Med Biol 601:123–31.

Atkins MB, Lotze MT, Dutcher JP, Fisher RI, Weiss G, Margolin K, Abrams J, Sznol M, Parkinson D, Hawkins M, et al. (1999), High-dose recombinant interleukin 2 therapy for patients with metastatic melanoma: analysis of 270 patients treated between 1985 and 1993. J Clin Oncol 17:2105–16.

Atkins MB, Sparano J, Fisher RI, Weiss GR, Margolin KA, Fink KI, Rubinstein L, Louie A, Mier JW, Gucalp R, et al. (1993), Randomized phase II trial of high-dose interleukin-2 either alone or in combination with interferon alfa-2b in advanced renal cell carcinoma. J Clin Oncol 11:661–70.

Attia P, Maker AV, Haworth LR, Rogers-Freezer L & Rosenberg SA (2005), Inability of a fusion protein of IL-2 and diphtheria toxin (Denileukin Diftitox, DAB389IL-2, ONTAK) to eliminate regulatory T lymphocytes in patients with melanoma. J Immunother 28:582–92.

Bai Y, Liu J, Wang Y, Honig S, Qin L, Boros P & Bromberg JS (2002), L-selectin-dependent lymphoid occupancy is required to induce alloantigen-specific tolerance. J Immunol 168: 1579–89.

Bao S, Wu Q, Li Z, Sathornsumetee S, Wang H, McLendon RE, Hjelmeland AB & Rich JN (2008), Targeting cancer stem cells through L1CAM suppresses glioma growth. Cancer Res 68:6043–8.

Bao S, Wu Q, McLendon RE, Hao Y, Shi Q, Hjelmeland AB, Dewhirst MW, Bigner DD & Rich JN (2006a), Glioma stem cells promote radioresistance by preferential activation of the DNA damage response. Nature 444:756–60.

Bao S, Wu Q, Sathornsumetee S, Hao Y, Li Z, Hjelmeland AB, Shi Q, McLendon RE, Bigner DD & Rich JN (2006b), Stem cell-like glioma cells promote tumor angiogenesis through vascular endothelial growth factor. Cancer Res 66:7843–8.

Barclay AN & Brown MH (2006), The SIRP family of receptors and immune regulation. Nat Rev Immunol 6:457–64.

Barker N, Ridgway RA, Van Es JH, Van De Wetering M, Begthel H, Van Den Born M, Danenberg E, Clarke AR, Sansom OJ & Clevers H (2009), Crypt stem cells as the cells-of-origin of intestinal cancer. Nature 457:608–11.

Bauer S, Groh V, Wu J, Steinle A, Phillips JH, Lanier LL & Spies T (1999), Activation of NK cells and T cells by NKG2D, a receptor for stress-inducible MICA. Science 285:727–9.

Becker JC, Brabletz T, Czerny C, Termeer C & Brocker EB (1993), Tumor escape mechanisms from immunosurveillance: induction of unresponsiveness in a specific MHC-restricted CD4+ human T cell clone by the autologous MHC class II+ melanoma. Int Immunol 5:1501–8.

Ben-Neriah Y, Daley GQ, Mes-Masson AM, Witte ON & Baltimore D (1986), The chronic myelogenous leukemia-specific P210 protein is the product of the bcr/abl hybrid gene. Science 233:212–4.

Beyth S, Borovsky Z, Mevorach D, Liebergall M, Gazit Z, Aslan H, Galun E & Rachmilewitz J (2005), Human mesenchymal stem cells alter antigen-presenting cell maturation and induce T-cell unresponsiveness. Blood 105:2214–9.

Biernacki MA, Marina O, Zhang W, Liu F, Bruns I, Cai A, Neuberg D, Canning CM, Alyea EP, Soiffer RJ, et al. (2010), Efficacious immune therapy in chronic myelogenous leukemia (CML) recognizes antigens that are expressed on CML progenitor cells. Cancer Res 70:906–15.

Bonnet D & Dick JE (1997), Human acute myeloid leukemia is organized as a hierarchy that originates from a primitive hematopoietic cell. Nat Med 3:730–7.

Bonneville M & Scotet E (2006), Human Vgamma9Vdelta2 T cells: promising new leads for immunotherapy of infections and tumors. Curr Opin Immunol 18:539–46.

Brahmer JR, Drake CG, Wollner I, Powderly JD, Picus J, Sharfman WH, Stankevich E, Pons A, Salay TM, McMiller TL, et al. (2010), Phase I Study of Single-Agent Anti-Programmed Death-1 (MDX-1106) in Refractory Solid Tumors: Safety, Clinical Activity, Pharmacodynamics, and Immunologic Correlates. J Clin Oncol 28:3167–75.

Brocker EB, Suter L & Sorg C (1984), HLA-DR antigen expression in primary melanomas of the skin. J Invest Dermatol 82:244–7.

Brown CE, Starr R, Martinez C, Aguilar B, D'Apuzzo M, Todorov I, Shih CC, Badie B, Hudecek M, Riddell SR, et al. (2009), Recognition and killing of brain tumor stem-like initiating cells by CD8+ cytolytic T cells. Cancer Res 69:8886–93.

Bruce WR & Van Der Gaag H (1963), A Quantitative Assay For The Number Of Murine Lymphoma Cells Capable Of Proliferation In Vivo. Nature 199:79–80.

Bubenik J (2003), Tumour MHC class I downregulation and immunotherapy (Review). Oncol Rep 10:2005–8.

Burnet M (1957a), Cancer; a biological approach. I. The processes of control. Br Med J 1:779–86.

Burnet M (1957b), Cancer: a biological approach. III. Viruses associated with neoplastic conditions. IV. Practical applications. Br Med J 1:841–7.

Cabrera T, Lara E, Romero JM, Maleno I, Real LM, Ruiz-Cabello F, Valero P, Camacho FM & Garrido F (2007), HLA class I expression in metastatic melanoma correlates with tumor development during autologous vaccination. Cancer Immunol Immunother 56:709–17.

Carretero R, Romero JM, Ruiz-Cabello F, Maleno I, Rodriguez F, Camacho FM, Real LM, Garrido F & Cabrera T (2008), Analysis of HLA class I expression in progressing and regressing metastatic melanoma lesions after immunotherapy. Immunogenetics 60:439–47.

Casiraghi F, Azzollini N, Cassis P, Imberti B, Morigi M, Cugini D, Cavinato RA, Todeschini M, Solini S, Sonzogni A, et al. (2008), Pretransplant infusion of mesenchymal stem cells prolongs the survival of a semiallogeneic heart transplant through the generation of regulatory T cells. J Immunol 181:3933–46.

Castor A, Nilsson L, Astrand-Grundstrom I, Buitenhuis M, Ramirez C, Anderson K, Strombeck B, Garwicz S, Bekassy AN, Schmiegelow K, et al. (2005), Distinct patterns of hematopoietic stem cell involvement in acute lymphoblastic leukemia. Nat Med 11:630–7.

Chan KS, Espinosa I, Chao M, Wong D, Ailles L, Diehn M, Gill H, Presti J Jr, Chang HY, Van De Rijn M, et al. (2009), Identification, molecular characterization, clinical prognosis, and therapeutic targeting of human bladder tumor-initiating cells. Proc Natl Acad Sci USA 106:14016–21.

Cho RW, Wang X, Diehn M, Shedden K, Chen GY, Sherlock G, Gurney A, Lewicki J & Clarke MF (2008), Isolation and molecular characterization of cancer stem cells in MMTV-Wnt-1 murine breast tumors. Stem Cells 26:364–71.

Clark RA, Huang SJ, Murphy GF, Mollet IG, Hijnen D, Muthukuru M, Schanbacher CF, Edwards V, Miller DM, Kim JE, et al. (2008), Human squamous cell carcinomas evade the immune response by down-regulation of vascular E-selectin and recruitment of regulatory T cells. J Exp Med 205:2221–34.

Clarke MF, Dick JE, Dirks PB, Eaves CJ, Jamieson CH, Jones DL, Visvader J, Weissman IL & Wahl GM (2006), Cancer stem cells – perspectives on current status and future directions: AACR Workshop on cancer stem cells. Cancer Res 66:9339–44.

Cox CV, Evely RS, Oakhill A, Pamphilon DH, Goulden NJ & Blair A (2004), Characterization of acute lymphoblastic leukemia progenitor cells. Blood 104:2919–25.

Cox CV, Martin HM, Kearns PR, Virgo P, Evely RS & Blair A (2007), Characterization of a progenitor cell population in childhood T-cell acute lymphoblastic leukemia. Blood 109:674–82.

Curiel TJ, Coukos G, Zou L, Alvarez X, Cheng P, Mottram P, Evdemon-Hogan M, Conejo-Garcia JR, Zhang L, Burow M, et al. (2004), Specific recruitment of regulatory T cells in ovarian carcinoma fosters immune privilege and predicts reduced survival. Nat Med 10:942–9.

Dalerba P, Dylla SJ, Park IK, Liu R, Wang X, Cho RW, Hoey T, Gurney A, Huang EH, Simeone DM, et al. (2007), Phenotypic characterization of human colorectal cancer stem cells. Proc Natl Acad Sci USA 104:10158–63.

Dannull J, Su Z, Rizzieri D, Yang BK, Coleman D, Yancey D, Zhang A, Dahm P, Chao N, Gilboa E, et al. (2005), Enhancement of vaccine-mediated antitumor immunity in cancer patients after depletion of regulatory T cells. J Clin Invest 115:3623–33.

Deshpande AJ, Cusan M, Rawat VP, Reuter H, Krause A, Pott C, Quintanilla-Martinez L, Kakadia P, Kuchenbauer F, Ahmed F, et al. (2006), Acute myeloid leukemia is propagated by a leukemic stem cell with lymphoid characteristics in a mouse model of CALM/AF10-positive leukemia. Cancer Cell 10:363–74.

Di Ianni M, Del Papa B, De Ioanni M, Moretti L, Bonifacio E, Cecchini D, Sportoletti P, Falzetti F & Tabilio A (2008), Mesenchymal cells recruit and regulate T regulatory cells. Exp Hematol 36:309–18.

Di Tomaso T, Mazzoleni S, Wang E, Sovena G, Clavenna D, Franzin A, Mortini P, Ferrone S, Doglioni C, Marincola FM, et al. (2010), Immunobiological characterization of cancer stem cells isolated from glioblastoma patients. Clin Cancer Res 16:800–13.

Diefenbach A, Jensen ER, Jamieson AM & Raulet DH (2001), Rae1 and H60 ligands of the NKG2D receptor stimulate tumour immunity. Nature 413:165–71.

Diehn M, Cho RW, Lobo NA, Kalisky T, Dorie MJ, Kulp AN, Qian D, Lam JS, Ailles LE, Wong M, et al. (2009), Association of reactive oxygen species levels and radioresistance in cancer stem cells. Nature 458:780–3.

Djouad F, Charbonnier LM, Bouffi C, Louis-Plence P, Bony C, Apparailly F, Cantos C, Jorgensen C & Noel D (2007), Mesenchymal stem cells inhibit the differentiation of dendritic cells through an interleukin-6-dependent mechanism. Stem Cells 25:2025–32.

Djouad F, Plence P, Bony C, Tropel P, Apparailly F, Sany J, Noel D & Jorgensen C (2003), Immunosuppressive effect of mesenchymal stem cells favors tumor growth in allogeneic animals. Blood 102:3837–44.

Dong H, Strome SE, Matteson EL, Moder KG, Flies DB, Zhu G, Tamura H, Driscoll CL & Chen L (2003), Costimulating aberrant T cell responses by B7-H1 autoantibodies in rheumatoid arthritis. J Clin Invest 111:363–70.

Dong H, Strome SE, Salomao DR, Tamura H, Hirano F, Flies DB, Roche PC, Lu J, Zhu G, Tamada K, et al. (2002), Tumor-associated B7-H1 promotes T-cell apoptosis: a potential mechanism of immune evasion. Nat Med 8:793–800.

Du R, Lu KV, Petritsch C, Liu P, Ganss R, Passegue E, Song H, Vandenberg S, Johnson RS, Werb, Z, et al. (2008), HIF1alpha induces the recruitment of bone marrow-derived vascular modulatory cells to regulate tumor angiogenesis and invasion. Cancer Cell 13:206–20.

Du W, Wong FS, Li MO, Peng J, Qi H, Flavell RA, Sherwin R & Wen L (2006), TGF-beta signaling is required for the function of insulin-reactive T regulatory cells. J Clin Invest 116:1360–70.

Dudley ME, Wunderlich J, Nishimura MI, Yu D, Yang JC, Topalian SL, Schwartzentruber DJ, Hwu P, Marincola FM, Sherry R, et al. (2001), Adoptive transfer of cloned melanoma-reactive T lymphocytes for the treatment of patients with metastatic melanoma. J Immunother 24:363–73.

Dunn GP, Bruce AT, Ikeda H, Old LJ & Schreiber R D (2002), Cancer immunoediting: from immunosurveillance to tumor escape. Nat Immunol 3:991–8.

Dylla SJ, Beviglia L, Park IK, Chartier C, Raval J, Ngan L, Pickell K, Aguilar J, Lazetic S, Smith-Berdan S, et al. (2008), Colorectal cancer stem cells are enriched in xenogeneic tumors following chemotherapy. PLoS One 3:e2428.

Fadok VA, Bratton DL & Henson PM (2001), Phagocyte receptors for apoptotic cells: recognition, uptake, and consequences. J Clin Invest 108:957–62.

Flaherty LE, Atkins M, Sosman J, Weiss G, Clark JI, Margolin K, Dutcher J, Gordon MS, Lotze M, Mier J, et al. (2001), Outpatient biochemotherapy with interleukin-2 and interferon alfa-2b in patients with metastatic malignant melanoma: results of two phase II cytokine working group trials. J Clin Oncol 19:3194–202.

Fong L & Small EJ (2008), Anti-cytotoxic T-lymphocyte antigen-4 antibody: the first in an emerging class of immunomodulatory antibodies for cancer treatment. J Clin Oncol 26:5275–83.

Frank NY, Margaryan A, Huang Y, Schatton T, Waaga-Gasser AM, Gasser M, Sayegh MH, Sadee W & Frank MH (2005), ABCB5-mediated doxorubicin transport and chemoresistance in human malignant melanoma. Cancer Res 65:4320–33.

Frank NY, Schatton T & Frank MH (2010), The therapeutic promise of the cancer stem cell concept. J Clin Invest 120:41–50.

Freeman GJ, Long AJ, Iwai Y, Bourque K, Chernova T, Nishimura H, Fitz, LJ, Malenkovich N, Okazaki T, Byrne MC, et al. (2000), Engagement of the PD-1 immunoinhibitory receptor by a novel B7 family member leads to negative regulation of lymphocyte activation. J Exp Med 192:1027–34.

Gao Q, Wang, XY, Qiu SJ, Yamato I, Sho M, Nakajima Y, Zhou J, Li BZ, Shi YH, Xiao YS, et al. (2009), Overexpression of PD-L1 significantly associates with tumor aggressiveness and postoperative recurrence in human hepatocellular carcinoma. Clin Cancer Res 15:971–9.

Gorelik L & Flavell RA (2001), Immune-mediated eradication of tumors through the blockade of transforming growth factor-beta signaling in T cells. Nat Med 7:1118–22.

Grulich AE, Van Leeuwen MT, Falster MO & Vajdic CM (2007), Incidence of cancers in people with HIV/AIDS compared with immunosuppressed transplant recipients: a meta-analysis. Lancet 370:59–67.

Gupta PB, Chaffer CL & Weinberg RA (2009a), Cancer stem cells: mirage or reality? Nat Med 15:1010–2.

Gupta PB, Onder TT, Jiang G, Tao K, Kuperwasser C, Weinberg RA & Lander ES (2009b), Identification of selective inhibitors of cancer stem cells by high-throughput screening. Cell 138: 645–59.

Hahne M, Rimoldi D, Schroter M, Romero P, Schreier M, French LE, Schneider P, Bornand T, Fontana A, Lienard D, et al. (1996), Melanoma cell expression of Fas(Apo-1/CD95) ligand: implications for tumor immune escape. Science 274:1363–6.

Hallermalm K, De Geer A, Kiessling R, Levitsky V & Levitskaya J (2004), Autocrine secretion of Fas ligand shields tumor cells from Fas-mediated killing by cytotoxic lymphocytes. Cancer Res 64:6775–82.

Hamanishi J, Mandai M, Iwasaki M, Okazaki T, Tanaka Y, Yamaguchi K, Higuchi T, Yagi H, Takakura K, Minato N, et al. (2007), Programmed cell death 1 ligand 1 and tumor-infiltrating CD8+ T lymphocytes are prognostic factors of human ovarian cancer. Proc Natl Acad Sci U S A 104:3360–5.

Hamburger AW & Salmon SE (1977), Primary bioassay of human tumor stem cells. Science 197:461–3.

Hanahan D & Weinberg RA (2000), The hallmarks of cancer. Cell 100:57–70.

Hasegawa H, Inoue A, Muraoka M, Yamanouchi J, Miyazaki T & Yasukawa M (2007), Therapy for pneumonitis and sialadenitis by accumulation of CCR2-expressing CD4+CD25+ regulatory T cells in MRL/lpr mice. Arthritis Res Ther 9:R15.

Held MA, Curley DP, Dankort D, McMahon M, Muthusamy V & Bosenberg MW (2010), Characterization of melanoma cells capable of propagating tumors from a single cell. Cancer Res 70:388–97.

Herfs M, Herman L, Hubert P, Minner F, Arafa M, Roncarati P, Henrotin Y, Boniver J & Delvenne P (2009), High expression of PGE2 enzymatic pathways in cervical (pre)neoplastic lesions and functional consequences for antigen-presenting cells. Cancer Immunol Immunother 58:603–14.

Hermann PC, Huber SL, Herrler T, Aicher A, Ellwart JW, Guba M, Bruns CJ & Heeschen C (2007), Distinct populations of cancer stem cells determine tumor growth and metastatic activity in human pancreatic cancer. Cell Stem Cell 1:313–23.

Hirano F, Kaneko K, Tamura H, Dong H, Wang S, Ichikawa M, Rietz C, Flies DB, Lau JS, Zhu G, Et Al. (2005), Blockade of B7-H1 and PD-1 by monoclonal antibodies potentiates cancer therapeutic immunity. Cancer Res 65:1089–96.

Hodi FS, O'Day SJ, Mcdermott DF, Weber RW, Sosman JA, Haanen JB, Gonzalez R, Robert C, Schadendorf D, Hassel JC, et al. (2010), Improved Survival with Ipilimumab in Patients with Metastatic Melanoma. N Engl J Med 363:711–23.

Hogquist KA, Baldwin TA & Jameson SC (2005), Central tolerance: learning self-control in the thymus. Nat Rev Immunol 5:772–82.

Hombach AA, Kofler D, Hombach A, Rappl G & Abken H (2007), Effective proliferation of human regulatory T cells requires a strong costimulatory CD28 signal that cannot be substituted by IL-2. J Immunol 179:7924–31.

Hori S, Nomura T & Sakaguchi S (2003), Control of regulatory T cell development by the transcription factor Foxp3. Science 299:1057–61.

Huntly BJ, Shigematsu H, Deguchi K, Lee BH, Mizuno S, Duclos N, Rowan R, Amaral S, Curley D, Williams IR, et al. (2004), MOZ-TIF2, but not BCR-ABL, confers properties of leukemic stem cells to committed murine hematopoietic progenitors. Cancer Cell 6:587–96.

Inge TH, Hoover SK, Susskind BM, Barrett SK & Bear HD (1992), Inhibition of tumor-specific cytotoxic T-lymphocyte responses by transforming growth factor beta 1. Cancer Res 52:1386–92.

Ishikawa F, Yoshida S, Saito Y, Hijikata A, Kitamura H, Tanaka S, Nakamura R, Tanaka T, Tomiyama H, Saito N, et al. (2007), Chemotherapy-resistant human AML stem cells home to and engraft within the bone-marrow endosteal region. Nat Biotechnol 25:1315–21.

Iwai Y, Terawaki S & Honjo T (2005), PD-1 blockade inhibits hematogenous spread of poorly immunogenic tumor cells by enhanced recruitment of effector T cells. Int Immunol 17:133–44.

Jager E, Gnjatic S, Nagata Y, Stockert E, Jager D, Karbach J, Neumann A, Rieckenberg J, Chen YT, Ritter G, et al. (2000), Induction of primary NY-ESO-1 immunity: CD8+ T lymphocyte and antibody responses in peptide-vaccinated patients with NY-ESO-1+ cancers. Proc Natl Acad Sci USA 97:12198–203.

Jaiswal S, Chao MP, Majeti R & Weissman IL (2010), Macrophages as mediators of tumor immunosurveillance. Trends Immunol 31:212–9.

Jaiswal S, Jamieson CH, Pang WW, Park CY, Chao MP, Majeti R, Traver D, Van Rooijen N & Weissman IL (2009), CD47 is upregulated on circulating hematopoietic stem cells and leukemia cells to avoid phagocytosis. Cell 138:271–85.

Jamieson CH, Ailles LE, Dylla SJ, Muijtjens M, Jones C, Zehnder JL, Gotlib J, Li K, Manz MG, Keating A, et al. (2004), Granulocyte-macrophage progenitors as candidate leukemic stem cells in blast-crisis CML. N Engl J Med 351:657–67.

Jenkins MK, Taylor PS, Norton SD & Urdahl KB (1991), CD28 delivers a costimulatory signal involved in antigen-specific IL-2 production by human T cells. J Immunol 147:2461–6.

Jensen JB & Parmar M (2006), Strengths and limitations of the neurosphere culture system. Mol Neurobiol 34:153–61.

Jiang XX, Zhang Y, Liu B, Zhang SX, Wu Y, Yu XD & Mao N (2005), Human mesenchymal stem cells inhibit differentiation and function of monocyte-derived dendritic cells. Blood 105:4120-6.

Jones E, Dahm-Vicker M, Simon AK, Green A, Powrie F, Cerundolo V & Gallimore A (2002), Depletion of CD25+ regulatory cells results in suppression of melanoma growth and induction of autoreactivity in mice. Cancer Immu 2:1.

Kappler JW, Roehm N & Marrack P (1987), T cell tolerance by clonal elimination in the thymus. Cell 49:273–80.

Kawakami Y, Dang N, Wang X, Tupesis J, Robbins PF, Wang RF, Wunderlich JR, Yannelli JR & Rosenberg SA (2000), Recognition of shared melanoma antigens in association with major HLA-A alleles by tumor infiltrating T lymphocytes from 123 patients with melanoma. J Immunother 23:17–27.

Kawasaki BT, Mistree T, Hurt EM, Kalathur M & Farrar WL (2007), Co-expression of the toleragenic glycoprotein, CD200, with markers for cancer stem cells. Biochem Biophys Res Commun 364:778–82.

Khong HT, Wang QJ & Rosenberg SA (2004), Identification of multiple antigens recognized by tumor-infiltrating lymphocytes from a single patient: tumor escape by antigen loss and loss of MHC expression. J Immunother 27:184–90.

Kim E & Deppert W (2004), Transcriptional activities of mutant p53: when mutations are more than a loss. J Cell Biochem 93:878–86.

Kirkwood JM, Tarhini AA, Panelli MC, Moschos SJ, Zarour HM, Butterfield LH & Gogas HJ (2008), Next generation of immunotherapy for melanoma. J Clin Oncol 26:3445–55.

Krambeck AE, Thompson RH, Dong H, Lohse CM, Park ES, Kuntz SM, Leibovich BC, Blute ML, Cheville JC & Kwon ED (2006), B7-H4 expression in renal cell carcinoma and tumor vasculature: associations with cancer progression and survival. Proc Natl Acad Sci USA 103:10391–6.

Krivtsov AV, Twomey D, Feng Z, Stubbs MC, Wang Y, Faber J, Levine JE, Wang J, Hahn WC, Gilliland DG, et al. (2006), Transformation from committed progenitor to leukaemia stem cell initiated by MLL-AF9. Nature 442:818–22.

Kroczek RA, Mages HW & Hutloff A (2004), Emerging paradigms of T-cell co-stimulation. Curr Opin Immunol 16:321–7.

Kuipers H, Muskens F, Willart M, Hijdra D, Van Assema FB, Coyle AJ, Hoogsteden HC & Lambrecht BN (2006), Contribution of the PD-1 ligands/PD-1 signaling pathway to dendritic cell-mediated CD4+ T cell activation. Eur J Immunol 36:2472–82.

Lahn M, Kloeker S & Berry BS (2005), TGF-beta inhibitors for the treatment of cancer. Expert Opin Investig Drugs 14:629–43.

Lapidot T, Sirard C, Vormoor J, Murdoch B, Hoang T, Caceres-Cortes J, Minden M, Paterson B, Caligiuri MA & Dick JE (1994), A cell initiating human acute myeloid leukaemia after transplantation into SCID mice. Nature 367:645–8.

Lathia JD, Gallagher J, Heddleston JM, Wang J, Eyler CE, Macswords J, Wu Q, Vasanji A, McLendon RE, Hjelmeland AB, et al. (2010), Integrin alpha 6 regulates glioblastoma stem cells. Cell Stem Cell 6:421–32.

Le Blanc K & Ringden O (2007), Immunomodulation by mesenchymal stem cells and clinical experience. J Intern Med 262:509–25.

Le Blanc K, Tammik C, Rosendahl K, Zetterberg E & Ringden O (2003), HLA expression and immunologic properties of differentiated and undifferentiated mesenchymal stem cells. Exp Hematol 31:890–6.

Lee PP, Yee C, Savage PA, Fong L, Brockstedt D, Weber JS, Johnson D, Swetter S, Thompson J, Greenberg PD, et al. (1999), Characterization of circulating T cells specific for tumor-associated antigens in melanoma patients. Nat Med 5:677–85.

Li C, Heidt DG, Dalerba P, Burant CF, Zhang L, Adsay V, Wicha M, Clarke MF & Simeone DM (2007), Identification of pancreatic cancer stem cells. Cancer Res 67:1030–7.

Li W, Jian-Jun W, Xue-Feng Z & Feng Z (2010), CD133(+) human pulmonary adenocarcinoma cells induce apoptosis of CD8(+) T cells by highly expressed galectin-3. Clin Invest Med 33:E44-53.

Li, X., Lewis, M. T., Huang, J., Gutierrez, C., Osborne, C. K., Wu, M. F., Hilsenbeck, S. G., Pavlick A, Zhang X, Chamness GC, et al. (2008), Intrinsic resistance of tumorigenic breast cancer cells to chemotherapy. J Natl Cancer Inst 100:672–9.

Li XC, Rothstein DM & Sayegh MH (2009a), Costimulatory pathways in transplantation: challenges and new developments. Immunol Rev 229:271–93.

Li Z, Bao S, Wu Q, Wang H, Eyler C, Sathornsumetee S, Shi Q, Cao Y, Lathia J, McLendon RE, et al. (2009b), Hypoxia-inducible factors regulate tumorigenic capacity of glioma stem cells. Cancer Cell 15:501–13.

Liu J, Lu XF, Wan L, Li YP, Li SF, Zeng LY, Zeng YZ, Cheng LH, Lu YR & Cheng JQ (2004), Suppression of human peripheral blood lymphocyte proliferation by immortalized mesenchymal stem cells derived from bone marrow of Banna Minipig inbred-line. Transplant Proc 36:3272–5.

Liu K & Rosenberg SA (2001), Transduction of an IL-2 gene into human melanoma-reactive lymphocytes results in their continued growth in the absence of exogenous IL-2 and maintenance of specific antitumor activity. J Immunol 167:6356–65.

Liyanage UK, Moore TT, Joo HG, Tanaka Y, Herrmann V, Doherty G, Drebin JA, Strasberg SM, Eberlein TJ, Goedegebuure PS, et al. (2002), Prevalence of regulatory T cells is increased in peripheral blood and tumor microenvironment of patients with pancreas or breast adenocarcinoma. J Immunol 169:2756–61.

Lynch DH (2008), The promise of 4-1BB (CD137)-mediated immunomodulation and the immunotherapy of cancer. Immunol Rev 222:277–86.

Majeti R, Chao MP, Alizadeh AA, Pang WW, Jaiswal S, Gibbs KD Jr, Van Rooijen N & Weissman IL (2009), CD47 is an adverse prognostic factor and therapeutic antibody target on human acute myeloid leukemia stem cells. Cell 138:286–99.

Mannie MD, Prevost KD & Marinakis CA (1995), Prostaglandin E2 promotes the induction of anergy during T helper cell recognition of myelin basic protein. Cell Immunol 160:132–8.

Mapara MY & Sykes M (2004), Tolerance and cancer: mechanisms of tumor evasion and strategies for breaking tolerance. J Clin Oncol 22:1136–51.

Melkus MW, Estes JD, Padgett-Thomas A, Gatlin J, Denton PW, Othieno FA, Wege AK, Haase AT & Garcia JV (2006), Humanized mice mount specific adaptive and innate immune responses to EBV and TSST-1. Nat Med 12:1316–22.

Mine T, Matsueda S, Li Y, Tokumitsu H, Gao H, Danes C, Wong KK, Wang X, Ferrone S & Ioannides CG (2009), Breast cancer cells expressing stem cell markers CD44+ CD24 lo are eliminated by Numb-1 peptide-activated T cells. Cancer Immunol Immunother 58:1185–94.

Miyatake T, Tringler B, Liu W, Liu SH, Papkoff J, Enomoto T, Torkko KC, Dehn DL, Swisher A & Shroyer KR (2007), B7-H4 (DD-O110) is overexpressed in high risk uterine endometrioid adenocarcinomas and inversely correlated with tumor T-cell infiltration. Gynecol Oncol 106:119–27.

Moretta A (2002), Natural killer cells and dendritic cells: rendezvous in abused tissues. Nat Rev Immunol 2:957–64.

Mugler KC, Singh M, Tringler B, Torkko KC, Liu W, Papkoff J & Shroyer KR (2007), B7-h4 expression in a range of breast pathology: correlation with tumor T-cell infiltration. Appl Immunohistochem Mol Morphol 15:363–70.

Namba K, Kitaichi N, Nishida T & Taylor AW (2002), Induction of regulatory T cells by the immunomodulating cytokines alpha-melanocyte-stimulating hormone and transforming growth factor-beta2. J Leukoc Biol 72:946–52.

Nathan C & Muller WA (2001), Putting the brakes on innate immunity: a regulatory role for CD200? Nat Immunol 2:17–9.

Neuber K & Eidam B (2006), Expression of Fas ligand (CD95L) in primary malignant melanoma and melanoma metastases is associated with overall survival. Onkologie 29:361–5.

Nishimura MI, Avichezer D, Custer MC, Lee CS, Chen C, Parkhurst MR, Diamond RA, Robbins PF, Schwartzentruber DJ & Rosenberg SA (1999), MHC class I-restricted recognition of a melanoma antigen by a human CD4+ tumor infiltrating lymphocyte. Cancer Res 59:6230–8.

Nishizuka Y & Sakakura T (1969), Thymus and reproduction: sex-linked dysgenesia of the gonad after neonatal thymectomy in mice. Science 166:753–5.

Nomi T, Sho M, Akahori T, Hamada K, Kubo A, Kanehiro H, Nakamura S, Enomoto K, Yagita H, Azuma M, et al. (2007), Clinical significance and therapeutic potential of the programmed death-1 ligand/programmed death-1 pathway in human pancreatic cancer. Clin Cancer Res 13:2151–7.

Nowell PC (1976), The clonal evolution of tumor cell populations. Science 194:23–8.

O'Brien CA, Pollett A, Gallinger S & Dick JE (2007), A human colon cancer cell capable of initiating tumour growth in immunodeficient mice. Nature 445:106–10.

Ohm JE, Gabrilovich DI, Sempowski GD, Kisseleva E, Parman KS, Nadaf S & Carbone DP (2003), VEGF inhibits T-cell development and may contribute to tumor-induced immune suppression. Blood 101:4878–86.

Ostroukhova M, Qi Z, Oriss TB, Dixon-Mccarthy B, Ray P & Ray A (2006), Treg-mediated immunosuppression involves activation of the Notch-HES1 axis by membrane-bound TGF-beta. J Clin Invest 116:996–1004.

Park CH, Bergsagel DE & Mcculloch EA (1971), Mouse myeloma tumor stem cells: a primary cell culture assay. J Natl Cancer Inst 46:411–22.

Parmiani G, De Filippo A, Novellino L & Castelli C (2007), Unique human tumor antigens: immunobiology and use in clinical trials. J Immunol 178:1975–9.

Peng W, Wang HY, Miyahara Y, Peng G & Wang RF (2008), Tumor-associated galectin-3 modulates the function of tumor-reactive T cells. Cancer Res 68:7228–36.

Phan GQ, Yang JC, Sherry RM, Hwu P, Topalian SL, Schwartzentruber DJ, Restifo NP, Haworth LR, Seipp CA, Freezer LJ, et al. (2003), Cancer regression and autoimmunity induced by cytotoxic T lymphocyte-associated antigen 4 blockade in patients with metastatic melanoma. Proc Natl Acad Sci USA 100:8372–7.

Powell DJ Jr, De Vries CR, Allen T, Ahmadzadeh M & Rosenberg SA (2007), Inability to mediate prolonged reduction of regulatory T Cells after transfer of autologous CD25-depleted PBMC and interleukin-2 after lymphodepleting chemotherapy. J Immunother 30:438–47.

Prince ME, Sivanandan R, Kaczorowski A, Wolf GT, Kaplan MJ, Dalerba P, Weissman IL, Clarke MF & Ailles LE (2007), Identification of a subpopulation of cells with cancer stem cell properties in head and neck squamous cell carcinoma. Proc Natl Acad Sci USA 104:973–8.

Quintana E, Shackleton M, Sabel MS, Fullen DR, Johnson TM & Morrison SJ (2008), Efficient tumour formation by single human melanoma cells. Nature 456:593–8.

Radhakrishnan S, Nguyen LT, Ciric B, Flies D, Van Keulen VP, Tamada K, Chen L, Rodriguez M & Pease LR (2004), Immunotherapeutic potential of B7-DC (PD-L2) cross-linking antibody in conferring antitumor immunity. Cancer Res 64:4965–72.

Ramsdell F & Fowlkes BJ (1990), Clonal deletion versus clonal anergy: the role of the thymus in inducing self tolerance. Science 248:1342–8.

Ramsdell F & Fowlkes BJ (1992), Maintenance of in vivo tolerance by persistence of antigen. Science 257:1130–4.

Ramsdell F, Lantz T & Fowlkes BJ (1989), A nondeletional mechanism of thymic self tolerance. Science 246:1038–41.

Reuben JM, Lee BN, Li C, Gomez-Navarro J, Bozon VA, Parker CA, Hernandez IM, Gutierrez C, Lopez-Berestein G & Camacho LH (2006), Biologic and immunomodulatory events after CTLA-4 blockade with ticilimumab in patients with advanced malignant melanoma. Cancer 106:2437–44.

Reya T, Morrison SJ, Clarke MF & Weissman IL (2001), Stem cells, cancer, and cancer stem cells. Nature 414:105–11.

Ricci-Vitiani L, Lombardi DG, Pilozzi E, Biffoni M, Todaro M, Peschle C & De Maria R (2007), Identification and expansion of human colon-cancer-initiating cells. Nature 445:111–5.

Risau W (1997), Mechanisms of angiogenesis. Nature 386:671–4.

Rosenberg SA (1999), A new era for cancer immunotherapy based on the genes that encode cancer antigens. Immunity 10:281–7.

Rosenberg SA, Restifo NP, Yang JC, Morgan RA & Dudley ME (2008), Adoptive cell transfer: a clinical path to effective cancer immunotherapy. Nat Rev Cancer 8:299–308.

Rosenberg SA, Yang JC & Restifo NP (2004), Cancer immunotherapy: moving beyond current vaccines. Nat Med 10:909–15.

Ruiter DJ, Mattijssen V, Broecker EB & Ferrone S (1991), MHC antigens in human melanomas. Semin Cancer Biol 2:35–45.

Saikali S, Avril T, Collet B, Hamlat A, Bansard JY, Drenou B, Guegan Y & Quillien V (2007), Expression of nine tumour antigens in a series of human glioblastoma multiforme: interest of EGFRvIII, IL-13Ralpha2, gp100 and TRP-2 for immunotherapy. J Neurooncol 81:139–48.

Sakaguchi S, Sakaguchi N, Asano M, Itoh M & Toda M (1995), Immunologic self-tolerance maintained by activated T cells expressing IL-2 receptor alpha-chains (CD25). Breakdown of a single mechanism of self-tolerance causes various autoimmune diseases. J Immunol 155:1151–64.

Scadden DT (2006), The stem-cell niche as an entity of action. Nature 441:1075-9.

Schatton T & Frank MH (2008), Cancer stem cells and human malignant melanoma. Pigment Cell Melanoma Res 21:39-55.

Schatton T & Frank MH (2009), Antitumor immunity and cancer stem cells. Ann N Y Acad Sci 1176:154-69.

Schatton T, Frank NY & Frank MH (2009), Identification and targeting of cancer stem cells. Bioessays 31:1038-49.

Schatton T, Murphy GF, Frank NY, Yamaura K, Waaga-Gasser AM, Gasser M, Zhan Q, Jordan S, Duncan LM, Weishaupt C, et al. (2008), Identification of cells initiating human melanomas. Nature 451:345-9.

Schatton T, Schutte U, Frank NY, Zhan Q, Hoerning A, Robles SC, Zhou J, Hodi FS, Spagnoli GC, Murphy GF, et al. (2010), Modulation of T-cell activation by malignant melanoma initiating cells. Cancer Res 70:697-708.

Schuchter LM (2004), Adjuvant interferon therapy for melanoma: high-dose, low-dose, no dose, which dose? J Clin Oncol 22:7-10.

Schwartz RH (1990), A cell culture model for T lymphocyte clonal anergy. Science 248:1349-56.

Shah S & Qiao L (2008), Resting B cells expand a CD4+CD25+Foxp3+ Treg population via TGF-beta3. Eur J Immunol 38:2488-98.

Shankaran V, Ikeda H, Bruce AT, White JM, Swanson PE, Old LJ & Schreiber RD (2001), IFNgamma and lymphocytes prevent primary tumour development and shape tumour immunogenicity. Nature 410:1107-11.

Shipitsin M, Campbell LL, Argani P, Weremowicz S, Bloushtain-Qimron N, Yao J, Nikolskaya T, Serebryiskaya T, Beroukhim R, Hu M, et al. (2007), Molecular definition of breast tumor heterogeneity. Cancer Cell 11:259-73.

Singh SK, Hawkins C, Clarke ID, Squire JA, Bayani J, Hide T, Henkelman RM, Cusimano MD & Dirks PB (2004), Identification of human brain tumour initiating cells. Nature, *432*, 396-401.

Sioud M, Mobergslien A, Boudabous A & Floisand Y (2010), Evidence for the involvement of galectin-3 in mesenchymal stem cell suppression of allogeneic T-cell proliferation. Scand J Immunol 71:267-74.

Smith TR & Kumar V (2008), Revival of CD8+ Treg-mediated suppression. Trends Immunol 29:337-42.

Soria G & Ben-Baruch A (2008), The inflammatory chemokines CCL2 and CCL5 in breast cancer. Cancer Lett 267:271-85.

Sotomayor EM, Borrello I, Rattis FM, Cuenca AG, Abrams J, Staveley-O'Carroll K & Levitsky HI (2001), Cross-presentation of tumor antigens by bone marrow-derived antigen-presenting cells is the dominant mechanism in the induction of T-cell tolerance during B-cell lymphoma progression. Blood 98:1070-7.

Sotomayor EM, Borrello I, Tubb E, Rattis FM, Bien H, Lu Z, Fein S, Schoenberger S & Levitsky HI (1999), Conversion of tumor-specific CD4+ T-cell tolerance to T-cell priming through in vivo ligation of CD40. Nat Med 5:780-7.

Spaggiari GM, Capobianco A, Abdelrazik H, Becchetti F, Mingari MC & Moretta L (2008), Mesenchymal stem cells inhibit natural killer-cell proliferation, cytotoxicity, and cytokine production: role of indoleamine 2,3-dioxygenase and prostaglandin E2. Blood 111: 1327-33.

Staveley-O'Carroll K, Sotomayor E, Montgomery J, Borrello I, Hwang L, Fein S, Pardoll D & Levitsky H (1998), Induction of antigen-specific T cell anergy: An early event in the course of tumor progression. Proc Natl Acad Sci USA 95:1178-83.

Stockert E, Jager E, Chen YT, Scanlan MJ, Gout I, Karbach J, Arand M, Knuth A & Old LJ (1998), A survey of the humoral immune response of cancer patients to a panel of human tumor antigens. J Exp Med 187:1349-54.

Strand S, Hofmann WJ, Hug H, Muller M, Otto G, Strand D, Mariani SM, Stremmel W, Krammer PH & Galle PR (1996), Lymphocyte apoptosis induced by CD95 (APO-1/Fas) ligand-expressing tumor cells – a mechanism of immune evasion? Nat Med 2:1361-6.

Stumpfova M, Ratner D, Desciak EB, Eliezri YD & Owens DM (2010), The immunosuppressive surface ligand CD200 augments the metastatic capacity of squamous cell carcinoma. Cancer Res 70:2962–72.

Suva ML, Riggi N, Stehle JC, Baumer K, Tercier S, Joseph JM, Suva D, Clement V, Provero P, Cironi L, et al. (2009), Identification of cancer stem cells in Ewing's sarcoma. Cancer Res 69: 1776–81.

Theobald M, Biggs J, Hernandez J, Lustgarten J, Labadie C & Sherman LA (1997), Tolerance to p53 by A2.1-restricted cytotoxic T lymphocytes. J Exp Med 185:833–41.

Ting CC, Yang SS & Hargrove ME (1984), Induction of suppressor T cells by interleukin 2. J Immunol 133:261–6.

Todaro M, D'Asaro M, Caccamo N, Iovino F, Francipane MG, Meraviglia S, Orlando V, La Mendola C, Gulotta G, Salerno A, et al. (2009), Efficient killing of human colon cancer stem cells by gammadelta T lymphocytes. J Immunol 182:7287–96.

Tsukahara R, Takeuchi M, Akiba H, Kezuka T, Takeda K, Usui Y, Usui M, Yagita H & Okumura K (2005), Critical contribution of CD80 and CD86 to induction of anterior chamber-associated immune deviation. Int Immunol 17:523–30.

Uccelli A, Moretta L & Pistoia V (2008), Mesenchymal stem cells in health and disease. Nat Rev Immunol 8:726–36.

Van Belle P, Rodeck U, Nuamah I, Halpern AC & Elder DE (1996), Melanoma-associated expression of transforming growth factor-beta isoforms. Am J Pathol 148:1887–94.

Van Der Bruggen P, Traversari C, Chomez P, Lurquin C, De Plaen E, Van Den Eynde B, Knuth A & Boon T (1991), A gene encoding an antigen recognized by cytolytic T lymphocytes on a human melanoma. Science 254:1643–7.

Van Houdt IS, Sluijter BJ, Moesbergen LM, Vos WM, De Gruijl TD, Molenkamp BG, Van Den Eertwegh AJ, Hooijberg E, Van Leeuwen PA, Meijer CJ, et al. (2008), Favorable outcome in clinically stage II melanoma patients is associated with the presence of activated tumor infiltrating T-lymphocytes and preserved MHC class I antigen expression. Int J Cancer 123:609–15.

Wahl SM, Swisher J, Mccartney-Francis N & Chen W (2004), TGF-beta: the perpetrator of immune suppression by regulatory T cells and suicidal T cells. J Leukoc Biol 76:15–24.

Wang H, Lathia JD, Wu Q, Wang J, Li Z, Heddleston JM, Eyler CE, Elderbroom J, Gallagher J, Schuschu J, et al. (2009), Targeting interleukin 6 signaling suppresses glioma stem cell survival and tumor growth. Stem Cells 27:2393–404.

Wang L, Pino-Lagos K, De Vries VC, Guleria I, Sayegh MH & Noelle RJ (2008), Programmed death 1 ligand signaling regulates the generation of adaptive Foxp3+CD4+ regulatory T cells. Proc Natl Acad Sci USA 105:9331–6.

Wei J, Barr J, Kong LY, Wang Y, Wu A, Sharma AK, Gumin J, Henry V, Colman H, Priebe W, et al. (2010a), Glioblastoma cancer-initiating cells inhibit T-cell proliferation and effector responses by the signal transducers and activators of transcription 3 pathway. Mol Cancer Ther 9:67–78.

Wei J, Barr J, Kong LY, Wang Y, Wu A, Sharma AK, Gumin J, Henry V, Colman H, Sawaya R, et al. (2010b), Glioma-associated cancer-initiating cells induce immunosuppression. Clin Cancer Res 16:461–73.

Wing K, Onishi Y, Prieto-Martin P, Yamaguchi T, Miyara M, Fehervari Z, Nomura T & Sakaguchi S (2008), CTLA-4 control over Foxp3+ regulatory T cell function. Science, 322, 271–5.

Woo EY, Yeh H, Chu CS, Schlienger K, Carroll RG, Riley JL, Kaiser LR & June CH (2002), Cutting edge: Regulatory T cells from lung cancer patients directly inhibit autologous T cell proliferation. J Immunol 168:4272–6.

Wu A, Oh S, Wiesner SM, Ericson K, Chen L, Hall WA, Champoux PE, Low WC & Ohlfest JR (2008), Persistence of CD133+ cells in human and mouse glioma cell lines: detailed characterization of GL261 glioma cells with cancer stem cell-like properties. Stem Cells Dev 17:173–84.

Xu Q, Liu G, Yuan X, Xu M, Wang H, Ji J, Konda B, Black KL & Yu JS (2009), Antigen-specific T-cell response from dendritic cell vaccination using cancer stem-like cell-associated antigens. Stem Cells 27:1734–40.

Yang ZF, Ho DW, Ng MN, Lau CK, Yu WC, Ngai P, Chu PW, Lam CT, Poon RT & Fan ST (2008), Significance of CD90(+) Cancer Stem Cells in Human Liver Cancer. Cancer Cell 13: 153–66.

Yao Y, Wang X, Jin K, Zhu J, Wang Y, Xiong S, Mao Y & Zhou L (2008), B7-H4 is preferentially expressed in non-dividing brain tumor cells and in a subset of brain tumor stem-like cells. J Neurooncol 89:121–9.

Yi KH & Chen L (2009), Fine tuning the immune response through B7-H3 and B7-H4. Immunol Rev 229:145–51.

Yu F, Yao H, Zhu P, Zhang X, Pan Q, Gong C, Huang Y, Hu X, Su F, Lieberman J, et al. (2007), let-7 regulates self renewal and tumorigenicity of breast cancer cells. Cell 131:1109–23.

Zatloukal K, Schneeberger A, Berger M, Schmidt W, Koszik F, Kutil R, Cotten M, Wagner E, Buschle M, Maass G, et al. (1995), Elicitation of a systemic and protective anti-melanoma immune response by an IL-2-based vaccine. Assessment of critical cellular and molecular parameters. J Immunol 154:3406–19.

Zhang C, Zhang J, Wei H & Tian Z (2005), Imbalance of NKG2D and its inhibitory counterparts: how does tumor escape from innate immunity? Int Immunopharmacol, 5, 1099–111.

Zhang S, Balch C, Chan MW, Lai HC, Matei D, Schilder JM, Yan PS, Huang TH & Nephew KP (2008), Identification and characterization of ovarian cancer-initiating cells from primary human tumors. Cancer Res 68:4311–20.

Zheng G, Wang B & Chen A (2004), The 4-1BB costimulation augments the proliferation of CD4+CD25+ regulatory T cells. J Immunol 173:2428–34.

Zhu L, Gibson P, Currle DS, Tong Y, Richardson RJ, Bayazitov IT, Poppleton H, Zakharenko S, Ellison DW & Gilbertson RJ (2009), Prominin 1 marks intestinal stem cells that are susceptible to neoplastic transformation. Nature 457:603–7.

Index

A

ABC transporters. *See* ATP-binding cassette (ABC) transporters
Activated leukocyte cell adhesion molecule (ALCAM), 164, 165
Acute lymphoblastic leukemia (ALL), 4, 6
Acute myeloid leukemia (AML)
    CD34+ and CD38-populations, 20
    CSCs, 313
    remission rate improvement, 285
    stem cells isolation, 291
Acute promyelocytic leukemia (APL)
    all-trans-retinoic acid (ATRA), 261
    AML, 89
Adenomatous polyposis coli (APC)
    colon cancer cell, treatment, 175–176
    deficiency, 160
    stem cell compartment, 166
    tumour suppressor gene, 167
    WRE, 160
Adoptive cell transfer (ACT)
    approaches, 322–323
    cancer immunotherapeutic strategies, 319
AFP. *See* Alpha-fetoprotein
ALCAM. *See* Activated leukocyte cell adhesion molecule
Aldehyde dehydrogenase–1 (ALDH1)
    cell-surface markers, 55
    crypts, 172
    description, 165
    identification, CSCs, 56
Aldehyde dehydrogenase (ALDH), 21–22, 185, 188
ALDH1. *See* Aldehyde dehydrogenase–1
ALL. *See* Acute lymphoblastic leukemia
All-trans retinoic acid (ATRA)
    APL treatment, 261
    induced cell differentiation, 251
Alpha-fetoprotein (AFP), 184, 186, 187, 190, 191, 193–194
Anaplasia, CSC
    biomarkers
        CD34+CD38-, 8–9
        cellular evolution/adaptation, 10–11
        cellular metabolism, 12
        genetic instability, 12
        identification/target, 9
        instability, nucleotides, 11–12
        microarray analysis, 13
        miR–155, MMR proteins, 12
        mutations, 11
        nonclonal genomic rearrangements, 12
        research, human colon, 9
        side effects, 8
        stemness properties, 8–9
        telomere attrition, BFB cycles, 11
        therapeutic potential, 9
        tumor growth, 11
    chemoresistance, treatment, 1
    dedifferentiation, 2
    description, 1
    hierarchical manner, leukemic cells, 3
    morphologic changes, 2–3
    normal stem cell physiology, 1–2
    origin, progenitor cells, 3
    plasticity
        clonal evolution, 5
        CML, germ line programming, 6–7
        EGFR gene, 7
        EMT, 4
        fractionation, 5–6

Anaplasia, CSC (*cont.*)
    frequency and functional property, 6
    glioblastomas, 7
    H3K4 and JARID1B, 4
    mutant molecules, 6
    origin, cancer, 6
    pathophysiological role, 7–8
    Ph⁺, ALL, 4–5
    γ-secretase inhibitor, 7
    self-renewing, 6
    stage, disease, 6
    "stem-like" cells, 8
    subclones, 5
    transplanted cancer cell, 10
  research, 4
  self-renewal, 6
  subclones, 6
  tumor-maintaining/tumor-sustaining/
      tumor-propagating, 2
  xenograft assay
    CD44(+), 10
    xenotransplantation, 10
Anergy
  clonal, 308, 314–315
  induction, 315
  T-cell, 315, 316
Antigen-presenting cells (APCs), 315, 316
Antitumor immunity
  CSCs, 311, 317, 319, 323
  host, 308, 317, 319
  TAAs, 308
APC. *See* Adenomatous polyposis coli
APL. *See* Acute promyelocytic leukemia
ATP-binding cassette (ABC) transporters
  ABCB
    ABCB1, 274
    ABCB5, 275
    P-gp, cells apical surface, 274–275
  ABCB5
    human-to-mouse xenotransplantation,
        53–54
    novel molecular marker, 54
  ABCC
    ABCC1, 275, 276
    drug resistance, 276
  ABCG
    ABCG2/BCRP, 276–277
    anticancer drug substrates, 278
    CSC populations, 277
  ABCG2
    chemotherapy agents and substrates, 52
    MCF-7 and Cal-51 cell lines, 53
    tumorigenicity, 53
  ALDH1 (*see* Aldehyde dehydrogenase–1)

  classification
    antitumor drugs substrates class
        and MDR, 271
    NBDs and TMDs, 270–271
    structural features, 271
  CXCR4
    identification, brain cancer, 57
    SDF-1-CXCR4 interaction, 56
    transmembrane, GPCR, 56
  EpCAM
    characteristics, 54–55
    HCC growth and invasiveness, 54
    HEK 293 cells, 55
  inhibitors, 278–282
  proteins, 272
  SP cells, 58–59
  telomerase, 57
ATRA. *See* All-trans retinoic acid

B
Basal cell carcinomas (BCC), 300
Basic fibroblast growth factor (bFGF), 133, 217
BCC. *See* Basal cell carcinomas
bFGF. *See* Basic fibroblast growth factor
Biomarkers, CSCs
  ATP-binding cassette transporters
    ABCB5, 53–54
    ABCG2, 52–53
    ALDH1, 55–56
    CXCR4, 56–57
    EpCAM, 54–55
    SP cells, 58–59
    telomerase, 57
  CD24
    adult nonmalignant tissue, 50
    cancer cell expression, 51
  CD44
    multifunctional protein, 48
    positive staining, HCC, 49–50
    Wnt and prostaglandin E2, gastric
        cancer, 49
  CD133
    epithelial tumors, 47
    medulloblastomas and glioblastomas,
        46–47
    and mRNA, difference, 47–48
    preoperative chemoradiotherapy, 48
    spheroid cells, 47
  CD138, 51
  complexity and specificity, 52
  DCAMKL-1, 59
  hypothesis, 45
  isolation and characterization, 46

Index

LRCs, 60
malignancies, 46
NCI60 tumor cell line panel, 51–52
Nestin, 60
piwil2, 59–60
podocalyxin, 59
subpopulation, tumor cells, 45
Bmi1, 111
BMP. *See* Bone morphogenetic protein
Bone morphogenetic protein (BMP), 133
Brain tumor stem cell, 114
Breast cancer stem cells
  cellular origins and tumorigenesis
    asymmetrically and therapeutic eradication, 147
    deregulated pathways, 148
    mammary gland, EMT, 145, 146
    MSC and bone-marrow, 147
    symmetric division, 148
    transient amplifying cells, 145
    tumoral niche, 146, 147
    tumor-stroma interactions, 146
  CSC, 143
  definition, 143–144
  epithelial cell hierarchy
    anchorage-independent growth, 145
    CD, 145
    ER/PR, 145
    ESA and SMA, 144
    luminal and myoepithelial, 144
    NOD/SCID mice, 145
  experimental models
    BMI1, 149
    BRCA1 gene, 148
    MCF-10F, 148
    MMTV, 148
  heterogeneity, 151
  identification, feasability and utility
    ALDH1 immunoexpression group, 153
    Her2, 152
    Ki67 expression, 152
  isolation and characterization
    ALDH1, 150
    $CD44^+/CD24^{-/low}/lin^-$ phenotype, 149
    in vitro assays, 149
    side population technique, 150
    xenograft, 149
  metastasis, tumor dormancy, 151–152
  novel stem cells targeted therapies
    ADAM and MAML, 154
    hedgehog inhibitors, 153–154
    Her2 signaling and Notch pathway, 154
    Notch4, 154
    notch pathways inhibitors, 153
    oral hedgehog inhibitor, 153
    PTEN and PI3K/mTOR, 153–154
    trial design and rational endpoints, 154
  phenotypes, 143
  solid tissue, definition, 144
  treatment response, 152

C

CAF. *See* Cancer-associated fibroblasts
Cancer-associated fibroblasts (CAF)
  source, 70
  TAMs, 69, 80
Cancer stem cells (CSCs)
  cell-of-origin, 19
  characteristics
    chemotherapy resistance, 19
    invasion/metastatic activity, 20
    irradiation resistance, 19
  chemoresistance
    ABC transporters, 283–284
    leukemia and myeloma, 282, 283
  CNS (*see* Central nervous system (CNS) and CSCs)
  colon (*see* Colon CSCs)
  2-DE, 223–224
  definition, 17–18
  description, 303–304
  EMT, 74
  epigenetic changes and tumor microenvironment, 75–76
  ESC-specific proteins and ESC-derived proteins, 224
  FACS, 223
  glioblastoma (*see* Glioblastoma cancer stem cells (GCSC))
  ICAT and iTRAQ, 224
  and immunity
    immunogenic and self-tolerance, 308
    NOD/SCID, 307
    suppressor role, tumor, 309
    tumor antigens types, 308
    "tumor surveillance", 307
  immunomodulatory functions
    APC, 315–316
    class I and II MHC molecules, 310–311
    costimulatory molecules, 315–316
    galectin-3, 314
    hypothesis, 309
    macrophages, 313
    mechanisms, 311, 312
    MMIC, 310, 311
    NK, 311, 313–314
    PBMC, 310

Cancer stem cells (CSCs) (cont.)
  PD-L1, 314
  soluble mediator, 318–319
  TGF-β/PGE–2, 315
  Treg cells, 317
 mass spectrometry, 223
 models (see Mouse CSC model)
 "niche", 20
 pancreatic (see Pancreatic CSCs)
 preparation (see Tissue-specific stem cells)
 prologue, 17
 proteome
  benign and malignant, 229
  CD133+ and CD133-cells, 231
  ESCs and ECCs, 230
  GBM-SCs and T cell-based immunotherapies, 230
  hESCs and hECCs, 229
  isolation, 231
  microenvironmental factors, 229
  novel cell surface markers and colon tumour spheres, 231
  phenotypic heterogeneity and characteristics, 231
  plasma membrane and specific cell surface markers, 229
  side and non-side population cells, 231–232
  STAT3, 230–231
  tyrosine kinase signalling pathways, 232
 proteomic technologies, 224, 225
 RT-PCR/microarrays, 223
 SCID and proteins, 223
 signaling pathways
  Hh, 25
  notch, 23–24
  p53, 22
  Rb, 23
  receptor tyrosine kinase pathway, 23
  Wnt, 24–25
 stemness signalling pathways
  BMI–1 and chemoresistant proteins, 235
  CRC, 232–233
  GSIs, 234
  hepatic and peritoneal, 236
  Lu/B-CAM, 236
  molecular network and physiological processes, 236
  PP2A and anticancer therapies, 233
  PTEN, 235–236
  SKOV3, 234–235
  TCGA and proteomic approach, 233
  TNF-alpha and IRR cells, 234
  Wnt/beta-catenin, 232
  translational relevance, tumor immunotherapy
   ACT approaches, 322–323
   glioblastoma cells, 322
   IL–2 and IFN-α, 319–320
   immunization approaches, 321
   immunotherapeutic strategies, 319
   Treg cells, 319–320
   tumorigenic MMICs, 321
  tumorigenic process
   cell surface phenotype, human malignancies, 305
   definition, 304
   heterogeneity, 304
   model systems, CSC-driven immunomodulation, 306–307
   tumor-seeding properties, 304–305
   xenotransplantation studies, 74
Cancer therapeutics. See CSCs and therapeutic approaches
CCK-BR. See Cholecystokinin 2 receptor
CD. See Cluster of differentiation
Central nervous system (CNS) and CSCs
 developmental theories, tumorigenesis, 107–108
 GBM, 108–111
 pathways regulating proteins
  ABCG2 multidrug-resistance gene, 112
  Bmi1 and EZH2, 111
  c-MYC and STAT3, 113–114
  GSK3β, 114–115
  Nestin and Musashi, 114
  notch, 112–113
  SHH, 113
  SOX, 115
  TGF-β, 115–116
 stem cell niche, 108
 surface markers, 116
 therapy
  drugs and toxins, 117
  hypoxia, 116–117
Chemoresistance
 ABC transporters
  classification, 270–271
  inhibitors, 278–282
  and MDR, 272–278
 antineoplastic drugs, 270
 chemotherapy, 269
 CSCs, 282–284
 renal cancer cells, 284
Cholecystokinin 2 receptor (CCK-BR), 165
Chronic myeloid leukemia (CML), 6
Circulating tumor cells, 151

Index

Cluster of differentiation (CD), 145
CM. See Conditioned medium
CML. See Chronic myeloid leukemia
Colon CSCs
   ALDH1, 165
   CD44
      CD24, 173
      CD26, 172
      EpCAM, 172
   CD133, 162
   cell divisions, 157
   colorectal carcinogenesis
      adenoma carcinoma sequence model, 167–168
      APC, 167
      cancer development, 167
      tumor initiation, 168–169
   embryonal rest theory, 169
   gastrointestinal, 158
   intestinal
      ALCAM/CD166, 165
      ALDH1, 165
      BMI–1, 163
      CCK-BR, 165
      CD133, 162
      crypts, 161–162
      DCAMLK–1, 163–165
      Eph receptors, 165
      epithelium, 161
      OLFM4, 162–163
      quiescent, 161
      Sox9, 163
      spindle orientation, 166
   therapeutics
      drug resistance, 173
      IGF-IR and HH-GLI, 173–174
      IL–4, 174
      stem cell niche, 158
      Wnt signalling pathway, 176
   tissue, 157–158
   Wnt/beta-catenin signalling pathway
      NOTCH, 160
      role, 159
      stabilization, 159–160
Colorectal cancer (CRC), 232–233
Conditioned medium (CM), 228
Costimulation
   negative, 317
   positive, 315, 316
CRC. See Colorectal cancer
CSCs. See Cancer stem cells
CSCs and therapeutic approaches
   ABC drug inhibitors
      Dofequidar and Vandetanib, 260
      multifunctional efflux transporters, 259–260
      Salinomycin, 260
   defined, 241
   differentiation therapy
      ATRA, 261
      HDIs, 261–262
   inhibitors and potential targets, 242–245
   niche-targeted drugs, 258–259
   pharmacological research, 241–242
   signaling pathways
      Hh, 253–255
      notch, 255–257
      PI3Ks, 257
      TKIs, 249
      Wnt, 249–253
   surface markers
      bivatuzumab mertansine, 247
      CD44 and CD123, 246
      EpCAM, 247–248
      gemtuzumab ozogamicin, 247
      xenotransplantation assay, 242
   telomerase inhibitors, 258
Cytokine
   IL–2, 310, 320
   IL–10, 310, 317
Cytotoxic T lymphocytes (CTLs)
   MHC class I molecules, 311
   pp65-specific, 322
   p53-reactive, 309

D

DCAMLK–1. See Doublecortin CaM kinase-like–1
DCIS. See Ductal carcinoma in situ
Differentiation
   CD133-positive cells, 113
   GBM cell, 111
   glioma precursors, 117
DNA methyltransferases (DNMT1), 39
DNMT1. See DNA methyltransferases
Dormancy, 263
Doublecortin CaM kinase-like–1 (DCAMLK–1), 59, 163
Ductal carcinoma in situ (DCIS), 293
Dysregulated self-renewal pathways
   PcG
      PRC1 and PRC2, 191
      silencing bmi–1, 191–192
      target gene silencing, 191
   Wnt/ßcatenin signaling
      CD133+ liver CSCs, 192
      TGF-β–1, 193

E
ECM. *See* Extracellular matrix
EGF. *See* Epithelial growth factor
EGFR. *See* Epidermal growth factor receptor
EMT. *See* Epithelial-mesenchymal transition
Enhancer of zeste homologue 2 (EZH2), 111
EpCAM. *See* Epithelial cell adhesion molecule
Epidermal growth factor receptor (EGFR), 299–300
Epigenetics
　changes and tumor microenvironment, 75–76
　drugs, 261
　modifications, 262
　therapy, 80
Epithelial cell adhesion molecule (EpCAM), 247–248
Epithelial growth factor (EGF), 213, 217
Epithelial-mesenchymal transition (EMT), 4, 74, 206–207
Epithelial specific antigen (ESA), 144
ER. *See* Estrogen receptor
ESA. *See* Epithelial specific antigen
Estrogen receptor (ER), 145
Extracellular matrix (ECM)
　components, 69–70
　role, 77
EZH2. *See* Enhancer of zeste homologue 2

F
Fluorescence-activated cell sorting (FACS) analysis
　PDAC tumors, 201
　tumorspheres, 203

G
Gamma-secretase inhibitors (GSIs), 234, 300
GBM. *See* Glioblastoma multiforme
GBM-SCs. *See* Glioblastoma stem cells
GCSC. *See* Glioblastoma cancer stem cells
Genomics
　DNA sequencing, 39
　neoplastic and non-neoplastic stem cell, 40
　nuclear proteins, 36
Glioblastoma cancer stem cells (GCSC)
　biology, 128
　chemoradiation resistance, 129
　clinical implications
　　neuro-oncology, 135
　　therapeutic resistance, 135–136
　developmental markers, 128

gliomas
　classification and grading, 125–126
　clinical features, 126–127
　treatment, 127
　molecular pathways
　　BMP and Bmi1, 133–134
　　EGF-EGFR, 132–133
　　HIF, 134
　　Shh and notch, 134
　　STAT3 and bFGF, 133
　NSC, 127–128
　origin
　　criteria, 129–130
　　hierarchical and stochastic models, 130–131
　　INK4a-Arf disruption, 130
　　oncogenes, 130
　　xenograft models, 131–132
Glioblastoma multiforme (GBM)
　bevacizumab, 136
　brain CSCs
　　CD133-positive and negative cells, 110
　　p-GBM and c-GBM cells, 110–111
　chemoradiation resistance, 129
　described, 108–109
　patients survival, 125–126
Glioblastoma stem cells (GBM-SCs), 230
Glycogen synthase kinase 3β (GSK3β), 114–115
GSIs. *See* Gamma-secretase inhibitors

H
HCC. *See* Hepatocellular carcinoma
HDIs. *See* Histone deacetylase inhibitors
Hedgehog-Gli pathway, 292–293
Hedgehog (Hh) signaling pathways
　described, 253
　GDC–0449 inhibitor, 253–254
　IPI–926 drug, 254
　LDE225 and BMS–863923/XL139, 255
　pancreatic CSCs
　　ligand binding and components, 204
　　mammospheres, 204
　　metastasis prevention, 204–205
Hematopoietic microenvironment (HM)
　component, 88–89
　HSC niche hypothesis, 92
　LSC, 96
Hematopoietic stem cells (HSC)
　HM, 92
　LSC, 87
　progenitors, 88
　properties, 91

Index   339

Hematopoietic stem cell transplantation (HSCT), 300–301
Hepatocellular carcinoma (HCC), 183–196
HER2. *See* Human-epidermal growth factor receptor type 2
HIF. *See* Hypoxia inducible factors
Histone deacetylase inhibitors (HDIs), 261–262
HM. *See* Hematopoietic microenvironment
HSC. *See* Hematopoietic stem cells
HSCT. *See* Hematopoietic stem cell transplantation
Human-epidermal growth factor receptor type 2 (HER2), 299–300
Human Proteome Organization (HUPO), 228
Human tumors, 26
HUPO. *See* Human Proteome Organization
Hypoxia inducible factors (HIF), 134

I

ICAT. *See* Isotope-coded affinity tag
IL–4. *See* Interleukin–4
Immune evasion
  cells, tumor, 309
  CSC-driven, 314, 323
Immunomodulation
  CSC-driven, 306–307
  galectin–3, 314
Immunosuppressed non-obese diabetic/severe combined immunodeficiency mice (NOD/SCID mice), 145
Immunotherapy
  CSCs translational relevance
    ABCB5 antigen, 321–322
    active immunization approaches, 321
    ACT treatment efficacy, 322–323
    anti-CTLA–4 antibody, 320
    categories, 319
    human epidermal growth factor receptor 2 (HER2), 322
    IL–2 and IFN α, 319–320
  metastatic renal carcinoma, 213
Induced CSCs, 26, 27
Induced pluripotent stem (iPS), 294–295
Inhibitors, ABC transporters
  curcumin, 279–280
  imatinib, 282
  MDR, 278, 279
  P-gp inhibitors, cyclosporin and verapamil, 278, 279
  plant flavonoids modulatory effects, 279, 281
  tariquidar, zosuquidar, and elacridar, 279, 280
Interleukin–4 (IL–4), 174

International Society for Stem Cell Research (ISSCR), 228
iPS. *See* Induced pluripotent stem
Isobaric tag for relative and absolute quantitation (iTRAQ), 224
Isotope-coded affinity tag (ICAT), 224
ISSCR. *See* International Society for Stem Cell Research
iTRAQ. *See* Isobaric tag for relative and absolute quantitation

L

Let–7 regulated oncofetal genes (LOGs), 295–296
Leukemia stem cells (LSC)
  clonal evolution theory, 98–99
  definition, 87–88
  frequency and generation, 97–98
  HM, 92–94
  implications, diagnosis, prognosis and therapy
    arsenic trioxide, 96
    monoclonal antibodies, 95–96
    surrogate assays, 97
    therapeutic targeting, 95
    tumor therapy, 94–95
  origin
    cell populations, 90–91
    description, 88–89
    hierarchy, 90
    progenitor, 89
  properties
    cell-intrinsic mechanisms, 92
    quiescent state and cytotoxic agents, 91
    self-renewal pathways, 91–92
  research, 100
  xenograft models, 98
Lipid kinase phosphoinositide 3-kinase/mamalian target of rapamicine (PI3K/mTOR), 153–154
Liver tumor-initiating cells
  anticancer therapies, 183
  dysregulated self-renewal pathways
    Bmi–1, 191–192
    TGF-β, 193
    Wnt/βcatenin signaling, 192
  markers, liver CSC's
    ALDH, 188
    CD133+, 186–187
    CD90+ and CD90+CD44+, 189
    CD133+CD44+, 188
    EpCAM+/CD326+, 190
    OV6+, 190–191
  microarray analysis, 184

Liver tumor-initiating cells (cont.)
  miRNAs
    miR–181 and EpCAM, 193–194
    miR–130b and CD133, 194–195
    pathways mediating therapeutic resistance
      CD133, 195–196
      therapeutic implications, 196–197
  SP, 184
  stemness genes, 184
LOGs. See Let–7 regulated oncofetal genes
Long-term label retaining cells (LRCs), 60
LRCs. See Long-term label retaining cells
LSC. See Leukemia stem cells
Lu/B-CAM. See Lutheran/B-cell adhesion molecule
Lutheran/B-cell adhesion molecule (Lu/B-CAM), 236
Lymphocyte activation, 93, 246

M
Malignant glioma
  patient survival, 127
  therapeutic resistance, 135
Malignant melanoma-initiating cell (MMIC)
  ABCB5$^+$, 310, 311, 316, 318
  human malignant melanoma, 310
  tumorigenic, 317, 321
Markers, liver CSC's
  CD90$^+$ and CD90$^+$CD44$^+$
    anti-CD44, 189
    neutralizing antibody, 189
    tumor inoculation, 189
  CD133$^+$CD44$^+$
    β-catenin and Bmi–1, 189
    co-expression, 188
  EpCAM$^+$/CD326$^+$
    biomarker, HCC, 190
    Wnt/ßcatenin, 191
  flow cytometry, 186
  HCC
    IHC staining, 187
    PCR analysis, 187
    induce tumor formation, 186
    liver regeneration, 186
  OV6$^+$
    ductules and periportal parenchyma, 190
    miRNA, 190–191
  SCID/beige, 187
MB. See Medulloblastoma
Medulloblastoma (MB), 300
MEF, 228
Metastasis
  process, 260
  tumor, 246

Microenvironment. See Tumor microenvironment
microRNAs (mRNAs), posttranscriptional orchestration
  DNMT1 and miR–16, 39
  LIN28, 38
  manipulation, 39
  RISC, 38
Minimal residual disease (MRD), 95
MMTV. See Mouse mammary tumor virus
Molecular biology, CSCs
  biotechnological and pharmaceutical sectors, 41
  cancer therapeutics
    applied, 34
    and disease progression
    and disease progression: flow cytometry analyses, 33
    and disease progression: glioblastoma and breast cancer cells, 33–34
    stemness
    stemness: ectopic expression, pluripotency, 35–36
    stemness: posttranscriptional orchestration, microRNAs, 38–39
    stemness: self-renewal capacity, 36–37
    stemness: senescence, 37–38
  DNA sequencing, 39
  exon re-sequencing, key genes, 40
  genes and microRNAs, 40
  neoplastic and non-neoplastic stem cell, 40
Mouse CSC model
  in vitro, 26–27
  in vivo, 26
Mouse mammary tumor virus (MMTV), 148
Multidrug resistance (MDR) and ABC transporters
  ABCB, 274–275
  ABCC, 275–276
  ABCG, 276–278
  description, 272
  proteins, 272, 273
Multidrug resistance-associated protein (MRP)
  drug efflux and GSH system, 275
  physiological conditions, transported substrates, 275
Multiple myeloma (MM), 51

N
Natural killer (NK) cells, 311–312
Neural stem cells (NSCs), 227
Niche
  and anticancer therapies
    chemotherapy, 79

Index

epigenetic therapy, 80
factors, 80–81
description, 72
embryonal, 72
lymphvascular
EMILIN1, 77
lymphatic endothelium, 76–77
osteoblastic, 72–73
premetastatic, 78–79
vascular, 73
Non small-cell lung cancer (NSCLC), 276
Notch, signaling pathway
activation, 255
drug-induced modification, 256
MAML glutamine-rich nuclear protein, 256–257
MK–0752 and RO4929097 drug, 255–256
OMP–21M18, 256
NSCs. See Neural stem cells
Nucleotide binding domains (NBDs), 270, 271

P

Pancreatic CSCs
identification
CD133+ cells, 202
tumor-initiating potential, 201–202
tumorspheres, 202–203
xenografts and FACS analysis, 200–201
metastasis
CD133+/CXCR4+ cells, 205–206
EMT, 206–207
invasion potential, 206
PDAC, 199
resistance to therapy
CD133+ cells, 207
gemcitabine and ionizing radiation, 207
signaling pathways
Bmi–1, 205
developmental and canonical, 203
Hh, 204–205
theory, 200
therapeutics, 208
Pancreatic ductal adenocarcinoma (PDAC)
cell proliferation and invasion, 205
diagnosis and mortality, 199
FACS analysis, 201
gemcitabine drug, 208
tumors, 200
Pathways mediating therapeutic resistance, CD133
Akt/PKB and Bcl–2 pathway, 195–196
chemotherapy and radiotherapy, 184
PcG. See Polycomb group
PDAC. See Pancreatic ductal adenocarcinoma

Peripheral blood mononuclear cell (PBMC), 310, 318
Phosphatase and tensin homolog (PTEN), 153–154, 235–236
Phosphatidylinositol 3-kinases (PI3Ks)
signaling pathway, 257
PI3K/mTOR. See Lipid kinase phosphoinositide 3-kinase/mamalian target of rapamicine
Pluripotency, ectopic expression
LIN28, 36
mature cell transformation, 35
Oct4 expression, 35
tumorigenicity, 35
Polycomb group (PcG), 184, 191, 192, 297
PP2A. See Protein phosphatase 2A
PR. See Progesterone receptors
Primary brain tumor, 125–126
Progesterone receptors (PR), 145
Protein phosphatase 2A (PP2A), 233
PTEN. See Phosphatase and tensin homolog

R

Receptor tyrosine kinases (RTKs), 23
Regulatory T (Treg) cells
CSCs, 319
induction, 318–320
Renal carcinoma
adult stem cells
Bowman's capsule, 215
cortex, tubule/interstitium, 214
in vitro and in vivo, 214–215
CD105+
histologic type, origin, 216
magnetic cell sorting, 216
mutated stromal/mesenchymal/bone-marrow cells, 216–217
CD133+/CD34- cells, 215
endothelial differentiation, renal CSCs
clonal cell and multipotency, 218
tissue stem/progenitor cells, 218
tumor anti-angiogenic therapy, 218
vasculogenic properties, 218, 219
genetic/epigenetic, 213
G1 phase, cell cycle, 219
SP, 217
sphere-derived CSCs
complement-mediated cell killing, 218
EGF and bFGF, 217
tumorigenic population *vs.* non-tumorigenic-differentiated population, 218–220
urological tumor and inhibitors, 213
Wilm's tumor, 214

Resistance to therapy, 254, 260
Retinoblastoma (Rb), 23
RISC. *See* RNA-induced silencing complex
RNA-induced silencing complex (RISC), 38
RTKs. *See* Receptor tyrosine kinases

S

SCID. *See* Severe combined immunedeficient
Secreted frizzled-related proteins (SFRPs), 252–253
Self-renewal
    expression, E2F2, 36–37
    GADD45-β and GADD45-γ, down-regulation, 36
    mutations, 36
    signaling pathways, cancer, 36
Senescence
    DNA defense and cell cycle, 37
    ectopic expression, hTERT, 37
    ionizing radiation, 37–38
Severe combined immunedeficient (SCID), 223
SFRPs. *See* Secreted frizzled-related proteins
SHH. *See* Sonic hedgehog
Shh. *See* Sonic hedgehog
Side population (SP)
    ABC membrane transporters, 184
    non-SP and, 184
    PLC/PRF/5, 192
Signal transducer and activator of transcription 3 (STAT3), 113–114, 133, 230–231
Single nucleotide polymorphisms (SNPs), 276
SKOV3, 234–235
SMA. *See* Smooth muscle actin
Smooth muscle actin (SMA), 144
Sonic hedgehog (Shh), 113, 134, 297
SP. *See* Side population
STAT3. *See* Signal transducer and activator of transcription 3
Stem cell niche
    components, 241
    targeted drugs, 258–259
Stem cells and CSCs
    definition, 291
    myeloid leukemia, 291
    NOD/SCID, 291
    therapy
        BCC and MB, 300
        breast, 299
        cancer recurrence, 298, 299
        cell-cycle active chemotherapeutic agents, 298–299
        checkpoint kinases, 299
        EGFR and HER2, 299–300
        GSIs, 300
        HSCT, 300–301
        in vitro and in vivo, 300
        phase I and phase II, 300
        radiation and cytotoxic, 299
    tumoral
        Bmi-1, 297
        c-Myc and Ewing sarcoma, 296
        DCIS, 293
        dynamic regulation, chromatin/histone modifications, 297
        embryonic stem (ES) cells, 295
        epithelial-to-mesenchimal transition, 292
        Hedgehog-Gli pathway, 292–293
        iPS, 294–295
        Lin–28/Let–7 switch, 296
        LOGs, 295–296
        mammosphere and helix-loop-helix family, 293–294
        non-random reciprocal chromosomal translocation, 296
        notch signalling pathway, 293–294
        PcG and Shh, 297
        pluripotency reprogrammation, 294, 295
        regulation cell cycle, Bmi–1, 297, 298
        self-renewal pathways, 292
        signaling pathways, cell biology, 292, 293
        transcription factors, 294–295
        Wnt pathway, 294
Stem cells, proteome
    CM and MEF, 228
    foetal and neonatal, 228
    HUPO and ISSCR, 228
    life span and biological processes, 226
    low-abundance growth factors, 228
    NSCs and hESC populations, 227
    physiological/experimental conditions, 224–225
    plasma membrane protein, 227
    8-plex i-TRAQ labelling strategy, 227–228
    qualitative and quantitative changes, 228
    SDS-PAGE protocols and MS/MS fragmentation data, 226

T

TAM. *See* Tumor associated macrophages
Targeted intraoperative radiotherapy (TARGIT), 80
TARGIT. *See* Targeted intraoperative radiotherapy
TCGA. *See* The Cancer Genome Atlas
Telomerase, 57, 91, 258

TGF-β. *See* Transforming growth factor-β
The Cancer Genome Atlas (TCGA), 233
Therapy
    anticancer
        chemotherapy, 79
        epigenetic therapy, 80
        factors, 80–81
    chemotherapy, 74
Tissue-specific stem cells (TSCs)
    ALDH, 21–22
    block cell differentiation, 17
    cell surface markers, 20–21
    expression, markers, 18
    genetic alterations, 22
    "niche", 20
    NSCs and mammary gland stem cells, 22
    oncogenic mutation, 19
    RTKs maintenance, 23
    SP, 21
TKIs. *See* Tyrosine kinase inhibitors
Tolerance
    induction mechanism, 314
    tumor immunosurveillance and immunological, 307–309
Transforming growth factor-β (TGF-β), 115–116, 192, 193
Trans membrane domains (TMDs)
    half-transporter proteins, 271
    and NBDs, 270–271
    translocation pathway, transported substrates, 270
TSCs. *See* Tissue-specific stem cells
Tumor-associated antigens (TAAs)
    active immunization approaches, 321
    hypothesis, 308
    stem-like glioma cells, 311
Tumor associated macrophages (TAM)
    CAFs, 80
    role, 70
Tumor initiating cells, 200, 202
Tumor microenvironment
    description, 69
    ECM, 69–70
    TAM, 70–71
Tyrosine kinase inhibitors (TKIs)
    cellular signaling pathways, 249
    vandetanib, 260

W

Wilm's tumor, 214
Wnt responsive element (WRE), 160
Wnt signaling pathways
    β-catenin, 249–250
    COX–2 inhibitors, 251–252
    ICG–001 molecule, 252
    mAb and RNAi, 252
    SFRPs, 252–253
WRE. *See* Wnt responsive element